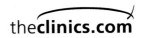

IMMUNOLOGY AND ALLERGY CLINICS OF NORTH AMERICA

Allergen-Specific Immunotherapy

GUEST EDITOR
Cezmi A. Akdis, MD

CONSULTING EDITOR
Rafeul Alam, MD, PhD

May 2006 • Volume 26 • Number 2

SAUNDERS

An Imprint of Elsevier, Inc.
PHILADELPHIA   LONDON   TORONTO   MONTREAL   SYDNEY   TOKYO

W.B. SAUNDERS COMPANY
A Division of Elsevier Inc.

Elsevier, Inc., 1600 John F. Kennedy Blvd., Suite 1800, Philadelphia, PA 19103-2899

http://www.theclinics.com

IMMUNOLOGY AND ALLERGY CLINICS
OF NORTH AMERICA   Volume 26, Number 2
May 2006   ISSN 0889-8561
Editor: Carla Holloway   ISBN 1-4160-3513-3

The ideas and opinions expressed in *Immunology and Allergy Clinics of North America* do not necessarily reflect those of the Publisher. The Publisher does not assume any responsibility for any injury and/or damage to persons or property arising out of or related to any use of the material contained in this periodical. The reader is advised to check the appropriate medical literature and the product information currently provided by the manufacturer of each drug to be administered to verify the dosage, the method and duration of administra-tion, or contraindications. It is the responsibility of the treating physician or other health care professional, relying on independent experience and knowledge of the patient, to determine drug dosages and the best treatment for the patient. Mention of any product in this issue should not be construed as endorsement by the contributors, editors, or the Publisher of the product or manufacturers' claims.

Immunology and Allergy Clinics of North America (ISSN 0889-8561) is published quarterly by Elsevier, Inc. Corporate and editorial Offices: Elsevier, Inc., 1600 John F. Kennedy Blvd., Suite 1800, Philadelphia, PA 19103-2899. Accounting and circulation offices: 6277 Sea Harbor Drive, Orlando, FL 32887-4800. Periodicals postage paid at Orlando, FL 32862, and addi-tional mailing offices. Subscription prices are $175.00 per year for US individuals, $280.00 per year for US institutions, $85.00 per year for US students and residents, $215.00 per year for Canadian individuals, $340.00 per year for Canadian institutions, $230.00 per year for international individuals, $340.00 per year for international institutions, $115 per year for Canadian and international students. To receive student/resident rate, orders must be accompanied by name of affiliated institution, date of term, and the *signature* of program/residency coordinator on institution letterhead. Orders will be billed at individual rate until proof of status is received. Foreign air speed delivery is included in all *Clinics* subscription prices. All prices are subject to change without notice. POSTMASTER: Send address changes to *Immunology and Allergy Clinics of North America*, W.B. Saunders Company, Periodicals Fulfillment, Orlando, FL 32887-4800. **Customer Service: 1-800-654-2452 (US). From outside of the US, call 1-407-345-4000. E-mail: hhspcs@wbsaunders.com**

Reprints. For copies of 100 or more, of articles in this publication, please contact the Commercial Reprints Department, Elsevier Inc., 360 Park Avenue South, New York, New York 10010-1710. Tel. (212) 633-3813 Fax: (212) 462-1935 e-mail: reprints@elsevier.com

Immunology and Allergy Clinics of North America is covered in *Index Medicus, Current Contents/Life Sciences, Science Citation Index, ISI/BIOMED, Chemical Abstracts,* and *EMBASE/Excerpta Medica*

Printed in the United States of America.

CONSULTING EDITOR

RAFEUL ALAM, MD, PhD, Veda and Chauncey Ritter Chair in Immunology; Professor and Director, Division of Allergy & Immunology, National Jewish Medical and Research Center; Co-Director, Allergy & Immunology, University of Colorado Health Sciences Center, Denver, Colorado

GUEST EDITOR

CEZMI A. AKDIS, MD, Head of Immunology, Swiss Institute of Allergy and Asthma Research, Davos, Switzerland

CONTRIBUTORS

CEZMI A. AKDIS, MD, Professor of Immunology, Swiss Institute of Allergy and Asthma Research, Davos, Switzerland

MÜBECCEL AKDIS, MD, PhD, Associate Professor of Immunology, Swiss Institute of Allergy and Asthma Research, Davos, Switzerland

NERIN N. BAHCECILER, MD, Associate Professor of Allergy, Division of Pediatric Allergy & Immunology, Marmara University Hospital, Istanbul, Turkey

ISIL BARLAN, MD, Professor of Pediatrics and Chief, Division of Pediatric Allergy and Immunology, Marmara University Hospital, Istanbul, Turkey

KURT BLASER, PhD, Professor, Swiss Institute of Allergy and Asthma Research (SIAF), Davos, Switzerland

BARBARA BOHLE, PhD, Institute of Pathophysiology, Center of Physiology and Pathophysiology, Medical University of Vienna, Vienna, Austria

RETO CRAMERI, PhD, Head Molecular Allergology, Swiss Institute of Allergy and Asthma Research (SIAF), Davos, Switzerland

OLIVER CROMWELL, PhD, Head of Research and Development, Allergopharma Joachim Ganzer KG, Reinbek, Germany

STEPHEN R. DURHAM, MD, Professor, Upper Respiratory Medicine, Imperial College, National Heart and Lung Institute, London, United Kingdom

HELMUT FIEBIG, PhD, Allergopharma Joachim Ganzer KG, Reinbek, Germany

JAMES N. FRANCIS, PhD, Upper Respiratory Medicine, Imperial College, National Heart and Lung Institute, London, United Kingdom

ERIKA JENSEN-JAROLIM, MD, Institute of Pathophysiology, Center of Physiology and Pathophysiology, Medical University of Vienna, Austria

MAREK JUTEL, MD, PhD, Professor of Medicine, Department of Internal Medicine and Allergy, Wroclaw Medical University, Wroclaw, Poland; Swiss Institute of Allergy and Asthma Research (SIAF), Davos, Switzerland

HELGA KAHLERT, PhD, Allergopharma Joachim Ganzer KG, Reinbek, Germany

JENS KETTNER, PhD, Allergopharma Joachim Ganzer KG, Reinbek, Germany

TAMARA KOPP, MD, Department of Dermatology, Division of Immunology, Allergy and Infectious Diseases, Medical University of Vienna, Vienna, Austria

MARK LARCHÉ, PhD, Reader in Respiratory Immunology, Department of Allergy and Clinical Immunology, Faculty of Medicine, Imperial College, London, United Kingdom

LAURENT MASCARELL, PhD, Research and Development, Stallergènes, Antony, France

PHILIPPE MOINGEON, PhD, Research and Development, Stallergènes, Antony, France

ANDREAS NANDY, PhD, Allergopharma Joachim Ganzer KG, Reinbek, Germany

ANNEMIE NARKUS, MD, Allergopharma Joachim Ganzer KG, Reinbek, Germany

JØRGEN NEDERGAARD LARSEN, PhD, Senior Scientist, ALK-Abelló, Hørsholm, Denmark

NATALIJA NOVAK, MD, Assistant Professor of Dermatology, Department of Dermatology, University of Bonn, Bonn, Germany

CARSTEN B. SCHMIDT-WEBER, PhD, Swiss Institute of Allergy and Asthma Research (SIAF), Davos, Switzerland

ISABELLA SCHÖLL, PhD, Institute of Pathophysiology, Center of Physiology and Pathophysiology, Medical University of Vienna, Vienna, Austria

MICHAEL D. SPANGFORT, PhD, Director of Research, ALK-Abelló, Hørsholm, Denmark

ROLAND SUCK, PhD, Allergopharma Joachim Ganzer KG, Reinbek, Germany

LAURENCE VAN OVERTVELT, PhD, Research and Development, Stallergènes, Antony, France

JOHAN VERHAGEN, PhD, Swiss Institute of Allergy and Asthma Research (SIAF), Davos, Switzerland

LOUISA K. WILCOCK, BSc, Upper Respiratory Medicine, Imperial College, National Heart and Lung Institute, London, United Kingdom

CONTENTS

Immunotherapy for allergic diseases represents an important but largely unmet medical need. Conventional immunotherapy suffers from several breakdowns related to the quality of the extracts used, the risk of inducing anaphylactic reactions, and the extremely long treatment time. Many of the problems associated with using natural allergenic products for allergy diagnosis and treatment can be overcome using genetically engineered recombinant allergens. New therapeutic strategies based on recombinant technology include peptide-based vaccines, engineered hypoallergens with reduced IgE-binding properties, nucleotide-conjugated vaccines that promote Th1 responses, and the possibility of developing prophylactic allergen vaccines.

In the 1970s and 1980s, scientific methods were introduced in the standardization of allergen vaccines and, in combination with improved documentation of the clinical benefits obtained using standardized vaccines, specific allergy treatment as a scientifically based, reproducible, and safe treatment for allergic disease was established. This article describes important issues in the control of source materials and vaccine preparation as part of the European standardization of allergen vaccines, and also includes a discussion of vaccines that are based on recombinant allergens, which may appear on the market in the near future.

Mechanisms of Allergen-Specific Immunotherapy: T-Regulatory Cells and More

Johan Verhagen, Kurt Blaser, Cezmi A. Akdis, and Mübeccel Akdis

Activation-induced cell death, anergy, or immune response modulation by regulatory T cells (Treg cells) are essential mechanisms of peripheral T-cell tolerance. Genetic predisposition and environmental instructions tune thresholds for the activation of T cells, other inflammatory cells, and resident tissue cells in allergic diseases. Skewing allergen-specific effector T cells to a Treg-cell phenotype seems to be crucial in maintaining a healthy immune response to allergens and successful allergen-specific immunotherapy. The Treg-cell response is characterized by an abolished allergen-specific T-cell proliferation and the suppressed secretion of T-helper 1– and T-helper 2–type cytokines. Suppressed proliferative and cytokine responses against allergens are induced by multiple suppressor factors, including cytokines such as interleukin-10 (IL-10) and transforming growth factor β (TGF-β), and cell surface molecules such as cytotoxic T-lymphocyte antigen-4, programmed death-1, and histamine receptor 2. The increased levels of IL-10 and TGF-β produced by Treg cells potently suppress IgE production while simultaneously increasing the production of noninflammatory isotypes IgG4 and IgA, respectively. In addition, Treg cells directly or indirectly suppress the activity of effector cells of allergic inflammation, such as mast cells, basophils, and eosinophils. In conclusion, peripheral tolerance to allergens is controlled by multiple active suppression mechanisms on T cells, regulation of antibody isotypes, and suppression of effector cells. The application of current knowledge of Treg cells and related mechanisms of peripheral tolerance may soon lead to more rational and safer approaches to the prevention and cure of allergic disease.

The Role of TGF-β in Allergic Inflammation

Carsten B. Schmidt-Weber and Kurt Blaser

The transforming growth factor β (TGF-β) plays a dual role in allergic disease. It is important in suppressing T cells and also mediates repair responses that lead to unwanted remodeling of tissues. Advances in the immunology of allergy indicate that allergens cause overreactions in the lymphocyte compartment because of the lack or decreased number of suppressive, regulatory T cells. TGF-β was shown to induce regulatory T cells and participate directly in suppression of effector T cells. Therefore, TGF-β may help return reactivity to allergens to normal subsymptomatic activity. Whether chronic inflammatory diseases such as asthma profit from TGF-β–mediated suppression of specific immune responses or whether the TGF-β–mediated tissue remodeling aggravates diseases more than it helps control immune reactions is unclear. This article addresses these issues and future strategies in this field.

Implications for the design and development of improved allergy vaccines that could be used through such nonparenteral routes are discussed. Specifically, allergen presentation platforms and adjuvants facilitating the targeting of immune cells at mucosal surfaces to promote tolerance induction are reviewed.

Allergen immunotherapy is a well-established strategy for treating allergic diseases with the goal of inducing allergen-specific tolerance. Identified mechanisms contributing to the therapeutic effect of immunotherapy include a shift of T helper 2 (Th2)-type immune responses to a modified Th2 immune response, a change of the balance of IgE-producing B cells to the production of IgG subtypes, in addition to increased IL-10 and TGF-β secretion and activation of the suppressive functions of regulatory T-cells. Dendritic cells (DCs), which as outposts of the immune system are capable of T-cell priming through efficient allergen uptake by IgE receptors expressed on their cell surface. Most of the hypotheses concerning the function of DCs as facilitators of allergen-specific tolerance in allergen immunotherapy remain speculative. Therefore, studies must focus on the functional changes of DCs under immunotherapy to close the gap of knowledge about their exact role. These experimental data should help confirm the hypothesis of DCs as efficient silencers and potential target cells and take advantage of the bivalent character and tolerogenic properties of DCs.

Synthetic peptides representing T-cell epitopes of allergens and autoantigens have been employed to induce antigen-specific tolerance in vivo in experimental models and the clinical setting. Delivery of peptides orally or by injection leads to reduced reactivity to antigen accompanied by the induction of T cells with a regulatory phenotype. Peptide therapy may provide a safe, effective, and economically viable approach for disease-modifying therapy in autoimmune and allergic diseases.

IgE-facilitated allergen presentation (FAP) is an important pathogenic mechanism in allergic disease and represents a potential therapeutic target. Allergen immunotherapy is a highly effective therapy, particularly in patients with seasonal pollinosis who fail to respond to usual pharmacotherapy. Allergen immunotherapy induces "blocking" IgG antibodies that are detectable in serum and have been shown to inhibit IgE-FAP in vitro. This review summarizes the main components involved in IgE-FAP and the potential value of a validated functional assay of serum inhibitory antibodies for IgE-FAP for monitoring the clinical response to immunotherapy.

Although allergen immunotherapy is basically a story of success, it still needs improvement. The goal of this study was to optimize parenteral and oral allergen formulations through using the biocompatible polymer of lactic and glycolic acid (PLGA). Subcutaneous application of birch pollen allergen Bet v 1 encapsulated in nanoparticles biased the immune response toward Th1 in allergic mice and did not elicit granuloma formation in mice and in human volunteers. When oral immunotherapy of mice was tried with birch pollen–filled PLGA microparticles, mucosal targeting was indispensable for achieving any immune response, and targeting of M-cells was necessary for modulating an ongoing allergic response toward Th1. The authors suggest that biocompatible PLGA nano- or microparticles can be useful tools for upgrading therapy of type I allergy.

Based on the hygiene hypothesis association between atopy and bacillus Calmette-Guerin (BCG), purified protein derivative skin test reaction, mycobacterial disease, and environmental mycobacteria are summarized. The role of mycobacterial species in the activation of the innate immune response through Toll-like receptors is mentioned. The implications and perspectives of BCG as a potential therapeutic adjuvant in atopic disease are discussed.

FORTHCOMING ISSUES

RECENT ISSUES

VISIT THESE RELATED WEB SITES

Access your subscription at:
www.theclinics.com

ELSEVIER
SAUNDERS

Immunol Allergy Clin N Am
26 (2006) xi–xii

IMMUNOLOGY
AND ALLERGY
CLINICS
OF NORTH AMERICA

Foreword

Allergen-Specific Immunotherapy

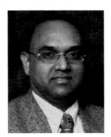

Rafeul Alam, MD, PhD
Consulting Editor

Until we succeed in primary prevention, immunomodulation will remain the most practical approach to controlling allergic diseases. Allergen immunotherapy is the most successful modality of immunomodulation. Although immunotherapy was introduced in early 20th century, its mechanism of action remains elusive. We have experienced evolving ideas—mast cell desensitization, IgE reduction, generation of IgG blocking antibodies, and a shift of Th2 to Th1. All of these ideas were subsequently supported by some experimental evidence. However, none of them really provided a comprehensive and complete understanding of the mechanism of allergen immunotherapy. Some exciting new developments have occurred in this field in recent years. One is the re-emergence of the concept of immunosuppression. Thanks to a better understanding of their origin, phenotype, and activity, regulatory T cells (Treg) are now widely accepted as the major regulators of effector T cells. In this issue, the authors present the latest on the role of Tregs and their mediators in Th2 response and allergic phenotype. The authors also present a wide range of possible immune interventions that are now being tested in the laboratory and on patients. The concepts are innovative; they incorporate the latest technological and intellectual achievements. Most likely not all of them will succeed. Nonetheless, it is the desire of this series to keep the readership abreast of the exciting research in the field.

0889-8561/06/$ – see front matter © 2006 Elsevier Inc. All rights reserved.
doi:10.1016/j.iac.2006.02.014   *immunology.theclinics.com*

Rafeul Alam, MD, PhD
National Jewish Medical and Research Center
1400 Jackson Street K1003b
Denver, CO 80206, USA
E-mail address: alamr@njc.org

IMMUNOLOGY
AND ALLERGY
CLINICS
OF NORTH AMERICA

Immunol Allergy Clin N Am
26 (2006) xiii–xxii

Preface

Future of Allergen-Specific Immunotherapy: Better Understanding of the Mechanisms, Novel Treatments, and Long-Term Cure

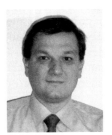

Cezmi A. Akdis, MD
Guest Editor

Current problems of conventional allergen-specific immunotherapy

Allergen-specific immunotherapy (allergen-SIT) has several problems related to vaccine content, type of adjuvant, route of application, duration of treatment, side effects, and limited efficacy. Currently, allergen-SIT uses vaccines based on allergen extracts. The vaccines are standardized in terms of total allergenic activity or potency and possibly the concentration of one individual major allergen, whereas product consistency is assessed in terms of protein and allergen profiles determined through various techniques, which are discussed by Spangfort elsewhere in this issue. An extract may contain many proteins and allergens, and also nonallergenic or even toxic proteins. The composition is determined largely by the quality of the raw material and method of extraction and purification. Raw materials are provided by certified suppliers and produced under controlled conditions, but differences still exist. For example, the allergen

The author's laboratory is supported by the Swiss National Science Foundation Grant No: 32-105865 and Global Allergy and Asthma European Network (GA²LEN).

doi:10.1016/j.iac.2006.02.013   *immunology.theclinics.com*

content of mold cultures is highly dependent on the time and conditions of culture. Climatic factors or pollution can influence the allergenicity of pollen. Some manufacturers use whole cultures of house dust mites, including the nutrient medium and fecal particles, whereas others use purified mite bodies. In addition, many extracts derived from natural materials contain innate immune response–triggering substances, such as lipopolysaccharide, which is detectable and can be eliminated. However, lipopolysaccharide accompanies several other innate immune response–triggering substances that are not detectable through conventional methods. Administration of allergen extracts can cause severe, often life-threatening anaphylactic reactions and new IgE sensitization to other antigens contained in the extract. Many of the problems associated with the use of natural allergens and extracts for diagnosing and treating allergy can be overcome using recombinant allergens, as discussed by Crameri elsewhere in this issue. Another important problem is that current protocols of allergen-SIT require at least 3 years of clinical treatment, and efficacy is questionable in certain cases. Novel strategies based on technological developments in the engineering of recombinant allergens and the underlying immunologic mechanisms necessary to overcome the problems associated with allergen-SIT are reviewed in detail elsewhere in this issue.

Recent developments in mechanisms of specific immunotherapy that may lead to novel treatment strategies

Despite its use since the beginning of the century, the underlying immunologic mechanisms of allergen-SIT are continuously being elucidated. The induction of a tolerant state in peripheral T cells represents an essential step in allergen-SIT. This topic is further reviewed by Verhagen and colleagues elsewhere in this issue. Peripheral T-cell tolerance is characterized mainly by generation of allergen-specific T-regulatory (Treg) cells and suppressed proliferative and cytokine responses against the major allergen [1–5]. T-cell tolerance is initiated through autocrine action of interleukin (IL)-10, which is increasingly produced by antigen-specific T cells [2]. Studies of the mechanisms through which immune responses to nonpathogenic environmental antigens lead to either allergy or nonharmful immunity have shown that Treg cells are dominant in healthy individuals [6]. Treg cells use multiple suppressive mechanisms, IL-10, and transforming growth factor (TGF)-β as secreted cytokines, and cytotoxic T-lymphocyte antigen 4 and programmed death 1 as surface molecules. Individuals who are healthy and those who have allergies exhibit all three allergen-specific subsets (ie, Th1-, Th2-, and Tr1-type) in different proportions [6]. Accordingly, a change in the dominant subset and balance between Th2 and Treg cells may lead to either allergy development or recovery. IL-10 and TGF-β secreted from Treg cells directly or indirectly suppress Th2 cells, Th1 cells, mast cells, eosinophils, and basophils and regulate antibody isotypes in B cells. TGF-β plays a dual role in allergic disease: it suppresses allergen-specific T cells and plays a role in tissue remodeling. Whether the remodeling and suppressive role of TGF-β in allergic inflammation (discussed by Schmidt-Weber and colleagues elsewhere in this issue) show an imbalance that aggravates the disease rather than controls the immune response has not been elucidated.

A rise in allergen-blocking IgG antibodies, particularly of the IgG4 class, which block allergen and IgE-facilitated antigen presentation, represents an important event in allergen-SIT. See the article by Wilcock and colleagues elsewhere in this issue for further exploration of this topic. Antigen-presenting cells are able to focus very low concentrations of antigen through specific membrane immunoglobulins or surface receptor–bound immunoglobulins into endosomal compartments, a process that results in greatly enhanced cell activation. This receptor-mediated antigen focusing may occur at much lower antigen concentrations than those in nonspecific uptake [7]. Current data suggest that IgE- and FcεRII-facilitated allergen presentation is an important process that contributes to activation and exacerbation of inflammatory pathways in allergic diseases. The role of blocking antibodies in inhibiting this process in vivo is now emerging and is reviewed by Wilcock and colleagues elsewhere in this issue.

Sequential events in allergen-specific immunotherapy and the underlying mechanisms

Although definite decreases in IgE antibody levels and IgE-mediated skin sensitivity normally require years of SIT, most patients are already protected against bee stings at an early stage of venom–SIT. An important observation after the first injection is that an early decrease in mast cell and basophil activity for degranulation and systemic anaphylaxis occurs (Fig. 1). The mechanism of this desensitization effect is yet unknown. Studies have shown that mediators of anaphylaxis (histamine and leukotrienes) are released during SIT without inducing a systemic anaphylactic response. Particularly, ultrarush protocols induce significantly increased release of these mediators into circulation. Their piecemeal release may affect the threshold of mast cell and basophil activation. Although fluctuations occur and systemic anaphylaxis may develop during the course of allergen-SIT, the suppression of mast cells and basophils continues to be affected by changes in other immune parameters, such as generation of allergen-specific Treg cells and decreased specific IgE, particularly because these cells require T-cell cytokines for priming, survival, and activity, which are not efficiently provided by suppressed Th2 cells. In addition, Treg cells and their suppressor cytokines show direct or indirect suppression of effector cells. Long-term suppression of mast cell and basophil degranulation continues with the generation of blocking antibodies, which block cross-linking of FcεRI-bound IgE on their surface.

The second immunologic event in the early course of allergen-SIT is the generation of allergen-specific Treg cells and suppression of allergen-specific Th1 and Th2 cells. See the articles by Verhagen and colleagues and Schmidt-

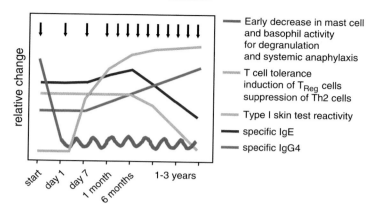

Fig. 1. Immunologic changes during the course of allergen-SIT. Although significant variation occurs between donors and protocols, an early decrease in mast cell and basophil activity and degranulation, and a decreased tendency for systemic anaphylaxis is observed starting from the first injection. The second immunologic event in the early course of allergen-SIT is the generation of allergen-specific Treg cells and suppression of allergen-specific Th1 and Th2 cells. A significant decrease in allergen-specific IgE/IgG4 ratio occurs after a few months, which is parallel to a decrease in type I skin test reactivity.

Weber and colleagues elsewhere in this issue for further discussion of this topic (see Fig. 1). Treg cells contribute to the control of allergen-specific immune responses in five major ways: (1) suppression of antigen-presenting cells that support the generation of effector Th2 and Th1 cells; (2) suppression of Th2 and Th1 cells; (3) suppression of allergen-specific IgE and induction of IgG4 or IgA; (4) suppression of mast cells, basophils, and eosinophils; and (5) interaction with resident tissue cells and remodeling [8]. These mechanisms are discussed in greater detail by Verhagen and colleagues and Schmidt-Weber and colleagues elsewhere in this issue. The decrease in IgE/IgG4 ratio during allergen-SIT is likely caused by skew from allergen-specific Th2 to Treg-cell predominance. However, although Treg-cell generation occurs within days, a significant decrease in IgE/IgG4 ratio occurs after years. The reason for the long gap between the change in T-cell subsets but not IgE/IgG4 levels can not be easily explained by the half-life of antibodies. In this context, the role of bone marrow–residing, IgE-producing memory B cells with very long life spans remains to be investigated.

Histamine regulates the immune response in allergen-specific immunotherapy

Many established G-protein–coupled receptor systems have been successfully exploited by the pharmaceutical industry to become the target for approximately 40% of the currently available drugs. As a small molecular weight monoamine that binds to four different G-protein–coupled receptors, histamine has been shown to regulate several essential events in the immune response [9]. The expression of these receptors on different cells and cell subsets is regulated, and apparently diverse effects of histamine on immune regulation are caused by differential expression of these receptors and their distinct intracellular signals. Histamine receptor 2 (HR2) represents a candidate molecule for the suppression of several features of allergic inflammation [10]. Histamine affects Treg cells and their suppressive properties through HR2. Increased IL-10 production in dendritic and T cells through HR2 may account for an important regulatory mechanism in the control of allergen-specific T cells through histamine. In accordance with this phenomenon, histamine supports the suppressive effect of TGF-β particularly on Th2 cells through HR2, as detailed elsewhere in this issue by Jutel and Akdis. Piecemeal release of histamine from mast cells and basophils during SIT in the induction phase of allergen-SIT needs further investigation. Moreover, histidine decarboxylase activity has been detected in other cells, and histamine production is not only a feature of mast cells and basophils [11].

Mucosal-specific immunotherapy routes: where are we?

Because of potentially severe, albeit infrequent, side effects associated with injection SIT, mucosal routes of administration are being investigated in allergenic desensitization. Because of its well-established safety profile, with more than 500 million doses administered to humans, sublingual immunotherapy (SLIT) is currently considered an alternative to subcutaneous SIT. Some of the immunologic mechanisms are known and some remain to be elucidated. This topic is discussed in greater detail by Mascarell and colleagues elsewhere in this issue. Novel approaches to the improvement of injection SIT, such as recombinant allergen-SIT vaccines, combination therapies, and novel adjuvants, are also applicable to SLIT. In addition, differences in antigen-presenting cells in the oral mucosa and adjuvants facilitating the targeting of immune cells at mucosal surfaces to promote tolerance induction might have key impacts in the improvement of SLIT. Several lines of evidence indicate that mucosal dendritic cells are potent inducers of tolerogenic immune responses after allergen challenge, which may play a crucial role in allergen immunotherapy, as discussed by Novak elsewhere in this issue.

Emerging specific immunotherapy vaccines and their underlying mechanisms

A basic requirement for an allergen vaccine to achieve successful SIT without risk for anaphylaxis is to express T-cell epitopes, which induce T-cell tolerance and lack antibody-binding sites that mediate IgE cross-linking [7]. Conformation dependence of B-cell epitopes and linearity of T-cell epitopes may induce a different regulation of allergen-specific T-cell cytokine toward a nonallergic phenotype [12]. Native allergens use IgE-facilitated antigen presentation by dendritic cells and B cells, which activates T cells to produce Th2-type cytokines and B cells to produce further IgE in a secondary response [7]. In contrast, B-cell epitope–deleted allergens, which do not bind IgE, do not initiate effector cell degranulation. These allergens use phagocytotic or pinocytic antigen-uptake mechanisms in dendritic cells, macrophages, and B cells. T cells may be subsequently induced to generate a balanced Th0/Th1-type cytokine pattern in lower quantities and T-cell tolerance, which involves Treg cells. Accordingly, targeting T cells and bypassing IgE through modified allergens enables the administration of higher doses of allergens, which is required to induce T-cell tolerance without risk for anaphylaxis [7].

Immunotherapy using peptides (PIT) is also an attractive approach for safe SIT. Short allergen peptides, either native sequences or altered peptide ligands, with amino acid substitutions do not contain epitopes for IgE cross-linking to induce anaphylaxis. Considerable rationale exists for targeting T cells with synthetic peptides based on such T-cell epitopes. As Larché discusses elsewhere in this issue, clinical trials of PIT have been performed in two allergies [13–15]. Long peptides of 27 and 35 amino acids of the major cat allergen Fel d 1 and a mixture of short T-cell epitope peptides spanning the whole protein sequence were used to treat allergy to cats, and induced tolerance in IL-4–producing cells and IL-10 production [14,15]. In bee venom phospholipase A2 peptide immunotherapy, induction of specific T-cell tolerance and a decrease in the specific IgE:IgG4 ratio against the whole allergen was observed [13].

A potential barrier to PIT is the apparent complexity of the allergen-specific T-cell response in terms of epitope use and dominant epitopes in humans and stability of peptides. To overcome these problems, genetically engineered recombinant hybrid molecules have been developed that span the whole T-cell repertoire but do not bind IgE. The construction of fusion proteins and hybrids is based on the exquisite conformational dependence of B-cell epitopes and the linearity of T-cell epitopes in allergenic molecules [12]. In cysteine-containing proteins, folding is complicated by the formation of intra- and intermolecular disulphide bonds, whereas any formed disulphide bond can fix the conformation and limit the freedom of further folding processes. With increased cysteines, the probability of a correct or native-like folding rapidly decreases because of the increased probability of incorrect disulphide-bound formation.

A fusion protein consisting of the two major allergens bee venom Api m 1 and Api m 2 has been generated to investigate this concept. Destroyed conformational B-cell epitopes but intact T-cell epitopes of the two allergens characterize this protein. Through providing decreased allergenicity with preserved T-cell tolerance–inducing capacity, the Api m [1/2] fusion protein represents a novel vaccine prototype for allergen-SIT [16].

Another interesting approach was to cut the major allergens to fragments and fuse them in a different order without missing any T-cell epitopes in one reassembled mosaic allergen [17]. In this study, two fragments of Api m 1, three fragments of Api m 2, and Api m 3 were reassembled in a different order with overlapping residues so no T-cell epitopes were missed. Single injection of the vaccines, which only target T cells, showed a preventive effect on IgE generation in mice. The advantage of these two approaches is that only one molecule has to be produced and purified instead of several recombinant allergens. T-cell epitopes are preserved and B-cell epitopes can be deleted or preserved depending on the type of fusion molecule.

A third approach was to use fragments and a trimer of major birch pollen allergen Bet v 1 to treat birch pollen allergy. A double-blind, placebo-controlled study was completed in three centers, showing improvement of clinical symptoms; increase in IgG1, IgG2, IgG4, and IgA; and suppression of seasonal increases of IgE [18,19].

A fourth approach was to use recombinant allergen vaccines, which combine different allergens of an extract similar to the native constitution. One study showed the effectiveness of a mixture of five recombinant grass pollen allergens in reducing symptoms and the need for symptomatic medication in patients allergic to grass pollen. In this study, which used well-defined recombinant allergen mixtures, all treated subjects developed strong allergen-specific IgG1 and IgG4 antibody responses [20]. Some patients were not sensitized to Phl p 5, although they nevertheless developed strong IgG– but not IgE–antibody responses to that allergen. In this issue, Cromwell and coworkers discuss the strategies and fruitful results from the first clinical studies involving recombinant allergens.

Adjuvants

The use of novel adjuvants that regulate immune responses in the desired way has been investigated. In most of the aforementioned vaccines, aluminium hydroxide was used as adjuvant, which may not be the most efficient. Administering allergens with bacterial lipopeptides to shift the balance toward Th1 and Treg cells through Toll-like receptor (TLR) 2 has been shown to be efficient in several different mouse models of allergy through suppressing IgE and eosinophilia [21]. Natural exposure to mycobacteria and the Bacillus-Calmette-Guerin vaccine has been suggested to influence the development and severity of allergic diseases, again probably related to innate immune response and TLRs, as reviewed by Barlan and colleagues elsewhere in this issue.

Oligodeoxynucleotides containing immunostimulatory CpG motifs that trigger TLR 9 linked to the allergen in ragweed allergy in humans have been used. Amb a 1–immunostimulatory DNA sequence conjugate SIT led to a prolonged shift from Th2 immunity toward Th1 immunity and appeared to be safe [22]. As a different immunologic approach, the fusion of allergens with human Fcγ has been reported to inhibit allergen-induced basophil and mast cell degranulation through cross-linking Fcγ and FcεRI receptors [23].

Carbohydrate-based adjuvants may begin to be more widely used because they do not induce tissue destruction, and they control the release of allergens [24]. In addition, lectins have been shown to target fucose residues on M cells in the intestine, resulting in sustained release of allergens [25]. In this issue, Schöll and coworkers discuss the use of biocompatible polymer of lactic and glycolic acid as an adjuvant for parenteral and oral application.

Summary

Peripheral T-cell tolerance is the key immunologic mechanism in the healthy immune response to self and noninfectious nonself antigens. Changes in the fine balance between allergen-specific Treg and Th2 or Th1 cells are crucial in the development and treatment of allergic diseases. In addition to treating established allergy, clinicians must also consider prophylactic approaches before initial sensitization takes place. Preventive vaccines that induce Treg responses could be developed and allergen-specific Treg cells, which will become predominant, may in turn dampen the Th1 and Th2 cells and their cytokines, ensuring a well-balanced immune response. Applying recent knowledge of peripheral tolerance mechanisms will allow the development of more rational and safer approaches to the treatment, prevention, and cure of allergic diseases.

New approaches to allergen-SIT, such as the use of recombinant proteins, peptides, fragments, and hybrid allergens, are promising but are only in an early stage of human clinical trials. Several essential requirements underlie novel strategies for the development of safe and more efficient SIT vaccines: (1) the vaccine should consist of perfectly well-standardized native proteins or recombinant allergens; (2) the vaccine should induce tolerance in allergen-specific effector T cells, suppress IgE production, and promote IgG4 or IgA isotype–blocking antibody production; (3) the vaccine should not induce severe side effects and should be well tolerated; (4) the vaccine should be easily administered, preferably through mucosal routes; (5) the treatment should achieve clinical success and long-term protection in a short time with few doses; and (6) early biologic markers to assess clinical success before the onset of the treatment should be identified. Intensive research is being undertaken to fulfill these requirements.

Acknowledgments

I thank Kurt Blaser for his true mentorship.

Cezmi A. Akdis, MD
Swiss Institute of Allergy and Asthma Research
Obere Strasse 22
CH-7270 Davos Platz
Switzerland
E-mail address: akdisac@siaf.unizh.ch

References

[1] Akdis CA, Akdis M, Blesken T, et al. Epitope-specific T cell tolerance to phospholipase A2 in bee venom immunotherapy and recovery by IL-2 and IL-15 in vitro. J Clin Invest 1996; 98(7):1676–83.

[2] Akdis CA, Blesken T, Akdis M, et al. Role of interleukin 10 in specific immunotherapy. J Clin Invest 1998;102(1):98–106.

[3] Jutel M, Akdis M, Budak F, et al. IL-10 and TGF-β cooperate in regulatory T cell response to mucosal allergens in normal immunity and specific immunotherapy. Eur J Immunol 2003;33: 1205–14.

[4] Francis JN, Till SJ, Durham SR. Induction of IL-10+ CD4+ CD25+ T cells by grass pollen immunotherapy. J Allergy Clin Immunol 2003;111(6):1255–61.

[5] Ling EM, Smith T, Nguyen XD, et al. Relation of CD4+ CD25+ regulatory T-cell suppression of allergen-driven T-cell activation to atopic status and expression of allergic disease. Lancet 2004;363(9409):608–15.

[6] Akdis M, Verhagen J, Taylor A, et al. Immune responses in healthy and allergic individuals are characterized by a fine balance between allergen-specific T regulatory 1 and T helper 2 cells. J Exp Med 2004;199(11):1567–75.

[7] Akdis CA, Blaser K. Bypassing IgE and targeting T cells for specific immunotherapy of allergy. Trends Immunol 2001;22:175–8.

[8] Akdis M, Blaser K, Akdis CA. T regulatory cells in allergy: novel concepts in the pathogenesis, prevention, and treatment of allergic diseases. J Allergy Clin Immunol 2005;116(5):961–8.

[9] Akdis CA, Blaser K. Histamine in the immune regulation of allergic inflammation. J Allergy Clin Immunol 2003;112:15–22.

[10] Jutel M, Watanabe T, Klunker S, et al. Histamine regulates T-cell and antibody responses by differential expression of H1 and H2 receptors. Nature 2001;413(6854):420–5.

[11] Szeberenyi JB, Pallinger E, Zsinko M, et al. Inhibition of effects of endogenously synthesized histamine disturbs in vitro human dendritic cell differentiation. Immunol Lett 2001;76(3):175–82.

[12] Akdis CA, Blesken T, Wymann D, et al. Differential regulation of human T cell cytokine patterns and IgE and IgG4 responses by conformational antigen variants. Eur J Immunol 1998;28: 914–25.

[13] Müller UR, Akdis CA, Fricker M, et al. Successful immunotherapy with T-cell epitope peptides of bee venom phospholipase A₂ induces specific T-cell anergy in patients allergic to bee venom. J Allergy Clin Immunol 1998;101:747–54.

[14] Marcotte GV, Braun CM, Norman PS, et al. Effects of peptide therapy on ex vivo T-cell responses. J Allergy Clin Immunol 1998;101(4 Pt 1):506–13.

[15] Oldfield WL, Larche M, Kay AB. Effect of T-cell peptides derived from Fel d 1 on allergic reactions and cytokine production in patients sensitive to cats: a randomised controlled trial. Lancet 2002;360:47–53.

[16] Kussebi F, Karamloo F, Rhyner C, et al. A major allergen gene-fusion protein for potential usage in allergen-specific immunotherapy. J Allergy Clin Immunol 2005;115(2):323–9.

[17] Karamloo F, Schmid-Grendelmeier P, Kussebi F, et al. Prevention of allergy by a recombinant multi-allergen vaccine with reduced IgE binding and preserved T cell epitopes. Eur J Immunol 2005;35(11):3268–76.

[18] Niederberger V, Horak F, Vrtala S, et al. Vaccination with genetically engineered allergens prevents progression of allergic disease. Proc Natl Acad Sci USA 2004;101(Suppl 2):14677–82.

[19] Gafvelin G, Thunberg S, Kronqvist M, et al. Cytokine and antibody responses in birch-pollen-allergic patients treated with genetically modified derivatives of the major birch pollen allergen Bet v 1. Int Arch Allergy Immunol 2005;138(1):59–66.

[20] Jutel M, Jaeger L, Suck R, et al. Allergen-specific immunotherapy with recombinant grass pollen allergens. J Allergy Clin Immunol 2005;116(3):608–13.

[21] Akdis CA, Kussebi F, Pulendran B, et al. Inhibition of T helper 2-type responses, IgE production and eosinophilia by synthetic lipopeptides. Eur J Immunol 2003;33(10):2717–26.

[22] Simons FE, Shikishima Y, Van Nest G, et al. Selective immune redirection in humans with ragweed allergy by injecting Amb a 1 linked to immunostimulatory DNA. J Allergy Clin Immunol 2004;113(6):1144–51.
[23] Zhu D, Kepley CL, Zhang K, et al. A chimeric human-cat fusion protein blocks cat-induced allergy. Nat Med 2005;11(4):446–9.
[24] Gronlund H, Vrtala S, Wiedermann U, et al. Carbohydrate-based particles: a new adjuvant for allergen-specific immunotherapy. Immunology 2002;107(4):523–9.
[25] Roth-Walter F, Scholl I, Untersmayr E, et al. Mucosal targeting of allergen-loaded microspheres by Aleuria aurantia lectin. Vaccine 2005;23(21):2703–10.

IMMUNOLOGY
AND ALLERGY
CLINICS
OF NORTH AMERICA

Immunol Allergy Clin N Am
26 (2006) 179–189

Allergy Diagnosis, Allergen Repertoires, and Their Implications for Allergen-Specific Immunotherapy

Reto Crameri, PhD

Molecular Allergology, Swiss Institute of Allergy and Asthma Research (SIAF), Obere Strasse 22, CH-7270 Davos, Switzerland

Allergic and asthmatic diseases represent a big health problem in industrialized countries where as many as 20% to 30% of the population sustain type I allergic symptoms such as rhinitis, conjunctivitis, atopic dermatitis, or bronchial asthma [1,2]. These diseases represent an important cause of morbidity and, occasionally, mortality [3]. Atopic disorders have become a relevant socioeconomic problem causing a health care burden to society in the order of billions of US dollars [4,5]. A common hallmark of these diseases is the production of allergen-specific IgE against normally innocuous environmental antigens. In sensitized individuals, allergen re-exposure induces cross-linking of high-affinity FcER1 receptor-bound IgE on effector cells and immediate release of anaphylactogenic mediators [6]. The clinical symptoms deriving from mild type I hypersensitivity reactions are not life threatening and manifest mainly as generalized urticaria, itching, constriction in the chest, nausea, vomiting, angioedema, and abdominal pain. Severe forms manifest as dyspnea, wheezing, and respiratory and cardiovascular symptoms up to shock with loss of consciousness and are associated with a risk of fatal reaction [7].

Current drugs for allergic diseases, such as antihistamines, corticosteroids, bronchodilators (β-adrenergic receptor antagonists), and anti-IgE antibody ther-

This work was supported by grants 31-63382.00/2 and 310000-112540 from the Swiss National Science Foundation and by the OPO-Stiftung, Zürich.

E-mail address: crameri@siaf.unizh.ch

apy, treat allergy symptoms and concomitant inflammatory reactions [8] and require a long-term recurrent administration of the drugs [9,10]. Allergen-specific immunotherapy (SIT) is the only treatment able to cure allergic diseases and has been shown to be successful in insect venom allergy [11] and patients sustaining allergic rhinitis [12] but not in other complex allergy syndromes such as eczema, food, or mold allergy [13]. There is a need for defining new therapeutic targets and strategies to allow a more efficient treatment of allergic diseases justified by the severely impaired quality of life of affected individuals and the annual costs related to the treatment of allergy and asthma [3–5]. Hyposensitization (immuno-therapy) is the practice of administrating gradually increasing quantities of an allergen extract to an allergic individual to ameliorate the symptoms associated with subsequent exposure to the causative allergen. Standardized allergen extracts have been designated "vaccines" in a recent World Health Organization position article on allergen immunotherapy [14]. Currently, allergen-SIT is performed using extracts from natural sources containing insufficiently characterized aller-gen mixtures and unwanted nonallergenic components. Immunotherapeutic treat-ment of allergic disease spans a period of 3 to 5 years. Unfortunately, allergen extract–based SIT can induce anaphylaxis as well as new IgE responses to aller-gens contained in the extract [15,16]. The development of new strategies for disease management requires a detailed understanding of the molecules able to elicit allergic reactions and the immunologic mechanisms underlying the pathol-ogy of type I hypersensitivity reactions.

Physiologic background of allergic diseases

The breakthrough in understanding hypersensitivity reactions was the discov-ery of the "reaginic antibody," termed *immunoglobulin E* (IgE), by Ishizaka and Ishizaka [17] more than 30 years ago. Allergy is caused by the overproduction of allergen-specific IgE in response to the exposure to allergens [1]. Pollens, foods, dust mites, animal dander, fungal spores, and insect venoms represent the most important sources of sensitization leading, after re-exposure, to a variety of dif-ferent clinical manifestations classified on the basis of their immunologic patho-genesis. The classification of hypersensitivity reactions into types I to IV [18] is widely accepted and used in clinical practice. In this context, the term *allergy* is used in a restricted sense to describe type I hypersensitivity reactions referring to damage caused by IgE antibody–mediated immune responses. IgE, a class of immunoglobulin normally present in the serum at low concentrations, is pro-duced by IgE-secreting plasma cells, which express the antibody on their surface at a certain stage of their maturation [19]. For reasons still not well understood, allergic individuals produce increased amounts of IgE with binding specificity for ordinarily innocuous antigens to which they are sensitive [20,21]. The allergen-specific IgE circulates in the blood and binds to IgE-specific receptors on the surface of basophils in the circulation and mast cells along mucosal linings and underneath the skin. During re-exposure, the inhaled or ingested allergens bind to IgE on mast cells and basophils, cross-link the IgE molecules, and aggregate the underlying receptors, triggering the effector cells to release histamine and other pharmacologic mediators causing symptomatic responses [22]. Systemic reactions to allergens may involve the cutaneous, gastrointestinal, respiratory, and cardiovascular systems, presenting in some cases as anaphylaxis [23].

Diagnosis of allergy and allergen repertoires

The diagnosis of an allergy is based on clinical history, skin test reactivity to the offending allergen, and in vitro determination of allergen-specific IgE antibodies in serum [24]. The results of in vivo and in vitro diagnostic procedures strongly depend on the allergen preparation used [25]. Despite many commercially available allergen extracts, only a few standardized extracts recognized by the US Food and Drug Administration are currently available [26]. The accuracy of skin tests in vivo and IgE determinations in vitro can be compromised if conducted with different protocols or with allergen extracts having insufficient quality control. Given the respective trajectories for technologic advancement, quantification, and quality control, recombinant allergens producible as single highly pure reagents offer a standardized approach for the diagnosis and treatment of allergic diseases [25]. Theoretically, single recombinant allergens can also be used as vaccines for an allergen-SIT; however, the success of such a treatment will depend on a patient-specific component-resolved diagnosis of the molecular structures to which a given individual is sensitized to avoid new sensitizations to additional allergens present in the extracts used for therapy [15].

The major allergens from the most prevalent allergenic sources (eg, pollens, mites, animal dander, food, molds, and insect venoms) have been identified and produced by recombinant DNA technology, allowing the assembly of panels of recombinant allergens reconstructing the epitope complexity of the corresponding allergen extracts [27–31]. The number of different allergenic structures present in different sources is highly variable. Some extracts such as grass and tree pollens or bee venoms contain only a few allergens, and it has been shown in both cases that a component-resolved allergy diagnosis based on recombinant allergens, approaching the sensitivity of the diagnoses obtained with commercially available allergen extracts, is feasible [32,33]. Other allergenic sources such as mites or molds contain complex allergen repertoires spanning several dozen different molecular structures [28,34,35]. *Aspergillus fumigatus* with an estimated allergen repertoire of more that 80 different structural entities represents the most complex system described thus far [36]. Nevertheless, sensitization to *A fumigatus* using skin tests and serology can be diagnosed with a high sensitivity and specificity using recombinant allergens [37,38].

In general, it is widely recognized that the diagnosis of allergic diseases based on recombinant allergens is superior to extract-based diagnosis in terms of specificity [39]. The technologic achievements in producing recombinant proteins will allow one to reconstruct the epitope complexity of natural extracts by mixing up panels of single recombinant allergens. The big challenge in view of diagnostic and therapeutic applications of recombinant allergens will be to estimate the size of the epitope repertoire needed to substitute allergen extracts. Bioinformatics analyses based on structural motifs [40] and BLAST similarity search methods [41] involving 101,602 and 135,850 protein entries deposited in the Swissprot database predict 4093 (4%) and 4768 (3.5%) different potential allergen structures, respectively; therefore, one can assume that the size of the allergen repertoire involved in eliciting allergic symptoms is in the range of 5000 different structures. Not all structures will be required for diagnostic and therapeutic applications, because many allergens can be grouped in pan-allergen families sharing cross-reactive epitopes [42–45]. Cross-reactivity will reduce drastically the number of epitopes needed for a careful diagnosis of allergic conditions. The rapidly increasing knowledge of primary and three-dimensional structures of allergens [46] will speed up theoretical and practical progress in defining the number of structures/epitopes needed for a component-resolved diagnosis of allergic diseases, forming the basis for the development of rational therapy approaches. Moreover, rapid progress in developing microchip-based diagnostic procedures [47,48] will allow parallel multiplexed analyses of serum samples at low cost, a prerequisite to establish the use of recombinant allergens in clinical routine assessments.

Current forms of allergy treatment

Current drugs for allergic diseases, such as antihistamines, corticosteroids, and bronchodilators (β-adrenergic receptor antagonists) treat allergic symptoms and concomitant inflammatory reactions [8]. Although pharmacotherapeutic ap-

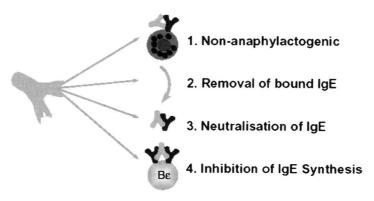

Fig. 1. Properties of antihuman IgE monoclonal antibodies used in passive anti-IgE therapy. (*Adapted from* Marti P. New perspectives for allergy diagnosis and therapy [PhD thesis]. University of Berne, 2006; with permission.)

proaches are effective in controlling symptoms, these therapies have a limited capacity to alter the natural course of allergic diseases, and discontinuation of medication results in the redevelopment of symptoms on re-exposure to the offending allergen. A new approach in treating allergic diseases and asthma consists of the administration of anti-IgE antibodies to out-compete IgE binding to the FcφRI and FcφRII receptors (Fig. 1), preventing cross-linking and release of mediators [9]. This type of treatment requires a long-term recurrent administration of the drug [10]. SIT, the only treatment to cure allergic diseases, is performed using allergen extracts [14]. Unfortunately, SIT can induce new IgE responses to allergens contained in the extract [15] as well as anaphylaxis [49]. A long-term therapy consisting of the practice of administrating subcutaneously gradually increasing doses of an allergen extract to an allergic individual, SIT is most efficiently used in allergies to insect venoms [11] and allergic rhinitis [12,50]. It is not efficient in other complex allergic syndromes, such as eczema, food, or mold allergy [13].

New trends in allergen-specific immunotherapy

Recent advances in understanding the immunologic mechanisms underlying allergic diseases and the molecular characterization of allergen repertoires have greatly expanded the potential therapeutic options for future use. Nevertheless, only a few new drugs have reached clinical application, and none provides long-term immunomodulatory effects [51]. Immunotherapy through its capacity to produce a long-lasting, antigen-specific, protective immune response is the only etiologic treatment that offers the possibility of curing or even preventing atopic diseases [52,53]; however, the potential for severe side effects associated with conventional immunotherapy using whole allergen extracts limits its widespread use, especially in highly sensitized individuals [7,54]. The major problem has been recognized to be related to IgE-facilitated allergen presentation mediated by allergen-specific B cells [55]. B cells can present low concentrations of allergen to T cells (Fig. 2), inducing high interleukin-4 (IL-4) but little or no interferon-γ (INF-γ), favoring Th2-biased immune responses. By contrast, the use of monocytes and macrophages as antigen-presenting cells and high doses of allergen results in high INF-γ but low IL-4 synthesis, favoring an immune deviation toward a balanced Th0/Th1 immune response associated with blocking antibodies [55,56]. As a consequence, the high doses required for successful immunotherapy might not be reached using native allergen extracts [55]. Novel strategies to minimize the side effects and improve the efficacy of immunotherapy are of considerable interest in the treatment of atopic diseases. Promising animal and human studies using approaches such as peptide immunotherapy, DNA vaccination, CpG oligonucleotides, and modified allergens suggest that it might be possible to prevent or cure atopic disorders in an efficient way [52,53]. Nevertheless, the actual vaccination concepts still suffer from an extremely long treatment period as true for classical SIT, and the development of improved and

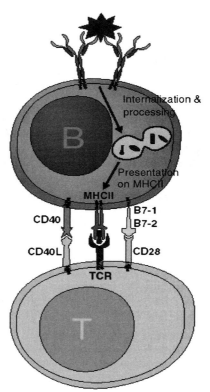

Fig. 2. B-cell–mediated antigen presentation. Antigen binding to B cells expressing allergen-specific IgE on their surface stimulates expression of the co-stimulatory molecules B7-1 and B7-2. Internalization and presentation of allergen-derived peptides on the MHC class II context to T helper cells results in T-cell activation and induction of CD40 ligand. CD40/CD40L interaction induces B-cell proliferation. Because new IgE-secreting plasma cells go through mIgE-expressing B-cell stages during differentiation, CD40/CD40L–mediated B-cell proliferation is an efficient way to stimulate allergen-specific serum IgE production. (*Adapted from* Inführ S, Crameri R, Lamers R, et al. Molecular and cellular targets of anti-IgE antibodies. Allergy 2005;60:981; with permission.)

safe allergy vaccines represents one of the most important challenges in allergy and asthma research.

Therapeutic approaches based on recombinant allergens

Recombinant DNA technology enables allergens to be produced with high quality in terms of purity, batch-to-batch consistency, composition, and dosage, satisfying the requirements for therapeutic applications in humans. Theoretically, there is also the possibility of formulating personalized vaccines including only allergens to which the patient is sensitized to, avoiding the risk of inducing new sensitizations during the time course of the therapy [57]. Moreover, the same technology allows the generation of allergens with reduced IgE-binding capacity [58–60], the production of multimeres [61], the fusion of vaccines containing different allergens [62] or epitopes [63], and the creation of unfolded recombinant molecules voided of IgE-binding epitopes [64,65]. Currently, all proposed concepts for improving SIT based on recombinant allergens remain highly speculative. To date, only two clinical studies involving vaccination with rBet v 1, the major birch pollen allergen, and a mixture of five recombinant *Phleum pratense* allergens are available from the literature [66,67]. Both studies show that recombinant allergen vaccines can be effective and safe, as least for the treatment of allergic rhinitis. Additionally, peptide-based immunotherapy using short synthetic peptides derived from Api m 1, the major bee venom allergen [68], and the major cat allergen Fel d 1 [69] has been clinically evaluated.

Although these studies indicate the possibility of using peptides containing the major T-cell epitopes of allergens for successful immunotherapy, the approach requires prior identification of the T-cell epitopes to be able to produce the synthetic peptides required for treatment. In view of the complexity of the allergen repertoire, it seems questionable that such an approach will be feasible on a large scale.

SIT is the only treatment available for allergic diseases that can cure patients, and recombinant allergens are suitable reagents that can induce long-lasting protection against the natural offending allergens. Open questions regarding successful applications of recombinant allergens for SIT are less related to scientific issues and more to financial and regulatory aspects. Because the regulatory requirements include cGMP material for human use, with the costs of production of vaccines based on a hundred different recombinant allergens, the therapy concept based on these substances is unlikely to be financially affordable. Only in a few exceptions, such as birch pollen or cat allergy, could one expect that a single allergen or a mixture of a few molecular structures would be sufficient to treat the majority of patients.

The most prominent problem in SIT is the dropout of patients in concomitance with the long treatment period required to obtain protection. Classical SIT requires approximately 30 to 80 injections with the respective allergen over 3 to 5 years, and at least 1 hour of medical supervision is required after every allergen injection. Although SIT from a medical perspective is clearly the best treatment for an allergy, few patients can afford or are willing to invest the time for 30 to 80 physician visits lasting more than 1 hour over several years. Patients' compliance for immunotherapy is likely to increase if the vaccination procedures can be drastically shortened. Research to enhance the efficiency of allergy vaccines is focused mainly on improving the adjuvant or the type and form of the antigen used, although some activities are devoted to studying the effects of the route of administration on therapy success. Allergy vaccines are generally administered subcutaneously or intradermally, from where they must reach secondary lymphatic organs to induce an immune response. Recent studies show that direct injection of naked DNA vaccines [70], peptide vaccines [71], and adjuvant [72] into peripheral lymph nodes dramatically enhances the immunogenicity of the substances. In view of the fact that even large amounts of immunogenic antigens can be ignored by the immune system, as long as they remain outside organized lymphoid tissue [73], these results are not unexpected. The first clinical evaluations of the direct injection of bee venom extract and grass pollen extract into the lymph nodes of correspondingly sensitized patients have shown that three injections scattered over a period of 1 month are sufficient to confer a long-lasting protection against allergen re-exposure (T. Kündig, personal communication, 2006). If confirmed in a large number of patients, these results should have important implications for the clinical immunotherapy of allergic diseases.

Summary

The first two reports on SIT for birch and grass pollen allergy based on recombinant allergens show the feasibility of the approach. Recombinant allergen vaccines can be an effective and safe treatment to ameliorate the symptoms of allergic rhinitis and probably other forms of allergies including allergic asthma. Allergen repertoires can be cloned and characterized in a short time, and each single allergen can be produced at reasonable yields and of a quality satisfying the standards for applications in humans. Nevertheless, the two reports to date on allergen-specific SIT are based on procedures similar to those used in conventional SIT, which spans a long treatment period. To become more attractive, SIT needs to be optimized in terms of dosage, component-resolved composition according to the sensitization pattern of single individuals, and the number of injections required to achieve protection. In an optimal scenario, allergen vaccines would be effective after the administration of a few injections like in conventional vaccinations. The achievement of this goal would substantially decrease the costs related to SIT, increase the patient's compliance, and, consequently, result in a strong reduction of the dropouts associated with classical long-term SIT.

References

[1] Hopkin JM. Mechanisms of enhanced prevalence of asthma and atopy in developed countries. Curr Opin Immunol 1997;9:788–92.
[2] Sennhauser FH, Braun-Fahrlander C, Wildhaber JH. The burden of asthma in children: a European perspective. Paediatr Respir Rev 2005;6:2–7.
[3] Montanaro A, Bardana Jr EJ. The mechanisms, causes, and treatment of anaphylaxis. J Invest Allergol Clin Immunol 2002;12:2–11.
[4] Law AW, Reed SD, Sundy JS, et al. Direct costs of allergic rhinitis in the United States: estimates from the 1996 Medical Expenditure Panel Survey. J Allergy Clin Immunol 2003;111:296–300.
[5] Gupta R, Sheikh A, Strachan DP, et al. Burden of allergic disease in the UK: secondary analyses of national databases. Clin Exp Allergy 2004;34:520–6.
[6] Turner H, Kinet JP. Signalling through the high-affinity IgE receptor FcφRI. Nature 1999;402(Suppl. 6760):B24–30.

[7] Rusznak C, Peebles Jr RS. Anaphylaxis and anaphylactoid reactions: a guide to prevention, recognition, and emergent treatment. Postgrad Med 2002;111:101–4.
[8] Barnes PJ. Therapeutic strategies for allergic diseases. Nature 1999;402(Suppl. 6760):B31–8.
[9] Chang TW. The pharmacological basis of anti-IgE therapy. Nat Biotechnol 2000;18:157–62.
[10] Milgrom H. Anti-IgE therapy in allergic disease. Curr Opin Pediatr 2004;16:642–7.
[11] Müller UR. Recent developments and future strategies for immunotherapy of insect venom allergy. Curr Opin Allergy Clin Immunol 2003;3:299–303.
[12] Durham SR, Walker SM, Varga EM, et al. Long-term clinical efficacy of grass-pollen immunotherapy. N Engl J Med 1999;341:468–75.
[13] Burks W, Bannon G, Lehrer SB. Classic specific immunotherapy and new perspectives in specific immunotherapy for food allergy. Allergy 2001;56(Suppl. 67):121–4.
[14] Bousquet J, Lockey RR, Malling HJ. Allergen immunotherapy: therapeutic vaccines for allergic diseases. A WHO Position Paper. J Allergy Clin Immunol 1998;102:558–62.
[15] van Hage-Hamsten M, Valenta R. Specific immunotherapy—the induction of new IgE specificities? Allergy 2002;57:375–7.
[16] Gastaminza G, Algorta J, Audicana M, et al. Systemic reactions to immunotherapy: influence of composition and manufacturer. Clin Exp Allergy 2003;33:470–4.
[17] Ishizaka K, Ishizaka T. Identification of gamma-E antibodies as a carrier of reaginic activity. J Immunol 1967;99:1187–98.
[18] Coombs RRA, Gell PGH. The classification of allergic reactions underlying disease. In: Gell PGH, Coombs RRA, editors. Clinical aspects of immunology. Philadelphia: F.A. Davis; 1963. p. 333.
[19] Inführ S, Crameri R, Lamers R, et al. Molecular and cellular targets of anti-IgE antibodies. Allergy 2005;60:977–85.
[20] O'Hehir RE, Graman RD, Greenstein JL, et al. The specificity and regulation of T-cell responsiveness to allergens. Annu Rev Immunol 1991;9:67–95.
[21] Leung DY. Molecular basis of allergic diseases. Mol Genet Metab 1998;63:157–67.
[22] Sutton BJ, Gould HJ. The human IgE network. Nature 1993;366:421–8.
[23] Greineder DK. Risk management in allergen immunotherapy. J Allergy Clin Immunol 1996; 98:330–4.
[24] Krouse JH, Stachler RJ, Shah A. Current in vivo and in vitro screens for inhalant allergy. Otolaryngol Clin North Am 2003;36:855–68.
[25] Chapman MD, Smith AM, Vailes LD, et al. Recombinant allergens for diagnosis and therapy of allergic disease. J Allergy Clin Immunol 2002;106:409–18.
[26] American Academy of Allergy, Asthma and Immunology. Position statement: the use of standardized allergen extracts. J Allergy Clin Immunol 1997;99:583–6.
[27] Andersson K, Lidholm J. Characteristics and immunobiology of grass pollen allergens. Int Arch Allergy Immunol 2003;130:87–107.
[28] Thomas WR, Smith W. Towards defining the full spectrum of important house dust mite allergens. Clin Exp Allergy 1999;29:896–904.
[29] Lorenz AR, Scheurer S, Haustein D, et al. Recombinant food allergens. J Chromatogr B Biomed Sci Appl 2001;756:255–79.
[30] Weichel M, Flückiger S, Crameri R. Molecular characterisation of mold allergens involved in respiratory complications. Recent Dev Resp Crit Care Med 2002;2:29–45.
[31] King TP, Spangfort MD. Structure and biology of stinging insect venom allergens. Int Arch Allergy Imunol 2000;123:183–95.
[32] Müller UR. New developments in the diagnosis and treatment of hymenoptera venom allergy. Int Arch Allegy Immunol 2001;124:447–53.
[33] Heiss S, Mahler V, Steiner R, et al. Component-resolved diagnosis (CRD) of type I allergy with recombinant grass and tree pollen allergens by skin testing. J Invest Dermatol 1999;113:830–7.
[34] Le Mao J, Mayer C, Peltre G, et al. Mapping of *Dermatophagoides farinae* mite allergens by two-dimensional immunoblotting. J Allergy Clin Immunol 1998;102:631–6.
[35] Crameri R, Weichel M, Flückiger S, et al. Fungal allergies: a yet unsolved problem. Chem Immunol Allergy 2006;91:121–33.

[36] Kodzius R, Rhyner C, Konthur Z, et al. Rapid identification of allergen-encoding cDNA clones by phage display and high density arrays. Combin Chem High Throughput Screen 2003;6: 147–54.

[37] Crameri R, Hemmann S, Ismail C, et al. Disease-specific recombinant allergens for the diagnosis of allergic bronchopulmonary aspergillosis. Int Immunol 1998;10:1211–6.

[38] Hemmann S, Nilolaizik WH, Schöni MH, et al. Differential IgE recognition of recombinant *Aspergillus fumigatus* allergens by cystic fibrosis patients with allergic bronchopulmonary aspergillosis or *Aspergillus* allergy. Eur J Immunol 1998;28:1155–60.

[39] Schmid-Grendelmeier P, Crameri R. Recombinant allergens for skin testing. Int Arch Allergy Immunol 2001;125:96–111.

[40] Stadler MB, Stadler BM. Allergenicity prediction by protein sequence. FASEB J 2003;17: 1141–3.

[41] Li KB, Issac P, Krishnan A. Predicting allergenic proteins using wavelet transform. Bioinformatics 2004;20:2572–8.

[42] Valenta R, Duchene M, Ebner C, et al. Profilins constitute a novel family of functional plant pan-allergens. J Exp Med 1992;175:377–85.

[43] Reese G, Ayuso R, Lehrer SB. Tropomyosin: an invertebrate pan-allergen. Int Arch Allergy Immunol 1999;119:247–58.

[44] Flückiger S, Fijten H, Whitley P, et al. Cyclophilins, a new family of cross-reactive allergens. Eur J Immunol 2002;32:10–7.

[45] Barral P, Batanero E, Palomares O, et al. A major allergen from pollen defines a novel family of plant proteins and shows intra- and interspecies cross-reactivity. J Immunol 2004;172:3644–51.

[46] Flückiger S, Limacher A, Glaser AG, et al. Structural aspects of cross-reactive allergens. Recent Res Dev Allergy Clin Immunol 2004;5:57–75.

[47] Hiller R, Laffer S, Harwanegg C, et al. Microarrayed allergen molecules: diagnostic gatekeepers for allergy treatment. FASEB J 2002;16:414–6.

[48] Deinhofer K, Sevcik H, Balic N, et al. Microarrayed allergens for IgE profiling. Methods 2004;32:249–54.

[49] Moverare R, Elfman L, Vesterinen E, et al. Development of new IgE specificities to allergic components in birch pollen extract during specific immunotherapy studied with immunoblotting and Pharmacia CAP System. Allergy 2002;57:423–30.

[50] DuBuske LM. Appropriate and inappropriate use of immunotherapy. Ann Allergy Asthma Immunol 2001;87(Suppl. 1):56–7.

[51] Walker C, Zuany-Amorim C. New trends in immunotherapy to prevent atopic diseases. Trends Pharmacol Sci 2001;22:84–90.

[52] Campbell D, DeKruiff RH, Umetsu DT. Allergen immunotherapy: novel approaches in the management of allergic diseases and asthma. Clin Immunol 2000;97:193–202.

[53] Valenta R, Kraft D. From allergen structure to new forms of allergen-specific immunotherapy. Curr Opin Immunol 2002;14:718–27.

[54] Nettis E, Giordano D, Ferrannini A, et al. Systemic reaction to allergen immunotherapy: a review of the literature. Immunopharmacol Immunotoxicol 2003;25:1–11.

[55] Akdis CA, Blaser K. Bypassing IgE and targeting T cells for specific immunotherapy of allergy. Trends Immunol 2001;24:175–8.

[56] Akdis CA, Blesken T, Wymann D, et al. Differential regulation of human T cell cytokine patterns and IgE and IgG4 responses by conformational antigen variants. Eur J Immunol 1998;28:914–25.

[57] Valenta R, Lidholm J, Niederberger V, et al. The recombinant allergen-based concept of component-resolved diagnostics and immunotherapy (CRD and CRIT). Clin Exp Allergy 1999; 29:896–904.

[58] Ferreira F, Ebner C, Kramer B, et al. Modulation of IgE reactivity of allergens by site-directed mutagenesis: potential use of hypoallergenic variants for immunotherapy. FASEB J 1998;12:231–42.

[59] Chapman MD, Smith AM, Vailes LC, et al. Recombinant allergens for immunotherapy. Allergy Asthma Proc 2002;23:5–8.

[60] Saarne T, Kaiser L, Grönlund H, et al. Rational design of hypoallergens applied to the major cat allergen Fel d 1. Clin Exp Allergy 2005;35:657–63.

[61] Vrtala S, Hintenlehrer K, Susani M, et al. Genetic engineering of a hypoallergenic trimer of the major birch pollen allergen Bet v 1. FASEB J 2001;15:2045–7.

[62] Kussebi F, Karamloo F, Rhyner C, et al. A major allergen gene-fusion protein for potential usage in allergen-specific immunotherapy. J Allergy Clin Immunol 2005;115:323–9.

[63] Linhard B, Hartl A, Jahn-Schmid B, et al. A hybrid molecule resembling the epitope spectrum of grass pollen for allergy vaccination. J Allergy Clin Immunol 2005;115:1010–6.

[64] Neudecker P, Lehmann K, Nerkamp J, et al. Mutational epitope analysis of Pur av 1 and Api g 1, the major allergens of cherry (*Prunus avium*) and celery (*Apium graveolens*): correlating IgE reactivity with three dimensional structure. Biochem J 2003;376:97–107.

[65] Crameri R. Correlating IgE with three-dimensional structure. Biochem J 2003;376:e1–2.

[66] Niederberger V, Horak F, Vrtala S, et al. Vaccination with genetically engineered allergens prevents progression of allergic disease. Proc Natl Acad Sci USA 2004;101(Suppl. 2): 14677–82.

[67] Jutel M, Jaeger L, Suck R, et al. Allergen-specific immunotherapy with recombinant grass pollen allergens. J Allergy Clin Immunol 2005;60:1459–70.

[68] Müller U, Akdis CA, Fricker M, et al. Successful immunotherapy with T-cell epitope peptides of bee venom phospholipase A_2 induces specific T-cell anergy in patients allergic to bee venom. J Allergy Clin Immunol 1998;101:747–54.

[69] Pene J, Besroches A, Paradis L, et al. Immunotherapy with Fel d 1 peptides decreases IL-4 release by peripheral blood T cells of patients allergic to cats. J Allergy Clin Immunol 1998;102: 571–8.

[70] Maloy KJ, Erdmann I, Basch V, et al. Intralymphatic immunization enhances DANN vaccination. Proc Natl Acad Sci USA 2001;98:3299–303.

[71] Johansen P, Haffner AC, Koch F, et al. Direct intralymphatic injection of peptide vaccine enhances immunogenicity. Eur J Biochem 2005;35:568–74.

[72] von Beust BR, Johansen P, Smith KA, et al. Improving the therapeutic index of CpG oligodeoxynucleotides by intralymphatic administration. Eur J Immunol 2005;35:1869–76.

[73] Zinkernagel RM, Ehl S, Aichele P, et al. Antigen localisation regulates immune responses in a dose- and time-dependent fashion: a geographical view of immune reactivity. Immunol Rev 1997;156:199–209.

ELSEVIER
SAUNDERS

Immunol Allergy Clin N Am
26 (2006) 191–206

IMMUNOLOGY
AND ALLERGY
CLINICS
OF NORTH AMERICA

Standardization of Allergen-Specific Immunotherapy Vaccines

Michael D. Spangfort, PhD*, Jørgen Nedergaard Larsen, PhD

ALK-Abelló, Bøge Allé 6-8, DK – 2970 Hørsholm, Denmark

History of standardization

Specific allergy treatment (ie, specific immunotherapy or specific allergy vaccination) has been performed for almost a century since Noon [1] first described it in 1911. The discovery in 1967 of the IgE molecule [2,3] and the central role of IgE in allergy gradually led to a better understanding of the immunologic mechanisms, improved diagnostic tools, and a consolidation of the concept of specific allergy diagnosis and treatment. In the 1970s and 1980s, scientific methods were introduced in the standardization of allergen vaccines [4] and, in combination with improved documentation of the clinical benefits obtained using standardized vaccines, specific allergy treatment as a scientifically based, reproducible, and safe treatment for allergic disease was established.

The first international initiative on allergen standardization was the preparation of the Nordic Guidelines [5], which were based on the Danish Allergen Standardization 1976 program. These guidelines established the first regulatory demands for allergen vaccines. The guidelines introduced the biological unit (BU) based on skin testing for potency measures. In Europe, current regulations in agreement with the Nordic Guidelines recommend that each manufacturer produces an in-house reference preparation (IHRP) and use it for batch-to-batch control using scientifically based laboratory testing [6]. The significance of the major allergen content for biologic activity was recognized in the early 1990s, and is now established in the World Health Organization (WHO) recommendations [7] and the European pharmacopoeia [8].

---

* Corresponding author.
E-mail address: msp@dk.alk-abello.com (M.D. Spangfort).

0889-8561/06/$ – see front matter © 2006 Elsevier Inc. All rights reserved.
doi:10.1016/j.iac.2006.02.012   *immunology.theclinics.com*

In the United States, the regulation of allergen extracts is much different from that of Europe. The Food and Drug Administration (FDA) issues common standards and assays for all manufacturers to use [9]. This system is more transparent but also more rigid.

This article describes important issues in the control of source materials and vaccine preparation as part of the European standardization of allergen vaccines, and also includes a discussion of vaccines that are based on recombinant allergens, which may appear on the market in the near future.

Standardization of allergen vaccines

Allergen vaccines are complex mixtures of antigenic components. They are produced through extraction of naturally occurring source materials that are known to vary considerably in composition, depending on time and place. Without intervention, this variation would be reflected in the final products.

Source materials

The source materials for allergy vaccines should represent the material to which humans are exposed, and selected with attention to the need for specificity and inclusion of all relevant allergens in sufficient amounts [10]. The collection of the source materials should be performed by qualified personnel, and reasonable measures must be used by the producer of allergenic vaccines to ensure that collector qualifications and collection procedures are appropriate for verifying the identity and quality of the source materials. Only specifically identified allergenic source materials that do not contain avoidable foreign substances should be used in the manufacture of allergenic vaccines. Means of identification and limits of foreign materials should meet established acceptance criteria for each source material. Processing and storage of source materials should prevent decomposition and ensure that no unintended substances, including microbial organisms, are introduced into the materials.

Strategy for standardization

The production process leading to allergen extracts is basically an aqueous extraction of source materials followed by purification and adjustment of potency. The nature of the active ingredient imposes several constraints on the selection of source materials and physicochemical conditions used during the extraction procedure. The process must neither denature the proteins/allergens nor significantly alter the composition, including the quantitative ratio among soluble components.

Standardization of allergen vaccines is complicated because of the complexity of the allergen vaccines, the allergen molecules, and their epitopes. Acquired immune responses are driven by contact with epitopes, which are structural elements of the allergens (antigens). T-cell epitopes are linear fragments of the polypeptide chain, whereas B-cell epitopes (ie, antibody-binding epitopes) are sections of the surface structure present only in the native conformation of the allergen. T- and B-cell epitopes are apparently essential for effective initiation and stimulation of immune responses to immunotherapy.

The allergens themselves are complex mixtures of isoallergens and variants that differ in amino acid sequence. Some allergens are composed of two or more subunits, the association and dissociation of which affect IgE binding. In addition, partial denaturation or degradation, which may be imposed by physical or chemical conditions in the production process, is difficult to assess and may have a significant effect on the conformation of the allergens.

Another complicating aspect is the complexity of the immune responses of individual patients. Patients respond individually to allergen sources with respect to specificity and potency. Allergens are proteins, and all proteins are potential allergens. A *major allergen* is statistically defined as an allergen that is frequently recognized by serum IgE when a larger panel of patient sera is analyzed. Less frequent IgE-binding allergens (less than 50%) are termed *minor allergens* [11]. Furthermore, patients respond individually to B- and T-cell epitopes and hence to isoallergens and variants.

A major aspect of allergen vaccine standardization, therefore, is to ensure an adequate complexity in vaccine composition. Knowledge of all essential allergens is a precondition to ensure their presence in the final products.

The other important aspect of standardization is the control of the total allergenic potency. The total IgE-binding activity is intimately related to the content of major allergen [12], and control of the content of major allergen is essential for an optimal standardization procedure.

Various techniques are available to assess allergen vaccine complexity and potency. Most of these techniques use antibodies as reagents, adding another level of complexity to the standardization procedure. Human IgE and antibodies raised through immunization of animals are subject to natural variation and may change over time.

These problems are handled by the establishment of reference and control standards. International collaboration is necessary to ensure that manufacturers, control authorities, clinicians, and research laboratories worldwide refer to the same preparations when comparing the results of quality control studies and potency estimates for different allergen vaccines. Ideally, standards for reagents should also be established in international collaborations.

The establishment and use of international standards

In 1980 to 1981, a subcommittee under the International Union of Immunological Societies (IUIS) formulated guidelines for the establishment of international standards. The collaboration and joint authority of WHO was assumed to be essential for international acceptance. In the following years, the subcommittee selected, characterized, and produced international standards from several allergenic sources, including *Ambrosia artemisiifolia* (short ragweed) [13], *Phleum pratense* (timothy grass) [14], *Dermatophagoides pteronyssinus* (house dust mite) [15], *Betula verrucosa* (birch) [16], and *Canis familiaris* (dog) [17]. Additional standards were planned but terminated prematurely because of lack of general acceptance.

Each of these standard reference vaccines has been thoroughly investigated in collaborative studies involving laboratories and clinics worldwide. The results of the characterization and comparison of several coded vaccines, which were made available by allergen manufacturers on a voluntary basis, and the selection of the international standards have been published and are available. Each international standard was produced in 3000 to 4000 lyophilized, glass-sealed ampules, which can be obtained from the National Institute of Biological Science and Control located in Herts, United Kingdom.

Recently, the WHO-IUIS Allergen Standardization Committee has taken an initiative, funded by the European Union, to develop certified reference materials (CRMs) based on purified natural and recombinant allergens (ie, the CREATE Project) [18].

Depending on the success of this initiative, the existence and availability of allergen CRMs will enable a major allergen content to be assigned in common units to the internal reference preparations that are being used in different laboratories of manufacturers, allergen research groups, or control authorities.

The establishment and use of in-house reference preparations

In an established production process, including control of raw material, batch-to-batch standardization is performed relative to an IHRP. The IHRP must be thoroughly characterized through in vitro laboratory methods to show an adequate complexity and appropriate content of relevant major allergens. The potency of the IHRP must be determined through in vivo methods, such as skin testing, and the content of major allergens must be determined in absolute amounts. Furthermore, the IHRP should be efficacious in clinical trials of specific allergy vaccination.

The IHRP serves as a blueprint of the allergy vaccine to be matched by every following batch in all aspects. Specific activities of the IHRP should be compared with international standards. Using this method, measures from different manufacturers can be compared and consistency in internal standardization can be achieved [19].

Batch-to-batch standardization

In the production of routine batches of allergen vaccines, assessments of the clinical effect on every batch are impossible to make. In practical standardization, the batches are compared with the IHRP through a combination of different in vitro techniques to achieve a constant composition, content of major allergen, and potency. Proper performance of these controls ensures a constant clinical efficacy.

The standardization can be performed using the following three-step procedure:

1. Determination of allergen composition to ensure that all important allergens are present
2. Quantification of specific allergens to ensure that essential allergens are present in constant ratios
3. Quantification of the total allergenic activity to ensure that the overall potency of the vaccine is constant (in vivo or in vitro)

Methods for the assessment of allergen vaccine quality

The quality of an allergen extract is a measure of the composition complexity, including the concentration of each constituent. Having established a careful control of raw materials and a robust production process, a constant ratio among individual components can be achieved by quantifying only one or two components independently (ie, the major allergens).

The complexity of the composition of allergen extracts can be assessed using several techniques. These techniques are standard separation techniques in biochemistry and traditional immunochemistry. Crossed immunoelectrophoresis (CIE) [20] is a nondenaturing technique and is therefore well suited for batch-to-batch control. The technique is dependent on the availability of broadly reactive polyspecific rabbit antibodies, but yields information on the relative concentrations of several important antigens in a single experiment.

Quantification of specific allergens

Having determined an adequate complexity in composition, an allergen extract may theoretically still be deficient in the content of major allergen (Fig. 1).

The content of major allergens must be assessed independently, especially for allergen extracts used for allergy vaccination. The maintenance dose in effective allergy vaccination contains a well-defined amount of major allergen (ie, 5–20 μg, regardless of species [7]), and the major allergen content is therefore a usable measure relating vaccine potency and therapeutic effect.

The importance of controlling individual allergens in every batch has only been acknowledged by a few manufacturers of allergen vaccines, but the principle is gaining more weight among control authorities and clinicians. Allergen vaccine manufacturers currently have access to the published purification procedures of most major allergens, and the purified major allergens can be used for the production of antibodies for independent quantification, even in complex mixtures such as allergen vaccines. For this purpose, polyspecific or monospecific polyclonal rabbit antibodies or murine monoclonal antibodies are used most often.

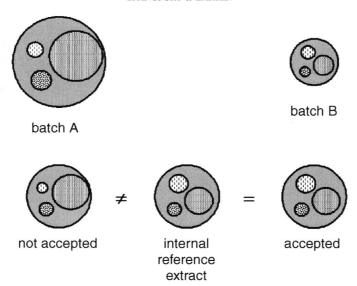

Fig. 1. Standardization of allergen extracts. Complexity of allergen extracts represented by a model with three major allergens. The area of shaded circles represents the relative potency of individual components. The area of outer circles represents the total allergenic potency of the extracts. The total allergenic potency of batch A and B may be adjusted through dilution or concentration, but the composition of the extracts may still vary, emphasizing the significance of the measurement of individual components.

Allergen vaccine potency

The potency of an allergen extract is the total allergen activity (ie, the sum of the contribution to allergenic activity from any individual IgE molecule specific for any epitope on any molecule in the allergen extract). Potency measures will therefore always depend on the serum pool or patient panel selected and the methodology used.

Methods used for the assessment of allergen vaccine potency may be divided into either in vitro or in vivo techniques.

The dominating in vitro technique for estimating relative allergenic potency is radioallergosorbent test inhibition [21] or related methods. Other techniques include enzyme-linked immunosorbent assay [22] and histamine release from washed human leukocytes [23]. Because histamine release tests are dependent on freshly drawn blood samples from a panel of individuals who have allergies, their practical application in routine determination of allergen extract potency is diminished.

Direct skin testing of human allergic subjects has been the predominant in vivo method for assessing allergen extract potency [24]. For ethical reasons, in vivo testing in humans cannot be used as a routine assay for batch release in production. However, through suitable in vitro methods, production batches may be compared with internal reference vaccines, the in vivo activity of which has been established. The patient selection criteria are important because all in vivo methods are dependent on the patient panel.

Skin testing in humans is the principle underlying the establishment of biologic units of allergen vaccine potency. Several units are in use.

In Europe, the potency unit is based on the dose of allergen vaccine resulting in a weal comparable in size with the weal produced through administration of a given concentration of histamine. This unit was originally called *histamine equivalent potency* (*HEP*), and is now expressed as a BU according to the Nordic Guidelines [5].

Determination of clinical efficacy

The potency of allergen vaccines used for specific allergy vaccination ideally should be expressed in units describing clinical efficacy rather than a skin-testing effect. In the United States and Europe, and expressed through the WHO, approaches to relate vaccine potency and clinical efficacy have been performed. For several standardized vaccines, the clinical effect was determined after extensive clinical trials, and the mean maintenance dose of the vaccine was used to quantify it.

However, determinations of clinical effect are extremely laborious. They can only be performed using highly standardized vaccines, which have been described in detail with respect to composition and in vitro and in vivo potency (eg, IHRPs).

Chemically modified allergen vaccines

Chemical modification of allergen extracts is based on the observation that successful allergy vaccination is accompanied by an increase in allergen-specific IgG. Thus, modifying the allergen to reduce allergenic reactivity (ie, through IgE binding) while preserving immunogenicity would theoretically allow higher doses to be administered without risk for systemic reactions.

Formaldehyde was used for vaccine development in detoxification of bacterial toxins until 1970 when Marsh and coworkers [25] applied formaldehyde treatment of allergens for allergy vaccination. The allergens are incubated with formaldehyde yielding the so-called "allergoids," high molecular weight covalently coupled allergen complexes. Compounds with similar immunologic properties can be produced using glutaraldehyde instead of formaldehyde. The chemical modification of individual amino acids inactivates B- and T-cell epitopes irreversibly, however, and this effect seems to dilute epitopes and hence decrease allergenicity and immunogenicity, explaining why higher doses of allergoid are needed to achieve clinical efficacy.

Contrary to expectation, chemical modification using formaldehyde does not increase safety in practical allergy vaccination, as documented in a report from the German Federal Agency for Sera and Vaccines that analyzed all reported adverse reactions to allergen vaccines during a 10-year period from 1991 to 2000, including 555 life-threatening, nonfatal events [26].

Another approach is based on allergens chemically coupled to biodegradable polymers, such as methoxypolyethylene glycol or a copolymer of D-glutamic acid and D-lysine, or other nonimmunogenic polymers. From mouse experiments, such compounds were expected to suppress IgE biosynthesis in humans [27]. However, clinical studies in humans were discouraging. An aspect of this approach is the use of extremely high doses of these compounds, rendering their clinical use in humans problematic.

Most of the techniques used to characterize and standardize allergen vaccines are not applicable to modified allergen vaccines. Experts therefore recommend that standardization be completed using the intermediate allergen preparation before modification, and that the reproducibility of the modification process be documented through methods specific to the procedure in question.

Standardization and allergy vaccination in Europe and the United States

Regulations of standardization of allergy vaccines in Europe according to the European Pharmacopoeia are remarkably different from those in the United States according to the FDA. In Europe, allergy vaccine consistency is maintained primarily through the use of in-house standards and international references, whereas in the United States the FDA issues detailed standardization procedures and reagents to be used by all manufacturers. The advantage of the European system is that the doctor is able to choose from different products and manufacturers can continuously improve product quality, documentation, and development. The American system, on the other hand, has the advantage of being more conservative and resistant to new developments and having a higher degree of consistency among manufacturers.

Another difference between Europe and the United States is the allergy vaccine formulations. Aqueous vaccines are commonly used in the United States, whereas mostly alum-adsorbed vaccines, either chemically modified or native, are used in Europe. Theoretically, this practice should result in a higher frequency of anaphylactic side reactions in the United States compared with Europe. The reason why this does not occur can be ascribed to a third difference in current procedures. Common practice in the United States is to mix a cocktail of all relevant allergen sources when treating patients who have multiple allergies, thereby reducing the therapeutic dose and increasing the risk for proteolytic degradation. In Europe, the current practice is to treat the most severe allergy first or, if more than one treatment is conducted simultaneously, to distribute the injection sites between both arms of the patient, ensuring the optimal maintenance dose is reached. Retrospective studies have shown coherence between the optimal maintenance dose and the major allergen content in absolute amounts when comparing different allergen sources. This coherence has been acknowledged by the WHO, but unfortunately not by the FDA.

Formulation of allergen vaccines

Formulation for injection therapy

The efficacy of specific allergy vaccination is related to the dose of vaccine administered, but the inherent allergenic properties of the vaccine imply a risk for inducing anaphylactic side reactions. In traditional allergy vaccination, this conflict is handled by administering repeated injections over extended periods after an initial up-dosing period. Formulation of the vaccine can further reduce the risk for side effects. Most vaccines on the market are formulated through adsorption of the allergens to inorganic gels, such as aluminum hydroxide [Al(OH)$_3$], to attain a depot effect characterized by a slow release of the allergens.

Formulation with Al(OH)$_3$ has long been used for vaccination in human and veterinary medicine [28]. The advantages are based on two characteristics of the complexes: the depot effect and the adjuvant effect. The allergens bind firmly but noncovalently to the inorganic complexes, causing slow release of the proteins and thereby lowering the concentration of allergen in the tissue and reducing the risk for systemic side effects. Given optimized formulation conditions, allergens seem to preserve their native configuration on association with Al(OH)$_3$. Furthermore, the depot effect reduces the number of injections needed in the course of specific allergy vaccination. Although the significance of the adjuvant effect is unclear, higher levels of IgG antibodies have been observed when alum-adsorbed vaccines were used in specific allergy vaccination compared with aqueous vaccine [29]. Compared with aqueous vaccine, patients receiving depot preparations experience fewer side reactions [30].

Formulations for sublingual allergy vaccination

In sublingual allergy vaccination, the allergen vaccine is administered directly on the mucous membrane under the tongue, avoiding the use of needles and injections. Because of its high safety profile, virtually no anaphylactic events have been reported. Sublingual allergy vaccination is potentially useful in children, although clinical documentation in children should be improved. Vaccines used for sublingual vaccination are aqueous extracts, or 50% glycerol may be added to stabilize the allergens. The concept of sublingual therapy emerged as a practice among clinicians in the 1980s, and several studies addressing safety and efficacy were published in the early 1990s. The documentation of clinical efficacy among the studies is variable [31], likely because of the variability in protocols, treatment durations, extracts, and doses used. Allergen manufacturers have recently offered products that allow more convenient sublingual allergy vaccination, such as single-dose containers that improve uniform dosing and allow self-treatment.

The latest development in sublingual allergy vaccination is the formulation of allergic extracts as sublingual tablets. Compared with drop-based application, tablets offer the advantage of standardized delivery, increased contact with sublingual mucosal surface, and more convenient handling. In a recently published safety study using a fast-dissolving tablet formulation, very high doses of grass pollen extract were tolerated without serious or systemic adverse events [32]. A dose corresponding to 15 μg of major allergen administered daily 10 weeks before and throughout the grass pollen season showed a 37% reduction in rhino-conjunctivitis symptom scores and a concomitant reduction of 41% in medication use compared with placebo [33]. Tablets were administrated without up-dosing, and no serious side effects were observed. The most prominent side effects were mild oral pruritus, nasopharyngitis, and throat irritation. Self-administration of the fast-dissolving grass allergen tablet was safe and efficacious and holds great promise for the future.

Recombinant allergens

Recombinant allergens were first described in 1988, when Thomas and colleagues [34] described the cloning and expression of Der p 1 in *Escherichia coli*. Since then, recombinant allergens have been accommodated in research of allergens and mechanisms of the allergic immune response with great success. Today, most important allergens from various sources have been cloned and sequenced, yielding insight into molecular characteristics and biologic function. The IUIS Allergen Nomenclature Sub-committee [35] maintains an updated official list of allergens, accessible at www.allergen.org.

Early studies of clinical use showed that recombinant allergens or cocktails of a limited number of recombinant allergens were efficient for in vitro diagnosis showing the presence of specific IgE in blood samples, and the idea of using similar cocktails for allergy vaccination was obvious [36]. A breakthrough in clinical use of recombinant allergens for therapy, however, is still awaited, although clinical proof-of-concept studies are in progress and one study has been completed [37]. Manufacturers are hesitating to follow strategies based on recombinant allergens for multiple reasons, including comprehensive regulatory requirements for clinical documentation, large investments in production capacity, uncertainty of clinical benefits, and unsolved technical difficulties. Despite these obstacles, recombinant allergens still play a central role in future scenarios of specific allergy vaccination because they have significant advantages, including certain supply of homogenous allergens, precision in physical–chemical standardization, improved reproducibility, and a stable regulatory situation. Other areas of vaccinology (eg, infectious disease) have moved toward more well-defined vaccine components [38].

Recombinant allergens for allergy vaccination

Recombinant so-called "wild type'" allergens are produced to resemble natural allergens in every detail. The term *wild type* was coined to distinguish these allergens from recombinant allergens that were deliberately modified to reduce

IgE-binding. Modified recombinant allergens are discussed below. This section discusses some difficulties and advantages of recombinant wild type allergens.

Although production of recombinant allergens identical to allergens from natural sources may be possible, the regulatory authorities will likely not recognize previous documentation based on allergens of natural origin. Market authorizations must therefore rely on comprehensive clinical safety and efficacy documentation developed using the recombinant product. On the other hand, the authorities are likely to welcome recombinant allergens because of the improved reproducibility of the products. Recombinant allergens represent chemical entities, the identity of which can be established through physical–chemical means and in absolute terms. Through peptide mapping combined with mass spectrometry, the entire amino acid sequence can be verified as batch-to-batch control. The uncertainties of traditional allergen standardization are thereby obviated.

How many and which allergens to include in a vaccine so as not to compromise efficacy compared with conventional extracts is important to determine. When mapping patient reactivity to individual allergens, a large heterogeneity is observed. Although most patients react to a limited number of major allergens, many minor allergens can be identified though screening large numbers of patients. Most of the techniques used, however, do not take quantitative aspects into consideration. Thus, even if a patient reacts to five different allergens in a grass pollen extract, for example, 99% of the IgE may theoretically be directed toward the major allergen. The observation that the recommended maintenance doses of different allergen vaccines contain similar quantities of major allergen (ie, 5–20 μg) shows the exceptional significance of the major allergens [7]. Therefore, a large portion of the clinical efficacy is likely mediated by the major allergens alone. A limited number of clinical studies comparing purified natural allergens with extracts seem to confirm this idea [39], although Østerballe [40] used a mixture of Phl p 5 and Phl p 6 in a grass pollen study, and not the optimal combination of Phl p 1 and Phl p 5.

Recombinant allergens should display the amino acid sequence of the natural allergen, or more precisely, one of its isoallergenic variants. Isoallergens and variants show differences in IgE-binding, and one variant that covers a broad range of IgE specificities directed toward the natural mixture of isoallergens should be selected. Any tags attached to the recombinant allergen for efficient expression or purification should be removed. Most of the recombinant allergens described in the literature are fusion proteins. A problem more difficult to assess is the conformation of the recombinant protein. An unfolded allergen is characterized by lack of (1) a stable, well-defined, three-dimensional structure, (2) antibody recognition, and (3) enzymatic activity. The folded state, on the other hand, displays full antibody-binding capacity and enzymatic activity showing authentic three-dimensional structure and a well-defined conformation. The binding of specific IgE and subsequent appearance of clinical symptoms of allergy are intimately connected with the three-dimensional folded structure of the allergen. The conformational nature of B-cell epitopes was shown by the crystal structural determination of the antibody–allergen complex Bet v 1– BV16 Fab [41].

Reduced activity of unfolded allergens with respect to IgE binding can therefore increase as a result of spontaneous or facilitated refolding when allergens are released in human tissues or fluids that have a risk for adverse systemic reactions. In many cases, the equilibrium between the folded and unfolded state is strongly shifted in favor of the folded state; however, handling and storage conditions (eg, lyophilization) of the purified protein, which pose a risk to denaturation, are important factors to control.

Modified recombinant allergens in allergy vaccination

Approaches to reduce the allergenicity of allergen vaccines have been attempted though disruption of the tertiary structure of allergen molecules using denatured [42] or degraded antigens or peptides [43]. However, these approaches have shown reduced efficacy in allergy vaccination compared with those involving native allergens.

The concept of using recombinant major allergens for specific allergy vaccination offers important opportunities for modifying the molecules through DNA recombinant technology to reduce IgE binding and potentially circumvent the inherent problem of current vaccines inducing IgE-mediated side effects. Different concepts have been proposed and are being pursued in laboratories worldwide [44]. Some concepts aim to completely disrupt the three-dimensional structure of the recombinant allergen, either through preventing the formation

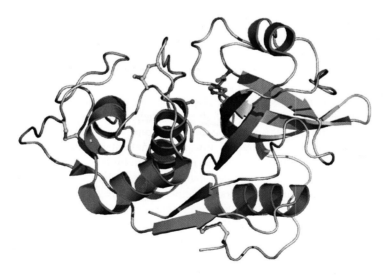

Fig. 2. Model of the crystal structure of mature Der p 1. The structure folds in two domains separated by the substrate cleft, which runs vertically down the center in the plane of the paper. Alpha-helices are colored red and beta-strands orange. The catalytic triad is highlighted as ball and stick model in light blue. (*From* Meno K, Thorsted PB, Ipsen H, et al. The crystal structure of recombinant proDer p 1, a major house dust mite proteolytic allergen. J Immunol 2005;175:3835–45; with permission.)

of disulphide bonds by substitution of the cysteines or by fragmenting the allergen molecule. The goal of other concepts is to modify IgE-binding conformational epitopes without a priori knowledge of the architecture of allergen molecular surface (eg, through gene shuffling) [45] or through determining the three-dimensional structure of the allergen (Figs. 2 and 3).

Once IgE-binding epitopes have been identified, antibody reactivity can be rationally modified by substituting critical amino acid residues on the molecular surface [46,47]. Such mutations may affect IgE reactivity but also may influence the stability and refolding properties of the mutated allergen. Thus, in the characterization of the mutated allergen, the immunochemical effects of the substitutions must be separated from the physicochemical effects. For this purpose, antibody-based assays are not always sufficient because detection often does not differentiate between unfolded protein and mutations aimed at decreasing specific serum IgE reactivity and antibody binding. Thus, with respect to the structural integrity of the mutated allergen, amino acid substitutions must always be analyzed through relevant assays and reagents.

One clinical trial of modified recombinant allergens has been performed. This trial included two concepts based on Bet v 1, the major allergen from birch pollen; a Bet v 1 molecule cleaved in two halves; and a trimer produced by consecutive connection of three Bet v 1 molecules [48]. Although the study reported clinical improvement, no underlying data are presented. Other concepts of modified recombinant allergens are currently in clinical trial or preclinical testing, and because of the fundamental differences among the concepts, the failure or success of one concept cannot be extrapolated to apply for others.

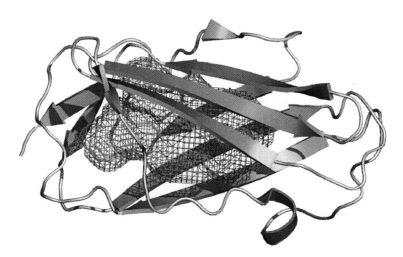

Fig. 3. Model of the crystal structure of Der f 2. The internal cavity is highlighted in light blue. Alpha-helices are colored red and beta-strands orange. (*Data from* Johannessen BR, Skov LK, Kastrup JS, et al. Structure of the house dust mite allergen Der f 2: implications for function and molecular basis of IgE cross-reactivity. FEBS Lett 2005;579:1208–12.)

SPANGFORT & LARSEN

Summary

The purpose of standardization is to minimize the qualitative and quantitative variation in the composition of the final products to obtain higher levels of safety, efficacy, accuracy, and simplicity in allergy diagnosis and allergy vaccination. The benefits of improved standardization of allergen vaccines for the clinician include easier differentiation between allergy and nonallergy, a more precise definition of the specificity and degree of allergy, and a more reliable and reproducible outcome of specific allergy vaccination.

Recombinant allergens, which are standardized in absolute terms through physical–chemical methods, will obviate the uncertainties of allergen standardization.

References

[1] Noon L. Prophylactic inoculation against hay fever. Lancet 1911;1:1572–3.
[2] Ishizaka K, Ishizaka T, Hornbrook MM. Physicochemical properties of reaginic antibody. V. Correlation of reaginic activity with gamma-E-globulin antibody. J Immunol 1966;97:840–53.
[3] Johansson SG, Bennich H. Immunological studies of an atypical (myeloma) immunoglobulin. Immunology 1967;13:381–94.
[4] Løwenstein H. Report on behalf of the International Union of Immunological Societies (I.U.I.S.) Allergen Standardization Subcommittee. Arb Paul Ehrlich Inst 1983;78:41–8.
[5] Nordic Council on Medicines. Registration of allergen preparations: Nordic Guidelines. NLN Publication No 1989;23:1–34.
[6] Larsen JN, Houghton CG, Løwenstein H, et al. Manufacturing and standardizing allergen extracts in Europe. Clin Allergy Immunol 2004;18:433–55.
[7] Allergen immunotherapy: therapeutic vaccines for allergic diseases. Geneva: January 27–29 1997. Allergy 1998;53(Suppl 44):1–42.
[8] Council of Europe. European Pharmacopoeia. European Treaty Series 50. Strasbourg: Council of Europe; 2001.
[9] Slater JE. Standardized allergen extracts in the United States. Clin Allergy Immunol 2004;18: 421–32.
[10] Løwenstein H. Selection of reference preparation. IUIS reference preparation criteria. Arb Paul Ehrlich Inst 1987;80:75–8.
[11] King TP, Hoffman D, Løwenstein H, et al. Allergen Nomenclature. J Allergy Clin Immunol 1995;96:5–14.
[12] Dreborg S, Einarsson R. The major allergen content of allergenic preparations reflects their biological activity. Allergy 1992;47:418–23.
[13] Helm RM, Gauerke MB, Baer H, et al. Production and testing of an international reference standard of short ragweed pollen extract. J Allergy Clin Immunol 1984;73:790–800.
[14] Gjesing B, Jäger L, Marsh DG, et al. The international collaborative study establishing the first international standard for timothy (*Phleum pratense*) grass pollen allergenic extract. J Allergy Clin Immunol 1985;75:258–67.
[15] Ford A, Seagroatt V, Platts-Mills TAE, et al. A collaborative study on the first international standard of *Dermatophagoides pteronyssinus* (house dust mite) extract. J Allergy Clin Immunol 1985;75:676–86.
[16] Arntzen FC, Wilhelmsen TW, Løwenstein H, et al. The international collaborative study on the first international standard of birch (*Betula verrucosa*) pollen extract. J Allergy Clin Immunol 1989;83:66–82.

[17] Larsen JN, Ford A, Gjesing B, et al. The collaborative study of the international standard of dog, *Canis domesticus*, hair/dander extract. J Allergy Clin Immunol 1988;82:318–30.

[18] van Ree R, Partnership CREATE. The CREATE project: EU support for the improvement of allergen standardization in Europe. Allergy 2004;59:571–4.

[19] Løwenstein H. Physico-chemical and immunochemical methods for the control of potency and quality of allergenic extracts. Arb Paul Ehrlich Inst 1980;75:122–32.

[20] Løwenstein H. Quantitative immunoelectrophoretic methods as a tool for the analysis and isolation of allergens. Prog Allergy 1978;25:1–62.

[21] Ceska M, Eriksson R, Varga JM. Radioimmunosorbent assay of allergens. J Allergy Clin Immunol 1972;49:1–9.

[22] Engvall E, Perlmann P. Enzyme-linked immunosorbent assay, ELISA. III. Quantitation of specific antibodies by enzyme-labelled anti-immunoglobulin in antigen-coated tubes. J Immunol 1972;109:129–35.

[23] Siraganian RP. Automated histamine analysis for *in vitro* allergy testing. II. Correlation of skin test results with *in vitro* whole blood histamine release in 82 patients. J Allergy Clin Immunol 1977;59:214–22.

[24] Platts-Mills TAE, Chapman MD. Allergen standardization. J Allergy Clin Immunol 1991;87: 621–5.

[25] Marsh DG, Lichtenstein LM, Campbell DH. Studies on 'allergoids' prepared from naturally occurring allergens. I. Assay of allergenicity and antigenicity of formalinized rye group I component. Immunol 1970;18:705–22.

[26] Lüderitz-Püchel U, Keller-Stanislawski B, Haustein D. Neubewertung des Risikos von Test- und Therapieallergenen. Bundesgesundheitsbl-Gesundheitsforsch-Gesundheitsschutz 2001;44: 709–18.

[27] Lee WY, Sehon AH. Abrogation of reaginic antibodies with modified allergens. Nature 1977; 267:618–9.

[28] Butler NR, Voyce MA, Burland WL, et al. Advantages of aluminium hydroxide adsorbed combined diphtheria, tetanus and pertussis vaccines for the immunization of infants. BMJ 1969; 1:663–6.

[29] Norman PS, Lichtenstein LM. Comparisons of alum-precipitated and unprecipitated aqueous ragweed pollen extracts in the treatment of hay fever. J Allergy Clin Immunol 1978;61:384–9.

[30] Mellerup MT, Hahn GW, Poulsen LK, et al. Safety of allergen-specific immunotherapy. Relation between dosage regimen, allergen extract, disease and systemic side-effects during induction treatment. Clin Exp Allergy 2000;30:1423–9.

[31] Wilson DR, Lima MT, Durham SR. Sublingual immunotherapy for allergic rhinitis: systematic review and meta-analysis. Allergy 2005;60:4–12.

[32] Kleine-Tebbe J, Ribel M, Herold DA. Safety of a SQ-standardised grass allergen tablet for sublingual immunotherapy: a randomized, placebo-controlled trial. Allergy 2006;61:181–4.

[33] Dahl R, Stender A, Rak S. Specific immunotherapy with SQ standardized grass allergen tablets in asthmatics with rhinoconjunctivitis. Allergy 2006;61:185–90.

[34] Thomas WR, Stewart GA, Simpson RJ, et al. Cloning and expression of DNA coding for the major house dust mite allergen Der p 1 in Escherichia coli. Int Arch Allergy Appl Immunol 1988;85:127–9.

[35] Chapman MD. Allergen nomenclature. Clin Allergy Immunol 2004;18:51–64.

[36] Valenta R, Kraft D. Recombinant allergens for diagnosis and therapy of allergic diseases. Curr Opin Immunol 1995;7:751–6.

[37] Jutel M, Jaeger L, Suck R, et al. Allergen-specific immunotherapy with recombinant grass pollen allergens. J Allergy Clin Immunol 2005;116:608–13.

[38] Edelman R. The development and use of vaccine adjuvants. Mol Biotechnol 2002;21:129–48.

[39] Norman PS, Winkenwerder WL, Lichtenstein LM. Immunotherapy of hay fever with ragweed antigen E: comparisons with whole pollen extract and placebos. J Allergy 1968;42:93–108.

[40] Østerballe O. Immunotherapy in hay fever with two major allergens 19, 25 and partially purified extract of timothy grass pollen. A controlled double blind study. In vivo variables, season I. Allergy 1980;35:473–89.

[41] Mirza O, Henriksen A, Ipsen H, et al. Dominant epitopes and allergic cross-reactivity: complex formation between a Fab fragment of a monoclonal murine IgG antibody and the major allergen from birch pollen Bet v 1. J Immunol 2000;165:331–8.

[42] Norman PS, Ishizaka K, Lichtenstein LM, et al. Treatment of ragweed hay fever with urea-denatured antigen E. J Allergy Clin Immunol 1980;66:336–41.

[43] Norman PS, Ohman Jr JL, Long AA, et al. Treatment of cat allergy with T-cell reactive peptides. Am J Respir Crit Care Med 1996;154:1623–8.

[44] Akdis CA, Blaser K. Regulation of specific immune responses by chemical and structural modifications of allergens. Int Arch Allergy Immunol 2000;121:261–9.

[45] Punnonen J. Molecular breeding of allergy vaccines and antiallergic cytokines. Int Arch Allergy Immunol 2000;121:173–82.

[46] Spangfort MD, Mirza O, Ipsen H, et al. Dominating IgE-binding epitope of Bet v 1, the major allergen of birch pollen, characterized by X-ray crystallography and site-directed mutagenesis. J Immunol 2003;171:3084–90.

[47] Holm J, Gajhede M, Ferreras M, et al. Allergy vaccine engineering: epitope modulation of recombinant Bet v 1 reduces IgE binding but retains protein folding pattern for induction of protective blocking-antibody responses. J Immunol 2004;173:5258–67.

[48] Niederberger V, Horak F, Vrtala S, et al. Vaccination with genetically engineered allergens prevents progression of allergic disease. Proc Natl Acad Sci USA 2004;101(Suppl 2):14677–82.

ELSEVIER
SAUNDERS

Immunol Allergy Clin N Am
26 (2006) 207–231

IMMUNOLOGY
AND ALLERGY
CLINICS
OF NORTH AMERICA

Mechanisms of Allergen-Specific Immunotherapy: T-Regulatory Cells and More

Johan Verhagen, PhD, Kurt Blaser, PhD,
Cezmi A. Akdis, MD, Mübeccel Akdis, MD, PhD*

Swiss Institute of Allergy and Asthma Research (SIAF), Obere Strasse 22, CH-7270 Davos, Switzerland

T-cell tolerance is characterized by the functional inactivation of the cell to antigen encounter while remaining alive for an extended period in an unresponsive state. In recognition of the importance of immunologic tolerance, the 1960 Nobel Prize in Physiology and Medicine was awarded to Medawar [1] for discovering that skin allografts in mice and chicken can be accepted if they are preinoculated during embryonic development with allogeneic lymphoid cells, and to Burnet [2,3] for first proposing that exposure to antigens before the development of immune response specifically abrogates the capacity to respond to that antigen in later life. During the past decade, this area of immunologic research has gained much attention and popularity. Overall, studies on T-cell unresponsiveness suggest that anergy, tolerance, and active suppression are not entirely distinct but rather represent linked mechanisms that may involve the same molecular events. The term *anergy* was first coined by Von Pirquet [4] in 1908 to describe the loss of delayed-type hypersensitivity to tuberculin in individuals infected with measles virus. The term has been clinically accepted to describe negative tuberculin skin test results in conditions in which they are expected to be positive. In 1980, *anergy* was redefined to describe the specific inactivation of B cells in mice by high doses of antigen [5]. It was subsequently used for T cells to describe a phenomenon in which antigen presentation to T-cell clones in the absence of professional antigen-presenting cells (APC) induced a

The authors' laboratories are supported by the Swiss National Foundation Grants: 32-105865, 32-100266, and Global Allergy and Asthma European Network (GA²LEN).

* Corresponding author.

E-mail address: akdism@siaf.unizh.ch (M. Akdis).

doi:10.1016/j.iac.2006.02.008
immunology.theclinics.com

hyporesponsive state characterized by subdued interleukin (IL)-2 production and proliferation on restimulation [6].

In early studies, which serve as the basis for the definition of anergy/tolerance, functional unresponsiveness was analyzed through nonsophisticated assays such as IL-2 measurement and the determination of total IgG production. In addition, until recently antigens used in mouse models contained high amounts of impurities, such as lipopolysaccharides and other innate immune response-triggering substances, which may influence the outcome of experiments. Although some biochemical steps overlap with anergy, activation-induced cell death induced through the triggering of death receptors and caspase activation represents a distinct physiologic response [7,8]. Target cells do not survive in an unresponsive state but are deleted through apoptosis.

Why exposure to allergens leads to atopic disorders in some individuals but not others is still not understood. However, a strong interaction between environmental and genetic factors is clearly involved. During allergic inflammation, four cardinal events involving memory/effector T cells and other effector cells, such as mast cells, eosinophils, and basophils, can be classified as (1) activation, (2) organ-selective homing, (3) prolonged survival and reactivation inside the allergic organs, (4) and effector functions [9,10]. T cells are activated by aeroallergens, food antigens, autoantigens, and bacterial superantigens in allergic inflammation [11,12]. They are under the influence of skin-, lung-, or nose-related chemokine networks and they show organ-selective homing [13–15]. A prolonged survival of the inflammatory cells and strong interaction with resident cells of the allergic organ and consequent reactivation are observed in the subepithelial tissues [16,17]. T cells play important effector roles in atopic dermatitis and asthma through the induction of hyper IgE production, eosinophil survival, and mucus hyperproduction (Fig. 1) [11,17,18]. In addition, activated T cells induce apoptosis of bronchial epithelial cells and keratinocytes as major tissue injury events [19–22]. Peripheral T-cell tolerance to allergens can overcome the pathologic events in allergic inflammation because they all require T-cell activation.

The initial event responsible for the development of allergic diseases is the generation of allergen-specific $CD4^+$ T helper cells. The current view is that under the influence of IL-4, naïve T cells activated by APC differentiate into T helper 2 (Th2) cells [23–25]. Once generated, effector Th2 cells produce IL-4, IL-5, and IL-13 and exert several regulatory and effector functions. These cytokines induce production of allergen-specific IgE by B cells, development and recruitment of eosinophils, production of mucus, and contraction of smooth muscles [23,24,26]. Furthermore, the degranulation of basophils and mast cells by IgE-mediated cross-linking of receptors is the key event in type I hypersensitivity, which may lead to chronic allergic inflammation. Although Th2 cells are responsible for the development of allergic diseases, T helper 1 (Th1) cells may contribute to chronicity and effector phase in allergic diseases [19–22,27,28]. Distinct Th1 and Th2 subpopulations of T cells counter-regulate each other and play a role in distinct diseases [23,24]. In addition, a further subtype of T cells that have immunosuppressive function and cytokine profiles distinct from either

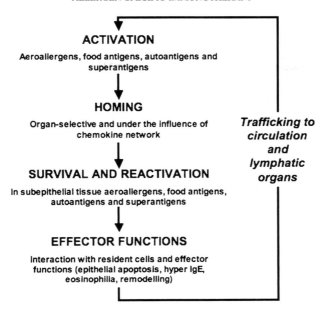

ACTIVATION

Aeroallergens, food antigens, autoantigens and
superantigens

HOMING

Organ-selective and under the influence of
chemokine network

Trafficking to circulation and lymphatic organs

SURVIVAL AND REACTIVATION

In subepithelial tissue aeroallergens, food antigens,
autoantigens and superantigens

EFFECTOR FUNCTIONS

Interaction with resident cells and effector
functions (epithelial apoptosis, hyper IgE,
eosinophilia, remodelling)

Fig. 1. The four sequential processes characterizing allergic inflammation. Various antigens or yet unidentified factors activate T cells; these cells then undergo organ-selective homing according to the influence of organ-related chemokine networks. T cells within subepithelial tissues show increased survival and are continuously stimulated. These activated T cells then trigger effector functions, including apoptosis, hyper IgE, and eosinophilia. Increasing allergen-specific Treg-cell numbers may abrogate all of these events and lead to a healthy immune response against allergens.

Th1 and Th2 cells, termed *regulatory/suppressor T cells* (*Treg*), has been described [29–34]. In addition to Th1 cells, Treg cells are able to inhibit the development of allergic Th2 responses [35] and play a major role in allergen-specific immunotherapy [32,36]. This article examines allergen-specific peripheral tolerance mechanisms in humans and discusses novel methods of T-cell suppression.

Peripheral T-cell tolerance to allergens in healthy immune response and allergen-specific immunotherapy

The symptoms of IgE-mediated allergic reactions, such as rhinitis, conjunctivitis, and asthma, can be alleviated through temporary suppression of inflammatory mediators and immune cells using agents such as antihistamines, antileukotrienes, β_2-adrenergic receptor agonists, and corticosteroids [37–40]. However, the only long-term solution is allergen-specific immunotherapy, which specifically restores normal immunity to allergens. Allergen-SIT is most efficiently used in allergy to insect venoms and allergic rhinitis [41–45]. In 1911, the original report of Noon [46] suggested that grass pollen extracts used for immunotherapy of hay fever induced a toxin that caused allergic symptoms. Researchers suggested that in response to injection of pollen extract, antitoxins develop and prevent the development of disease. Neutralizing antibodies have been shown to generate during allergen-specific immunotherapy [47,48]. Despite being used in clinical practice for nearly a century, the underlying immunologic mechanisms of allergen-specific immunotherapy are slowly being elucidated [36,49–54]. A rise in allergen-blocking IgG antibodies, particularly of the IgG4 class which supposedly block allergen and IgE-facilitated antigen presentation [55–57]; the generation of IgE-modulating CD8$^+$ T cells [58]; and a reduction in the numbers of mast cells and eosinophils, including the release of inflammatory mediators [59–61], were shown to be associated with successful allergen-specific immunotherapy. Furthermore, allergen-specific immunotherapy was found to be associated with a decrease in IL-4 and IL-5 production by CD4$^+$ T cells [45,62,63]. Also, a shift from a Th2 cytokine pattern toward increased interferon (IFN)-γ production in allergen-specific immunotherapy of allergy to bee venom, wasp venom, grass pollen, and house dust mite (HDM) has been observed [62,64]. The induction of a tolerant state in peripheral T cells, however, seems to represent the crucial step in allergen-specific immunotherapy (Fig. 2) [32,36,49,52]. Peripheral T-cell tolerance is characterized mainly by suppressed proliferative and cytokine responses against allergens and their isolated T-cell recognition sites (epitopes) [49]. T-cell tolerance is initiated by the autocrine action of IL-10, which is increasingly produced by antigen-specific T cells [32,52]. Tolerized T cells can be reactivated to produce either distinct Th1 or Th2 cytokine patterns, depending on the cytokines present in the tissue microenvironment, leading to either a successful or unsuccessful outcome in allergen-specific immunotherapy [49].

Most studies examined cultures of peripheral blood mononuclear cells (PBMCs). Whether these events reflect the changes in the immune response in the tissues is of interest. T-cell responses after grass pollen immunotherapy have been examined in nasal mucosal and skin tissue. Increased numbers of IL-10 mRNA–expressing cells were shown after allergen-specific immunotherapy with grass pollen during the pollen season. However, in contrast to the findings in peripheral blood, IL-10 was not increased in nonatopic subjects exposed during the pollen season. In addition, the studies showed reduced accumulation of T cells in skin and nose after allergen challenge but no decrease in T cell numbers during pollen season. Increased Th1 activity was shown in the skin and nasal mucosa [65–67], whereas increases in IFN-γ observed after allergen challenge outside the pollen season correlated with the clinical improvement [68]. During the summer pollen season, increases in the levels of IFN-γ and IL-5 were observed, with the ratio in favor of IFN-γ [69]. However, that modulation of peripheral immune responses is apparently pivotal for the effects of allergen-specific immunotherapy. Local tissue responses do not necessarily reflect peripheral tolerance and are dependent on several mechanisms, such as cell apoptosis, migration, homing, and survival signals, which are highly dependent on natural allergen exposure and environmental factors [10].

Individuals who are healthy and those who have allergies exhibit all three subsets of CD4$^+$ T cells, but in different proportions. In healthy individuals,

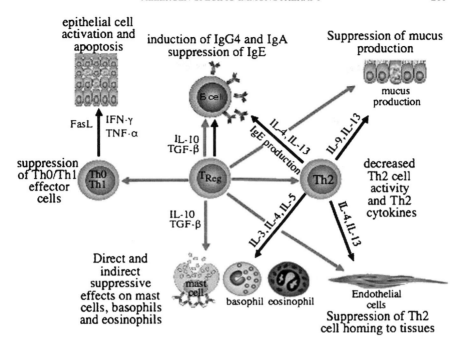

Fig. 2. Peripheral tolerance mechanisms in allergen-specific immunotherapy and healthy immune response to allergens. Immune deviation toward Treg-cell response is an essential step in allergen-specific immunotherapy and natural allergen exposure of individuals who are nonallergic. Treg cells use multiple suppressor factors that influence the final outcome of allergen-specific immunotherapy. IL-10 and TGF-β induce IgG4 and IgA, respectively, from B cells as noninflammatory Ig isotypes, and suppress IgE production. These two cytokines directly or indirectly suppress effector cells of allergic inflammation, such as mast cells, basophils, and eosinophils. In addition, Th2 cells, which are dominated by Treg cells, can no longer induce IgE through IL-4 and IL-13 and cannot provide cytokines such as IL-3, IL-4, IL-5, IL-9, and IL-13, which are required for the differentiation, survival, and activity of mast cells, basophils, and eosinophils and mucus-producing cells. In addition, migration of the inflammatory cells to the affected organs is controlled by Th2 cell–related chemokines and adhesion factors, which is also inhibited directly or indirectly by Treg cells and their cytokines. Moreover, suppression of the induction of Th0/Th1 cells abrogates tissue injury mechanisms, such as apoptosis of keratinocytes and bronchial epithelial cells, through interferon-γ, TNF-β, and Fas-ligand (FasL). The gray line designates suppression and the black line stimulation.

type 1 T regulatory (Tr1) cells represent the dominant subset for common environmental allergens, whereas a high frequency of allergen-specific IL-4 secreting (Th2) cells is found in individuals who are allergic [70]. Hence, a change in the dominant subset may lead to either the development of allergy or recovery from the disease. Peripheral tolerance to allergens involves multiple suppressive factors, such as IL-10, TGF-β, cytotoxic T-lymphocyte antigen-4 (CTLA-4), and programmed death-1 (PD-1) [70]. Accordingly, allergen-specific peripheral T-cell suppression mediated by IL-10 and TGF-β and other suppressive factors and a deviation toward a Treg-cell response were observed in normal immunity as key events in the healthy immune response to mucosal antigens. The analysis of other cytokines of the IL-10 family, such as IL-19, IL-20, IL-22, IL-24, and IL-26, showed that suppressor capacity for allergen/antigen-stimulated T cells is only a function of IL-10 in this family [71].

Unlike in mucosal allergies, no increase in TGF-β production was observed during specific immunotherapy in venom allergy. Differences in the control mechanisms that regulate the immune response to venoms and aeroallergens might be caused by different routes of natural allergen exposure and the induction of chronic events of allergic inflammation, leading to tissue injury and remodeling in the latter case. In humans, increasing evidence suggests that Treg cells play a major role in the inhibition of allergic disorders. Reports have shown that IL-10 levels in the bronchoalveolar-lavage fluid of patients who have asthma are lower than in healthy controls, and T cells in children who have asthma also produce less IL-10 mRNA than do T cells in healthy children [72,73]. Although some reports imply a role for TGF-β in the pathogenesis of asthma, particularly in remodeling of injured lung tissue in humans [74], a recent report indicates that the increased allergic inflammation observed after blocking CTLA-4 is clearly associated with decreased TGF-β levels in the bronchoalveolar-lavage fluid of mice [75].

Peripheral T-cell tolerance to allergens is associated with regulation of antibody isotypes and suppression of effector cells

The serum levels of specific IgE and IgG4 antibodies delineate allergic and normal immunity to allergen. Although peripheral tolerance has been shown in specific T cells, the capacity of B cells to produce specific IgE and IgG4 antibodies was not abolished during specific immunotherapy [49]. In fact, specific serum levels of both isotypes increased during the early phase of treatment. However, the increase in antigen-specific IgG4 was more pronounced and the ratio of specific IgE to IgG4 decreased by 10 to 100 fold. Also, the in vitro production of phospholipase A$_2$-specific IgE and IgG4 antibodies in PBMCs changed concomitantly with the serum levels of specific isotypes. A similar change in specific isotype ratio was observed in specific immunotherapy of various allergies. Moreover, the production of IL-10, which is induced and increases during allergen-specific immunotherapy, seems to counter-regulate antigen-specific IgE and IgG4 antibody synthesis [32]. IL-10 is a potent suppressor of total and allergen-specific IgE, while simultaneously increasing IgG4 production [32,76]. Thus, IL-10 not only generates tolerance in T cells but also regulates specific isotype formation and skews the specific response from an IgE- to an IgG4-dominated phenotype (see Fig. 2). The healthy immune response to *Dermatophagoides pteronyssinus* (Der p 1) showed increased specific IgA and IgG4, small amounts of IgG1, and almost undetectable IgE antibodies in serum [36]. Although HDM-specific immunotherapy did not significantly change specific IgE levels after 70 days of treatment, a significant increase in specific IgA, IgG1, and IgG4 was observed [36]. The increase of specific IgA and IgG4 in serum coincides with increased TGF-β and IL-10, respectively. These coincident increases may account for the role of IgA, TGF-β, IgG4, and IL-10 in peripheral mucosal immune responses to allergens in healthy individuals [32,77].

As early as the 1930s, Cooke and colleagues [47] suggested the induction of blocking antibodies through specific immunotherapy. Lichtenstein and colleagues [48] assigned these blocking antibodies to the IgG subclass. Research focusing on the subclasses of IgG antibodies suggested that IgG4 in particular captures the allergen before reaching the effector cell–bound IgE, thereby preventing the activation of mast cells and basophils. In fact, many studies showed increases in specific IgG4 levels in association with clinical improvement [78,79]. In the case of venom allergy, the rise of antivenom IgG correlates, at least at the onset of desensitization, with protection achieved through the treatment [80,81]. The concept of blocking antibodies has recently been reevaluated. Blocking antibodies seem to inhibit not only allergen-induced release of inflammatory mediators from basophils and mast cells but also IgE-facilitated allergen presentation to T cells, and prevent allergen-induced boost of memory IgE production during high allergen exposure during pollen season. Grass pollen immunotherapy has been shown to induce allergen-specific, IL-10-dependent protective IgG4 responses [82]. The data established an absolute association between IgG4-dependent blocking of IgE-binding to B cells in patients who underwent immunotherapy, and a trend toward a correlation with clinical efficacy. Measuring the blocking activity of allergen-specific IgG rather than its crude levels in sera seems to be preferable. This preference can explain the lack of correlation between antibody concentration and degree of clinical improvement. However, IgG4 antibodies can be viewed as having the ability to modulate the immune response to allergens and thus the potential to influence the clinical response. In a study using well-defined recombinant allergen mixtures, all treated subjects developed strong allergen-specific IgG1 and IgG4 antibody responses [83]. Some patients were not sensitized to *Phleum pratense* (Phl p 5) but nevertheless developed strong IgG antibody responses to that allergen. Researchers have suggested that subjects who do not have specific IgE against a particular allergen do not experience a significant IgG4 response [84], but recent studies do not support this view and are consistent with induction of a tolerant immune response together with induction of allergen-specific IgG4 [83].

An early effect of allergen-specific immunotherapy is an efficient modulation of the thresholds for mast cell and basophil degranulation. Although a definite decrease in IgE antibody levels and IgE-mediated skin sensitivity normally requires several years of allergen-specific immunotherapy, most patients are protected against bee stings already at an early stage of bee venom–specific immunotherapy. This early sensitivity occurs because effector cells of allergic inflammation, such as mast cells, basophils, and eosinophils, require T-cell cytokines for priming, survival, and activity [85, 86], but these cytokines are not efficiently provided by suppressed Th2 cells and generated Treg cells (see Fig. 2). In addition, IL-10 was shown to reduce proinflammatory cytokine release from mast cells [87]. IL-10 also down-regulates eosinophil function and activity and suppresses IL-5 production by human resting Th0 and Th2 cells [88]. Moreover, IL-10 inhibits endogenous granulocyte-macrophage colony-stimulating factor production and CD40 expression by activated eosinophils and enhances eosinophil cell death [89].

Peripheral T-cell tolerance by inhibition of T-cell costimulation

Inhibition of T-cell costimulatory molecules at the cell surface or through their intracellular signal transduction has repeatedly been reported to play an important role in T-cell tolerance [90–92]. T cells can be anergized in experimental animal models that bypass costimulatory signals [6,93,94]. The interaction between B7 and CD28 may determine whether a T-cell response develops. Blocking antibodies to B7-2 inhibits the development of specific IgE, pulmonary eosinophilia, and airway hyperresponsiveness in mice [95]. CTLA-4, a molecule on activated T cells, seems to act as an endogenous inhibitor of T-cell activation. CTLA-4-Ig, a soluble fusion-protein construct, is also effective in blocking airway hyperresponsiveness in mice [96]. Anti-CD28, anti-B7-2, and CTLA-4-Ig also block the proliferative response of T cells to allergen [97]. Furthermore, cytokine production by memory/effector T cells, particularly those of the Th2 subset, is highly dependent on costimulation through the ICOS/B7RP1 (ICOS-ligand) pathway. Blockage [98] or genetic disruption [99] of this costimulatory pathway markedly reduced allergen-induced asthma in mice. Thus, blockage of B7-2/CD28 and ICOS/B7RP1 interaction may be a promising approach for treating allergic disease in humans.

One mechanism of direct T-cell suppression by IL-10 is through inhibition of CD28 costimulation. IL-10 inhibits the proliferative T-cell response in PBMCs to various antigens, and the superantigen staphylococcal enterotoxin B [100]. However, IL-10 does not affect the proliferative responses of T cells stimulated with anti-CD3 monoclonal antibody (mAb). Analysis of the activity of T-cell receptors (TCRs) on T cells showed the essential requirement for costimulation in T-cell activation and its relation to the number of triggered TCRs [100]. IL-10 inhibited the T-cell proliferation within the range of triggered TCRs that require T-cell costimulation. T cells, which were stimulated with varying concentrations of anti-CD3, and a constant amount of anti-CD28 showed that low numbers of triggered TCRs required CD28 costimulation. Thus, IL-10 suppressed only those T cells that had low numbers of triggered TCRs and required CD28 for proliferation [100].

Stimulation of CD28 by B7 surface molecules leads to tyrosine phosphorylation of CD28. Ligation of IL-10 receptor (IL-10R) on CD28 stimulation inhibits tyrosine phosphorylation of CD28, as detected after 10 minutes [100,101]. The inhibitory effect of IL-10 on CD28 seemed to be specific for the CD28 pathway because IL-10 did not affect ZAP-70 tyrosine phosphorylation stimulated by CD3 cross-linking. As a consecutive event for signal transduction, the association of CD28 with the phosphatidylinositol 3-kinase (PI3-K) p85 molecule was inhibited by IL-10. This inhibition can be blocked specifically by preventing the binding of IL-10 to its receptor with an anti–IL-10R mAb. Binding of PI3-K to CD28 occurs through direct interaction between SH2 domain motifs of p85 PI3-K and a (p)YXXM motif in the cytoplasmic part [102]. This binding leads to a downstream signaling cascade in the transcription of various T-cell activation genes.

Although no clinical studies have related inhibition of costimulation to the specific treatment of allergy and asthma, it remains a fruitful approach to the treatment of autoimmunity and allergy.

T-regulatory cells

Since the mid-1990s, the concept of T-cell–mediated immune suppression has been strongly explored. Many types of suppressor T cells have been described in several systems, and their biology has been the subject of intensive investigation. Although many aspects of the mechanisms through which suppressor cells exert their effects have not been elucidated, it is well established that Treg cells suppress immune responses through cell-to-cell interactions or the production of suppressor cytokines (Table 1) [31,32,52,103].

Type-1 T regulatory cells

Tr1 cells are defined by their ability to produce high levels of IL-10 and TGF-β [31,103]. Tr1 cells specific for various antigens arise in vivo, but may also

Table 1
Regulatory/suppressor cells and their subsets

Regulatory/suppressor cells	Suppressor mechanism[a]
T cells	
Tr1	IL-10, TGF-β, CTLA-4, PD-1
Th3	TGF-β
CD4$^+$ CD25$^+$ Treg	IL-10, TGF-β, CTLA-4, PD-1, GITR
CD8$^+$ CD25$^+$ CD28$^-$ Treg	Same as CD4$^+$ CD25$^+$
CD4$^-$CD8$^-$ Treg	Induction of apoptosis
TCR-γ/δ Treg	IL-10, TGF-β
B-cell subset	IL-10
DC subset	IL-10
NK-cell subset[b]	IL-10
Macrophages	IL-10, TGF-β
Resident tissue cells[b]	IL-10, TGF-β

Abbreviations: DC, dendritic cell; NK, natural killer.
  [a] Multiple other suppressive mechanisms may exist.
  [b] NK cells and resident tissue cells are included in the table because these cells express suppressive cytokines.

differentiate from naïve CD4[+] T cells. Tr1 cells have a low proliferative capacity, which can be overcome by IL-15 [104]. Tr1 cells suppress naïve and memory Th1 and th2 responses through the production of IL-10 and TGF-β [103]. The use of Tr1 cells in identifying novel targets for the development of new therapeutic agents, and as a cellular therapy to modulate peripheral tolerance in allergy and autoimmunity, can be foreseen [52,105,106].

In vitro generation of Tr1 cells through stimulating naïve CD4[+] T cells in the presence of IL-10, IFN-α, or a combination of IL-4 and IL-10 has been reported [31,103]. To overcome problems in the cytokine profiles of Tr1 cells, a combination of vitamin D_3 and dexamethasone was shown to induce human and mouse naïve CD4[+] T cells to differentiate into Tr1 cells in vitro [107]. In contrast to the in vitro–derived CD4[+] T cells, these cells produced only IL-10 and no IL-5 and IFN-γ, retained strong proliferative capacity, and prevented central nervous system inflammation in an IL-10–dependent manner. Clear evidence now exists that IL-10– or TGF-β–producing Tr1 cells are generated in vivo in humans during the early course of allergen-specific immunotherapy, suggesting that high and increasing doses of allergens induce Tr1 cells in humans [32,36,108].

Regulatory/supressor T-cell clones have been induced through oral feeding of low doses of antigen in a TCR-transgenic experimental encephalitis model [29,109]. CD4[+] T-cell clones isolated from mesenteric lymph nodes in orally tolerated animals produced high levels of TGF-β and variable amounts of IL-4 and IL-10 on activation with appropriate antigen or anti-CD3 antibody [29]. These cells functioned in vivo to suppress encephalitis induction with myelin basic protein and were designated *Th3 cells*. TGF-β and IL-10 seemed critical because treatment with neutralizing antibodies abrogated the disease-protective effects of these cells. These Treg cells also exerted bystander immune suppression in vitro. The immunologic features of Th3 and Tr1 cells suggest that they can be of the same T-cell subset.

CD4+ CD25+ regulatory T cells

Clear evidence from various animal models and human studies shows an active mechanism of immune suppression whereby a distinct subset of T cells inhibits the activation of conventional T cells in the periphery [110–113]. This Treg cell population was determined to be CD4[+] CD25[+] T cells. CD4[+] CD25[+] T cells constitute 5% to 10% of peripheral CD4[+] T cells and express the IL-2 receptor α chain (CD25) [110] and the characteristic transcription factor FoxP3 [114]. They can prevent the development of autoimmunity, indicating that the normal immune system contains a population of professional Treg cells. Elimination of CD4[+] CD25[+] Treg cells leads to spontaneous development of various autoimmune diseases, such as gastritis or thyroiditis, in genetically susceptible hosts. In mice, these cells have been shown to express CD45RB[low] [30]. The CD38[−]CD25[+] CD4[+] CD45RB[low] subpopulation contains T cells that respond to recall antigens and produce high levels of cytokines in response to polyclonal stimulation. In contrast, the CD38[+] cells within this subpopulation do not proliferate or produce detectable levels of cytokines, and inhibit anti-CD3–induced proliferation by the CD38$^-$ population [115].

Other regulatory T cells

Researchers have proposed that, in addition to CD4$^+$ T cells, CD8$^+$ Treg cells may have a role in oral tolerance [116,117]. Recent efforts to generate suppressor cell lines in vitro resulted in a population of CD8$^+$ CD28$^-$ T cells, restricted by allogeneic class I HLA antigens, that were able to prevent up-regulation of B7 molecules induced by Th cells on APCs [118]. This outcome resulted in the suppression of CD4$^+$ T cells in an HLA-nonrestricted fashion [118]. The magnitude of a CD8$^+$ T-cell–mediated immune response to an acute viral infection is also subject to control by CD4$^+$ CD25$^+$ Treg cells. If natural Treg are depleted with specific anti-CD25 antibody before infection with virus, the resultant CD8$^+$ T-cell response is significantly enhanced, suggesting that controlling suppressor effects at vaccination could result in more effective immunity [119].

Double-negative (CD4$^-$ CD8$^-$) TCR$\alpha\beta^+$ Treg cells that mediate tolerance in several experimental autoimmune diseases have been described [120]. These double-negative T cells are specific for class I major histocompatibility complex molecules. The suppressive effect of these cells on the proliferation and cytotoxic activity of CD8$^+$ T cells with the same antigen specificity was not mediated by cytokines, but was instead attributed to Fas-mediated apoptosis of alloreactive T cells [121].

γ/δ T cells with regulatory functions have also been described. A population of γ/δ Treg cells with a cytokine profile reminiscent of Tr1 cell clones has been isolated from tumor-infiltrating lymphocytes [122]. These Treg cells could play a role in inhibiting immune responses to tumors [123]. Studies have also shown that aerosol delivery of protein antigens resulted in the differentiation of γ/δ T cells with regulatory functions [122]. Induction of tolerance through various doses of ovalbumin (OVA) has been shown to be abrogated in mice lacking TCRδ [124]. In contrast, TCRγ/δ-deficient mice have the same degree of IgE-specific unresponsiveness after aerosol priming and immunization with OVA [125].

Other regulatory cell types

One study has recently proposed a regulatory role for IL-10–secreting B cells [126]. These B cells prevented the development of arthritis, and their suppressive effect was particularly IL-10–dependent because the B cells isolated from IL-10–deficient mice did not protect from arthritis.

Some indications exist that dendritic cells (DCs) can induce peripheral T-cell tolerance and that a regulatory DC subset may exist. Pulmonary DCs from mice exposed to respiratory antigen transiently produce IL-10 [127]. These phenotypically mature pulmonary DCs, which were B7^{hi}, stimulated the development of

$CD4^+$ Tr1-like cells that also produced high amounts of IL-10. Adoptive transfer of pulmonary DCs from $IL-10^{+/+}$ but not $IL-10^{-/-}$ mice exposed to respiratory antigen induced antigen-specific unresponsiveness in recipient mice. In accordance with these findings, IL-10 inhibited the development of fully mature DCs, which induced a state of alloantigen-specific anergy in $CD4^+$ T cells [128]. These studies show that IL-10 production by DCs is critical for the induction of tolerance, and that phenotypically mature regulatory DCs may exist under certain circumstances.

Cells such as natural killer cells, epithelial cells, macrophages, and glial cells have been shown to express suppressor cytokines such as IL-10 and TGF-β. Although they have not been coined as professional regulatory cells, they may efficiently contribute to the generation and maintenance of a regulatory/suppressor-type immune response [129–134]. The expression of suppressor cytokines in resident tissue cells may also contribute to this process.

Mechanisms of regulatory T-cell generation

Two major hypotheses concern the generation of Treg cells. One suggests that Treg cells emerge from the thymus as a distinct subset of mature T cells with defined functions [110,112]. However, several studies have shown that Treg cells may differentiate from naïve T cells in the periphery when they encounter antigens in high concentrations [31,107,135]. Numerous studies suggest that thymic differentiation accounts for Treg cells that are specific for self-peptides and are devoted to the control of autoimmune responses, whereas peripheral differentiation may be required for environmental antigen-specific T cells for which an undesired immune response results in pathology. DCs not only control immunity but also maintain peripheral tolerance, two complementary functions that would ensure the integrity of the organism in an environment full of pathogens and allergens. The tolerogenic function of DCs depends on certain maturation stages and subsets of different ontogeny, and can be influenced by immunomodulatory agents. The differentiation of thymus-derived Treg cells does not depend on interaction with specialized DCs [136], whereas several studies support a role for DCs in the induction of Tr1 cells.

Immature DCs control peripheral tolerance through inducing Tr1-cell differentiation [34]. Related to prevention and development of asthma, airway DCs control the pulmonary immune response and determine tolerance and immunity to newly encountered antigens. Immature DCs are distributed throughout the lungs, capture allergens, and migrate to the T-cell area of mediastinal lymph nodes within 12 hours [137]. They express a partially mature phenotype with an intermediate array of costimulatory molecules and induce T-cell tolerance [138]. Antigen presentation by partially mature airway DCs that express IL-10 induce the formation of Tr1-like cells that inhibit subsequent inflammatory responses [127]. Moreover, depletion and adoptive transfer of pulmonary plasmacytoid DCs have shown that these cells have an important role in protection from allergen sensitization and asthma development in mice [139]. Although molecular mechanisms of Treg-cell generation have not been elucidated, some existing therapies for allergic diseases, such as treatment with glucocorticoids and β_2-agonists, might function to promote the numbers and function of IL-10–secreting Tr1-like cells [140,141].

Suppression mechanisms of regulatory T cells

Much uncertainty remains about the mechanisms of action of Treg cells. Initial studies have shown that Treg cells act as suppressor T cells, which inhibit the activation of effector cells and prevent inflammation in models of chronic infection, organ transplantation, and autoimmunity [29,31,142]. Treg cells have their suppressive functions only at certain stages of inflammation. Both Tr1 cells and $CD4^+ CD25^+$ Treg cells, which are highly capable of preventing allergen-induced activation and proliferation of effector T cells, cannot suppress the effector functions of preactivated T cells. This outcome was shown in a study of atopic dermatitis, where neither type of Treg cell could inhibit the apoptosis of keratinocytes induced by preactivated Th1 cells [143].

Most studies have failed to find a soluble factor as a suppressive mechanism of $CD4^+ CD25^+$ Treg cells. The suppression of antigen-induced proliferation of $CD4^+$ T cells was dramatically reduced after coculture with activated Treg clones that had been separated from the responding T cells by a Transwell (Corning Costar, Cambridge, MA) insert [144]. However, in Transwell membrane cultures that separate suppressor cells and target cells, the distance between two populations is approximately 2 mm, which may influence the concentration of suppressor cytokines. Membrane-bound TGF-β might be one of the mechanisms of suppression of $CD4^+ CD25^+$ Treg cells [145]. The suppressive effects of Tr1 cells were abrogated by the addition of neutralizing mAb directed against TGF-β and IL-10, implicating a role for suppressive cytokines in the mechanism of immune suppression in vitro and in vivo in different settings and different autoimmune and allergy models (Table 2) [31,36,100,145,146]. This suppression is a hallmark of Tr1 clones, because OVA-specific Th1 or Th2 clones derived from the same mice have no suppressive effects but rather enhanced OVA-induced proliferation of naïve $CD4^+$ T cells [35].

One group of $CD4^+ CD25^+$ Treg cells originates from the thymus as a distinctive subset [110,112,147]. Thymectomy at a very early stage of development induces various autoimmune diseases in genetically susceptible animals [148,149]. Furthermore, induction of autoimmune diseases in an immunodeficient animal model was prevented by adoptively transferred $CD4^+$ T cells or $CD4^+ CD8^-$ thymocytes isolated from normal syngeneic animals. In a rat model, $CD4^+$ Treg cells were found to be of the $CD45RC^{low}$ phenotype and to produce IL-2 and IL-4 but not IFN-γ on in vitro stimulation [148]. IL-4 and TGF-β are critical in preventing autoimmunity because neutralization of either of these cy-

Table 2
Mechanisms of action of IL-10 and TGF-β during allergen-SIT

IL-10	TGF-β
Suppresses allergen-specific IgE	Suppresses allergen-specific IgE
Induces allergen-specific IgG4	Induces allergen-specific IgA[a]
Blocks CD28 signal transduction pathway, suppresses allergen-specific Th1 and Th2 cells	Suppresses allergen-specific Th1 and Th2 cells
Inhibits DC maturation, leading to reduced class II major histocompatibility complex and costimulatory ligand expression, induces IL-10–producing DCs	Down-regulates FcεRI expression on Langerhans cells
Reduces release of proinflammatory cytokines by mast cells	Associated with CTLA-4 expression on T cells
Suppresses eosinophils, mast cells, and basophils[a]	Suppresses eosinophils, mast cells and basophils[a]
Suppresses endothelial cell expression of adhesion molecules and decreased inflammatory cell transmigration[a]	Suppresses endothelial cell expression of adhesion molecules and decreased inflammatory cell transmigration[a]
Induces IL-10 and TGF-β in T cells	Induces FoxP3 in T cells

[a] Most mechanisms have been shown in several studies, however, some are still under debate and their mechanisms remain to be further investigated.

tokines abrogates the protective response. In another study, CD4[+] CD25[+] Treg cells from thymus were shown to exert their suppressive function through the inhibition of IL-2Rα-chain in target T cells, induced by the combined activity of CTLA-4 and membrane TGF-β1 [150].

Studies of this activated CD4[+] T-cell subpopulation have shown that they do not proliferate on normal TCR-mediated stimulation, but they do suppress proliferation of other T cells. TCR stimulation was required for these cells to suppress other T cells. Such suppression, however, was not restricted to T cells specific for the same antigen. CD4[+] CD25[+] T cells are the only lymphocyte subpopulation in mice and humans that express CTLA-4 constitutively. The expression apparently correlates with the suppressor function of CTLA-4. The addition of anti–CTLA-4 antibody or its fragment of antigen binding reverses suppression in cocultures of CD4[+] CD25[+] and CD4[+] CD25[−] T cells [151]. Similarly, treating mice that were recipients of CD4[+] CD45RB[low] T cells with these agents abrogated the suppression of inflammatory bowel disease [152]. These studies indicate that signals resulting from the engagement of CTLA-4 with its ligands, CD80 and CD86, are required for the induction of suppressor activity. Under some circumstances, the engagement of CTLA-4 on the CD4[+] CD25[+] Treg cells with specific antibody or with CD80/CD86 might lead to inhibition of the TCR-derived signals that are required for the induction of suppressor activity.

PD-1 is an immunoreceptor tyrosine-based inhibitory motif (ITIM)–containing receptor expressed on T-cell activation. PD-1–deleted mice develop autoimmune diseases, suggesting an inhibitory role for PD-1 in immune responses [153]. Members of the B7 family, PD-L1 and PD-L2, are ligands for PD-1. PD-1: PD-L engagement on murine CD4 and CD8 T cells results in inhibition of proliferation and cytokine production. T cells stimulated with anti-CD3/PD-L1 display dramatically decreased proliferation and IL-2 production [154]. PD-1:PD-L interactions inhibit IL-2 production even in the presence of costimulation. Thus, after prolonged activation, the PD-1:PD-L inhibitory pathway dominates. Exogenous IL-2 is always able to overcome PD-L1–mediated inhibition, indicating that cells maintain IL-2 responsiveness.

Glucocorticoid-induced tumor necrosis factor receptor family-related gene (TNFRSF18, GITR) is expressed by $CD4^+$ $CD25^+$ alloantigen-specific and naturally occurring circulating Treg cells [155,156]. Stimulation of $CD4^+$ $CD25^+$ Treg cells through GITR breaks immunologic self-tolerance [156]. GITR is upregulated in $CD4^+$ $CD25^-$ T cells after TCR stimulation and also functions as a survival signal for activated cells [157]. In addition, CD103 ($\alpha_E\beta_7$ integrin) and CD122 (β chain of IL-2 receptor) are highly expressed on $CD4^+$ $CD25^+$ Treg cells, which correlates with their suppressive activity [158,159].

The X-linked forkhead/winged helix transcription factor FoxP3 is characteristic for $CD4^+$ $CD25^+$ Treg cells [160,161]. It is highly expressed in $CD4^+$ $CD25^+$ but not $CD4^+$ $CD25^-$ T cells [160,161]. It acts as a silencer of cytokine gene promoters and programs the development and function of $CD4^+$ $CD25^+$ Treg cells [160–163]. Mutations in the FoxP3 gene in humans leads to a severe immune dysregulation known as *IPEX syndrome* [164]. In addition, the absence of $FoxP3^+$ $CD4^+$ $CD25^+$ Treg cells in inflammatory and lesional skin suggests a mechanism for the development of eczematous lesions in atopic dermatitis observed in IPEX syndrome [143].

The failure of Treg cells to proliferate after TCR stimulation in vitro suggests that they are naturally anergic. However, Treg cells expressing a transgenic TCR were shown to proliferate and accumulate locally in response to transgenically expressed tissue antigen, whereas their $CD25^-$ counterparts are depleted at such sites [165].

Because the concept of professional suppressor cells is regaining interest in the immunologic community, how the manipulation of regulatory/suppressor T cells might be used clinically must now be considered. Sakaguchi and Sakaguchi [166] showed for first time that depletion of regulatory T cells from mice led to the development of autoimmune disease. Cotransfer of $CD4^+$ $CD25^+$ Treg cells together with effector, disease-causing, T cells prevented mice from developing multiple experimentally induced autoimmune diseases such as colitis, gastritis, type 1 diabetes, and thyroiditis [167–170]. Because tumor antigens are an important group of autoantigens, the depletion of Treg cells should result in an enhanced immune response to tumor vaccines. Several studies have shown that the antibody-mediated depletion of $CD25^+$ T cells facilitates the induction of tumor immunity [171,172].

Further studies are needed to show whether in vivo generation or adoptive transfer of Treg cells or their related suppressive cytokines may clinically change the course of allergy and asthma. Small molecular weight compounds that may generate Treg cells or increase their suppressive properties are an important target for use in not only allergy and asthma but also transplantation and autoimmunity.

Role of histamine receptor 2 in peripheral tolerance to allergens

As a small molecular weight monoamine that binds to four different G-protein–coupled receptors, histamine has recently been shown to regulate several essential events in the immune response [173,174]. Histamine receptor 2 (HR2) is coupled to adenylate cyclase, and studies in different species and several human cells have shown that inhibition of characteristic features of the cells primarily by cyclic adenosine monophosphate formation dominates in HR2-dependent effects of histamine [175]. Histamine enhances Th1-type responses by triggering the histamine receptor HR1, whereas Th1- and Th2-type responses are both negatively regulated by HR2. Human Th1 cells predominantly express HR1 and Th2 cells mostly express HR2, resulting in their differential regulation by histamine [38]. Histamine induces the production of IL-10 by DCs [176]. In addition, histamine induces IL-10 production by Th2 cells [177] and enhances the suppressive activity of TGF-β on T cells [178]. All three of these effects are mediated through HR2, which is highly expressed on Th2 cells and suppresses IL-4 and IL-13 production and T-cell proliferation [38]. These recent findings suggest that HR2 may represent an essential receptor that participates in peripheral tolerance or active suppression of inflammatory/immune responses. Histamine also regulates antibody isotypes, including IgE [38]. A high amount of allergen-specific IgE is induced in HR1-deleted mice. In contrast, deletion of HR2 leads to significantly lower amounts of allergen-specific IgE, probably caused by direct effect on B cells and indirect effect through T cells.

A double-blind, placebo-controlled trial analyzed the long-term protection from honeybee stings through terfenadine premedication during rush immunotherapy with honeybee venom [179]. After an average of 3 years, 41 patients were re-exposed to honeybee stings. Surprisingly, none of the 20 patients who had been given HR1-antihistamine premedication, but 6 of 21 who had been given placebo, had a systemic allergic reaction to the re-exposure through either a field sting or a sting challenge. This highly significant difference suggests that antihistamine premedication during the initial dose–increase phase may have enhanced the long-term efficacy of immunotherapy. Expression of HR1 on T lymphocytes is strongly reduced during ultrarush immunotherapy, which may lead to a dominant expression and function of tolerance-inducing HR2 [180]. Administration of antihistamines decreases the HR1/H2R expression ratio, which may enhance the suppressive effect of histamine on T cells. Further studies are required to substantiate these promising findings that support the use of antihistamine pretreatment in all patients undergoing venom-specific immunotherapy.

Summary

Peripheral T-cell tolerance is the key immunologic mechanism in the healthy immune response to self and noninfectious, nonself antigens. This phenomenon is clinically well documented in allergy, autoimmunity, transplantation, cancer, and infection. Changes in the fine balance between allergen-specific Treg cells and Th2 or Th1 cells are crucial in the development and treatment of allergic diseases. Strong evidence supports the role of Treg cells or immunosuppressive cytokines as a mechanism through which allergen-specific immunotherapy and healthy immune response to allergens are mediated (see Fig. 2).

In addition to the treatment of established allergy, prophylactic approaches must be considered before initial sensitization occurs. Allergen-specific Treg cells may in turn dampen the Th1 and Th2 cells and cytokines, ensuring a well-balanced immune response. Enhancement of the number and activity of Treg cells could be an obvious goal for the treatment of many diseases related to dysregulation of the immune response. Small molecular weight compounds that may generate Treg cells or increase their suppressive properties are an important target for use in not only allergy and asthma but also transplantation and autoimmunity. Treg cells may not always be responsible for a healthy immune response; several studies have shown that they may be responsible for the chronicity of infections and tumor tolerance. Treg-cell populations have proven difficult but not impossible to grow, expand, and clone in vitro. A crucial area for future study is the identification of drugs, cytokines, or costimulatory molecules that induce the growth while preserving the suppressor function of Treg cells. Applying current knowledge of Treg cells and related mechanisms of peripheral tolerance may lead to more rational and safer approaches to the prevention and cure of allergic disease in the near future.

References

[1] Billingham RE, Brent L, Medawar PB. Actively acquired tolerance of foreign cells. Nature 1953;172:603–6.
[2] Burnet F. The Nobel Lectures in Immunology. The Nobel Prize for Physiology or Medicine, 1960. Immunologic recognition of self. Scand J Immunol 1991;33:3–13.
[3] Burnet FM. The production of antibodies. Melbourne: Macmillan; 1949.
[4] Pirquet V. Das Verhalten der kutaanen Tuberkülin-reaktion wahrend der Masern. Munch Med Wochenschr 1908;34:1297–300.
[5] Nossal GJ, Pike BL. Clonal anergy: persistence in tolerant mice of antigen-binding B lymphocytes incapable of responding to antigen or mitogen. Proc Natl Acad Sci USA 1980;77: 1602–6.
[6] Lamb JR, Skidmore BJ, Green N, et al. Induction of tolerance in influenza virus-immune T lymphocyte clones with synthetic peptides of influenza hemagglutinin. J Exp Med 1983;157: 1434–47.
[7] Dhein J, Walczak H, Bäumler C, et al. Autocrine T-cell suicide mediated by APO-1(Fas/CD95). Nature 1995;373:438–41.
[8] Brunner T, Mogil RJ, LaFace D, et al. Cell-autonomous Fas (CD95)/Fas-ligand interaction mediates activation-induced apoptosis in T-cell hybridomas. Nature 1995;373:441–4.
[9] Akdis CA, Akdis M, Trautmann A, et al. Immune regulation in atopic dermatitis. Curr Opin Immunol 2000;12:641–6.
[10] Akdis CA, Blaser K, Akdis M. Apoptosis in tissue inflammation and allergic disease. Curr Opin Immunol 2004;16:717–23.

[11] Akdis M, Simon H-U, Weigl L, et al. Skin homing (cutaneous lymphocyte-associated antigen-positive) CD8 + T cells respond to superantigen and contribute to eosinophilia and IgE production in atopic dermatitis. J Immunol 1999;163:466–75.

[12] Abernathy-Carver KJ, Sampson HA, Picker LJ, et al. Milk-induced eczema is associated with the expansion of T cells expressing cutaneous lymphocyte antigen. J Clin Invest 1995;95:913–8.

[13] Klunker S, Trautmann A, Akdis M, et al. A second step of chemotaxis after transendothelial migration: keratinocytes undergoing apoptosis release IP-10, Mig and iTac for T cell chemotaxis towards epidermis in atopic dermatitis. J Immunol 2003;171:1078–84.

[14] Luster AD. The role of chemokines in linking innate and adaptive immunity. Curr Opin Immunol 2002;14:129–35.

[15] Gutierrez-Ramos JC, Lloyd C, Kapsenberg ML, et al. Non-redundant functional groups of chemokines operate in a coordinate manner during the inflammatory response in the lung. Immunol Rev 2000;177:31–42.

[16] Akdis M, Trautmann A, Klunker S, et al. T helper (Th) 2 predominance in atopic diseases is due to preferential apoptosis of circulating memory/effector Th1 cells. FASEB J 2003;17:1026–35.

[17] Simon H-U, Blaser K. Inhibition of programmed eosinophil death: a key pathogenic event for eosinophilia. Immunol Today 1995;16:53–5.

[18] Whittaker L, Niu N, Temann UA, et al. Interleukin-13 mediates a fundamental pathway for airway epithelial mucus induced by CD4 T cells and interleukin-9. Am J Respir Cell Mol Biol 2002;27:593–602.

[19] Trautmann A, Akdis M, Kleemann D, et al. T cell-mediated Fas-induced keratinocyte apoptosis plays a key pathogenetic role in eczematous dermatitis. J Clin Invest 2000;106:25–35.

[20] Trautmann A, Schmid-Grendelmeier P, Krüger K, et al. T cells and eosinophils cooperate in the induction of bronchial epithelial apoptosis in asthma. J Allergy Clin Immunol 2002;109:329–37.

[21] Trautmann A, Akdis M, Brocker EB, et al. New insights into the role of T cells in atopic dermatitis and allergic contact dermatitis. Trends Immunol 2001;22:530–2.

[22] Trautmann A, Akdis M, Schmid-Grendelmeier P, et al. Targeting keratinocyte apoptosis in the treatment of atopic dermatitis and allergic contact dermatitis. J Allergy Clin Immunol 2001;108:839–46.

[23] Romagnani S. Lymphokine production by human T cells in disease states. Annu Rev Immunol 1994;12:227–57.

[24] Mosmann TR, Sad S. The expanding universe of T-cell subsets: Th1, Th2 and more. Immunol Today 1996;17:142–6.

[25] Rincon M, Anguita J, Nakamura T, et al. Interleukin (IL)-6 directs the differentiation of IL-4-producing CD4 + T cells. J Exp Med 1997;185:461–9.

[26] Corry DB. IL-13 in allergy: home at last. Curr Opin Immunol 1999;11:610–4.

[27] Yssel H, Groux H. Characterization of T cell subpopulations involved in the pathogenesis of asthma and allergic diseases. Int Arch Allergy Immunol 2000;121:10–8.

[28] El Biaze M, Boniface S, Koscher V, et al. T cell activation, from atopy to asthma: more a paradox than a paradigm. Allergy 2003;58:844–53.

[29] Chen Y, Kuchroo VK, Inobe J, et al. Regulatory T cell clones induced by oral tolerance: suppression of autoimmune encephalomyelitis. Science 1994;265:1237–40.

[30] Powrie F, Correa-Oliveira R, Mauze S, et al. Regulatory interactions between CD45RB^{high} and CD45RB^{low} CD4 + T cells are important for the balance between protective and pathogenic cell- mediated immunity. J Exp Med 1994;179:589–600.

[31] Groux H, O'Garra A, Bigler M, et al. CD4 + T-cell subset inhibits antigen-specific T-cell responses and prevents colitis. Nature 1997;389:737–42.

[32] Akdis CA, Blesken T, Akdis M, et al. Role of IL-10 in specific immunotherapy. J Clin Invest 1998;102:98–106.

[33] Taams LS, Smith J, Rustin MH, et al. Human anergic/suppressive CD4(+)CD25(+) T cells: a highly differentiated and apoptosis-prone population. Eur J Immunol 2001;31:1122–31.

[34] Jonuleit H, Schmitt E, Schuler G, et al. Induction of interleukin 10-producing, nonproliferat-

ing CD4(+) T cells with regulatory properties by repetitive stimulation with allogeneic immature human dendritic cells. J Exp Med 2000;192:1213–22.

[35] Cottrez F, Hurst SD, Coffman RL, et al. T regulatory cells 1 inhibit a Th2-specific response in vivo. J Immunol 2000;165:4848–53.

[36] Jutel M, Akdis M, Budak F, et al. IL-10 and TGF-β cooperate in regulatory T cell response to mucosal allergens in normal immunity and specific immunotherapy. Eur J Immunol 2003;33: 1205–14.

[37] Bousquet J. Global initiative for asthma (GINA) and its objectives. Clin Exp Allergy 2000; 30(Suppl 1):2–5.

[38] Jutel M, Watanabe T, Klunker S, et al. Histamine regulates T-cell and antibody responses by differential expression of H1 and H2 receptors. Nature 2001;413:420–5.

[39] Holgate ST. Asthma: more than an inflammatory disease. Curr Opin Allergy Clin Immunol 2002;2:27–9.

[40] Kussebi F, Karamloo F, Akdis M, et al. Advances in immunological treatment of allergy. Curr Med Chem 2003;2:297–308.

[41] Müller UR, Mosbech H. Position paper: Immunotherapy with hymenoptera venoms. Allergy 1993;48:36–46.

[42] Bousquet J, Lockey R, Malling HJ, et al. Allergen immunotherapy: therapeutic vaccines for allergic diseases. World Health Organization. American academy of Allergy, Asthma and Immunology. Ann Allergy Asthma Immunol 1998;81:401–5.

[43] Walker SM, Varney VA, Gaga M, et al. Grass pollen immunotherapy: efficacy and safety during a 4-year follow- up study. Allergy 1995;50:405–13.

[44] Varney VA, Gaga M, Frew AJ, et al. Usefulness of immunotherapy in patients with severe summer hay fever uncontrolled by antiallergic drugs. BMJ 1991;302:265–9.

[45] Durham SR, Walker SM, Varga EM, et al. Long-term clinical efficacy of grass-pollen immuno-therapy. N Engl J Med 1999;341:468–75.

[46] Noon L. Prophylactic inoculation against hay fever. Lancet 1911;1:1572–3.

[47] Cooke R, Banard JH, Hebald S, et al. Serological evidence of immunity with coexisting sensitization in a type of human allergy (hay fever). J Exp Med 1935;62:733–51.

[48] Lichtenstein L, Norman PS, Winkenwerder WL, et al. In vitro studies of human ragweed allergy: changes in cellular and humoral activity associated with specific desensitization. J Clin Invest 1966;45:1126–36.

[49] Akdis CA, Akdis M, Blesken T, et al. Epitope-specific T cell tolerance to phospholipase A2 in bee venom immunotherapy and recovery by IL-2 and IL-15 in vitro. J Clin Invest 1996;98: 1676–83.

[50] Durham SR, Till SJ. Immunological changes associated with allergen immunotherapy. J Allergy Clin Immunol 1998;102:157–64.

[51] Rolland JM, Douglass J, O'Hehir RE. Allergen immunotherapy: current and new therapeutic strategies. Expert Opin Investig Drugs 2000;9:515–27.

[52] Akdis CA, Blaser K. IL-10-induced anergy in peripheral T cell and reactivation by micro-environmental cytokines: two key steps in specific immunotherapy. FASEB J 1999;13:603–9.

[53] Ebner C. Immunological mechanisms operative in allergen-specific immunotherapy. Int Arch Allergy Immunol 1999;119:1–5.

[54] Akdis CA, Blaser K. Mechanisms of allergen-specific immunotherapy. Allergy 2000;55:522–30.

[55] Flicker S, Steinberger P, Norderhaug L, et al. Conversion of grass pollen allergen-specific human IgE into a protective IgG(1) antibody. Eur J Immunol 2002;32:2156–62.

[56] Wetterwald A, Skvaril F, Muller U, et al. Isotypic and idiotypic characterization of anti-bee venom phospholipase A2 antibodies. Int Arch Allergy Appl Immunol 1985;77:195–7.

[57] van Neerven RJ, Wikborg T, Lund G, et al. Blocking antibodies induced by specific allergy vaccination prevent the activation of CD4 + T cells by inhibiting serum-IgE-facilitated allergen presentation. J Immunol 1999;163:2944–52.

[58] Rocklin RE, Sheffer A, Greineder DK, et al. Generation of antigen-specific suppressor cells during allergy desensitization. N Engl J Med 1980;302:1213–9.

[59] Creticos PS, Adkinson Jr NF, Kagey-Sobotka A, et al. Nasal challenge with ragweed pollen in hay fever patients. Effect of immunotherapy. J Clin Invest 1985;76:2247–53.

[60] Rak S, Lowhagen O, Venge P. The effect of immunotherapy on bronchial hyperresponsiveness and eosinophil cationic protein in pollen-allergic patients. J Allergy Clin Immunol 1988;82: 470–80.

[61] Otsuka H, Mezawa A, Ohnishi M, et al. Changes in nasal metachromatic cells during allergen immunotherapy. Clin Exp Allergy 1991;21:115–9.

[62] Jutel M, Pichler WJ, Skrbic D, et al. Bee venom immunotherapy results in decrease of IL-4 and IL-5 and increase of IFN-gamma secretion in specific allergen-stimulated T cell cultures. J Immunol 1995;154:4187–94.

[63] Secrist H, Chelen CJ, Wen Y, et al. Allergen immunotherapy decreases interleukin 4 production in CD4 + T cells from allergic individuals. J Exp Med 1993;178:2123–30.

[64] Bellinghausen I, Metz G, Enk AH, et al. Insect venom immunotherapy induces interleukin-10 production and a Th2- to-Th1 shift, and changes surface marker expression in venom-allergic subjects. Eur J Immunol 1997;27:1131–9.

[65] Varney VA, Hamid QA, Gaga M, et al. Influence of grass pollen immunotherapy on cellular infiltration and cytokine mRNA expression during allergen-induced late-phase cutaneous responses. J Clin Invest 1993;92:644–51.

[66] Varga EM, Wachholz P, Nouri-Aria KT, et al. T cells from human allergen-induced late asthmatic responses express IL-12 receptor beta 2 subunit mRNA and respond to IL-12 in vitro. J Immunol 2000;165:2877–85.

[67] Hamid QA, Schotman E, Jacobson MR, et al. Increases in IL-12 messenger RNA + cells accompany inhibition of allergen-induced late skin responses after successful grass pollen immunotherapy. J Allergy Clin Immunol 1997;99:254–60.

[68] Durham SR, Ying S, Varney VA, et al. Grass pollen immunotherapy inhibits allergen-induced infiltration of CD4 + T lymphocytes and eosinophils in the nasal mucosa and increases the number of cells expressing messenger RNA for interferon-gamma. J Allergy Clin Immunol 1996;97:1356–65.

[69] Wachholz PA, Nouri-Aria KT, Wilson DR, et al. Grass pollen immunotherapy for hayfever is associated with increases in local nasal but not peripheral Th1:Th2 cytokine ratios. Immunology 2002;105:56–62.

[70] Akdis M, Verhagen J, Taylor A, et al. Immune responses in healthy and allergic individuals are characterized by a fine balance between allergen-specific T regulatory 1 and T helper 2 cells. J Exp Med 2004;199:1567–75.

[71] Oral HB, Kotenko SV, Yilmaz M, et al. Regulation of T cells and cytokines by the interleukin-10 (IL-10)-family cytokines IL-19, IL-20, IL-22, IL-24 andIL-26. Eur J Immunol 2006; 36:380–8.

[72] Borish L, Aarons A, Rumbyrt J, et al. Interleukin-10 regulation in normal subjects and patients with asthma. J Allergy Clin Immunol 1996;97:1288–96.

[73] Koning H, Neijens HJ, Baert MR, et al. T cells subsets and cytokines in allergic and non-allergic children. II. Analysis and IL-5 and IL-10 mRNA expression and protein production. Cytokine 1997;9:427–36.

[74] Vignola AM, Chanez P, Chiappara G, et al. Transforming growth factor-beta expression in mucosal biopsies in asthma and chronic bronchitis. Am J Respir Crit Care Med 1997;156:591–9.

[75] Hellings PW, Vandenberghe P, Kasran A, et al. Blockade of CTLA-4 enhances allergic sensitization and eosinophilic airway inflammation in genetically predisposed mice. Eur J Immunol 2002;32:585–94.

[76] Punnonen J, De Waal Malefyt R, Van Vlasselaer P, et al. IL-10 and viral IL-10 prevent IL-4-indiced IgE synthesis by inhibiting the accessory cell function of monocytes. J Immunol 1993;151:1280–9.

[77] Sonoda E, Matsumoto R, Hitoshi Y, et al. Transforming growth factor beta induces IgA production and acts additively with interleukin 5 for IgA production. J Exp Med 1989;170: 1415–20.

[78] Flicker S, Valenta R. Renaissance of the blocking antibody concept in type I allergy. Int Arch Allergy Immunol 2003;132:13–24.

[79] Wachholz PA, Durham SR. Mechanisms of immunotherapy: IgG revisited. Curr Opin Allergy Clin Immunol 2004;4:313–8.

[80] Golden DB, Meyers DA, Kagey-Sobotka A, et al. Clinical relevance of the venom-specific immunoglobulin G antibody level during immunotherapy. J Allergy Clin Immunol 1982;69: 489–93.

[81] Müller UR, Helbling A, Bischof M. Predictive value of venom-specific IgE, IgG and IgG subclass antibodies in patients on immunotherapy with honey bee venom. Allergy 1989;44: 412–8.

[82] Nouri-Aria KT, Wachholz PA, Francis JN, et al. Grass pollen immunotherapy induces mucosal and peripheral IL-10 responses and blocking IgG activity. J Immunol 2004;172:3252–9.

[83] Jutel M, Jaeger L, Suck R, et al. Allergen-specific immunotherapy with recombinant grass pollen allergens. J Allergy Clin Immunol 2005;116:608–13.

[84] Rossi RE, Monasterolo G. Evaluation of recombinant and native timothy pollen (rPhl p 1, 2, 5, 6, 7, 11, 12 and nPhl p 4)- specific IgG4 antibodies induced by subcutaneous immunotherapy with timothy pollen extract in allergic patients. Int Arch Allergy Immunol 2004;135:44–53.

[85] Walker C, Virchow J-C, Bruijnzeel PLB, et al. T cell subsets and their soluble products regulate eosinophilia in allergic and nonallergic asthma. J Immunol 1991;146:1829–35.

[86] Schleimer RP, Derse CP, Friedman B, et al. Regulation of human basophil mediator release by cytokines. I. Interaction with anti-inflammatory steroids. J Immunol 1989;143:1310–27.

[87] Marshall JS, Leal-Berumen I, Nielsen L, et al. Interleukin (IL)-10 Inhibits long-term IL-6 production but not preformed mediator release from rat peritoneal mast cells. J Clin Invest 1996;97:1122–8.

[88] Schandane L, Alonso-Vega C, Willems F, et al. B7/CD28-dependent IL-5 production by human resting T cells is inhibited by IL-10. J Immunol 1994;152:4368–74.

[89] Ohkawara Y, Lim KG, Glibetic M, et al. CD40 expression by human peripheral blood eosinophils. J Clin Invest 1996;97:1761–6.

[90] Knechtle SJ, Hamawy MM, Hu H, et al. Tolerance and near-tolerance strategies in monkeys and their application to human renal transplantation. Immunol Rev 2001;183:205–13.

[91] Chambers CA. The expanding world of co-stimulation: the two-signal model revisited. Trends Immunol 2001;22:217–23.

[92] Schwartz RH. Models of T cell anergy: is there a common molecular mechanism? J Exp Med 1996;184:1–8.

[93] Faith A, Akdis CA, Akdis M, et al. Defective TCR stimulation in anergized type 2 T helper cells correlates with abrogated p56^{lck} and ZAP-70 tyrosine kinase activities. J Immunol 1997; 159:53–60.

[94] Hoyne GF, O'Hehir R, Wraith DC, et al. Inhibition of T cell and antibody responses to house dust mite allergen by inhalation of the dominant T cell epitope in naive and sensitized mice. J Exp Med 1993;178:1783–8.

[95] Haczku A, Takeda K, Redai I, et al. Anti-CD86 (B7.2) treatment abolishes allergic airway hyperresponsiveness in mice. Am J Respir Crit Care Med 1999;159:1638–43.

[96] Van Oosterhout AJ, Hofstra CL, Shields R, et al. Murine CTLA4-IgG treatment inhibits airway eosinophilia and hyperresponsiveness and attenuates IgE upregulation in a murine model of allergic asthma. Am J Respir Cell Mol Biol 1997;17:386–92.

[97] Van Neerven RJ, Van de Pol MM, Van der Zee JS, et al. Requirement of CD28–CD86 costimulation for allergen-specific T cell proliferation and cytokine expression. Clin Exp Allergy 1998;28:808–16.

[98] Gonzalo JA, Tian J, Delaney T, et al. ICOS is critical for T helper cell-mediated lung mucosal inflammatory responses. Nat Immunol 2001;2:597–604.

[99] Dong C, Juedes AE, Temann UA, et al. ICOS co-stimulatory receptor is essential for T-cell activation and function. Nature 2001;409:97–101.

[100] Akdis CA, Joss A, Akdis M, et al. A molecular basis for T cell suppression by IL-10: CD28-

associated IL-10 receptor inhibits CD28 tyrosine phosphorylation and phosphatidylinositol 3-kinase binding. FASEB J 2000;14:1666–9.

[101] Joss A, Akdis M, Faith A, et al. IL-10 directly acts on T cells by specifically altering the CD28 co-stimulation pathway. Eur J Immunol 2000;30:1683–90.

[102] Prasad KVS, Cai Y-C, Raab M, et al. T-cell antigen CD28 interacts with the lipid kinase phosphatidylinositol 3-kinase by a cytoplasmic Tyr(P)-Met-Xaa-Met motif. Proc Natl Acad Sci USA 1994;91:2834–8.

[103] Levings MK, Sangregorio R, Galbiati F, et al. IFN-alpha and IL-10 induce the differentiation of human type 1 T regulatory cells. J Immunol 2001;166:5530–9.

[104] Bacchetta R, Sartirana C, Levings MK, et al. Growth and expansion of human T regulatory type 1 cells are independent from TCR activation but require exogenous cytokines. Eur J Immunol 2002;32:2237–45.

[105] Roncarolo MG, Bacchetta R, Bordignon C, et al. Type 1 T regulatory cells. Immunol Rev 2001;182:68–79.

[106] Müller UR, Akdis CA, Fricker M, et al. Successful immunotherapy with T cell epitope peptides of bee venom phospholipase A_2 induces specific T cell anergy in bee sting allergic patients. J Allergy Clin Immunol 1998;101:747–54.

[107] Barrat FJ, Cua DJ, Boonstra A, et al. In vitro generation of interleukin 10-producing regulatory CD4(+) T cells is induced by immunosuppressive drugs and inhibited by T helper type 1 (Th1)- and Th2-inducing cytokines. J Exp Med 2002;195:603–16.

[108] Nasser SM, Ying S, Meng O, et al. Interleukin-10 levels increase in cutaneous biopsies of patients undergoing wasp venom immunotherapy. Eur J Immunol 2001;31:3704–13.

[109] Chen Y, Inobe J, Kuchroo VK, et al. Oral tolerance in myelin basic protein T-cell receptor transgenic mice: suppression of autoimmune encephalomyelitis and dose-dependent induction of regulatory cells. Proc Natl Acad Sci USA 1996;93:388–91.

[110] Sakaguchi S, Sakaguchi N, Asano M, et al. Immunologic self-tolerance maintained by activated T cells expressing IL-2 receptor alpha-chains (CD25). Breakdown of a single mechanism of self-tolerance causes various autoimmune diseases. J Immunol 1995;155:1151–64.

[111] Shevach EM. CD4 + CD25 + suppressor T cells: more questions than answers. Nat Rev Immunol 2002;2:389–400.

[112] Wood KJ, Sakaguchi S. Regulatory T cells in transplantation tolerance. Nat Rev Immunol 2003; 3:199–210.

[113] Read S, Powrie F. CD4(+) regulatory T cells. Curr Opin Immunol 2001;13:644–9.

[114] Hori S, Nomura T, Sakaguchi S. Control of regulatory T cell development by the transcription factor Foxp3. Science 2003;299:1057–61.

[115] Read S, Mauze S, Asseman C, et al. CD38 + CD45RB(low) CD4 + T cells: a population of T cells with immune regulatory activities in vitro. Eur J Immunol 1998;28:3435–47.

[116] Ke Y, Kapp JA. Oral antigen inhibits priming of CD8 + CTL, CD4 + T cells, and antibody responses while activating CD8 + suppressor T cells. J Immunol 1996;156:916–21.

[117] Weiner HL. Oral tolerance for the treatment of autoimmune diseases. Annu Rev Med 1997;48: 341–51.

[118] Ciubotariu R, Colovai AI, Pennesi G, et al. Specific suppression of human CD4 + Th cell responses to pig MHC antigens by CD8 + CD28- regulatory T cells. J Immunol 1998;161: 5193–202.

[119] Suvas S, Kumaraguru U, Pack CD, et al. CD4 + CD25 + T cells regulate virus-specific primary and memory CD8 + T cell responses. J Exp Med 2003;198:889–901.

[120] Strober S, Cheng L, Zeng D, et al. Double negative (CD4–CD8- alpha beta +) T cells which promote tolerance induction and regulate autoimmunity. Immunol Rev 1996;149:217–30.

[121] Zhang ZX, Yang L, Young KJ, et al. Identification of a previously unknown antigen-specific regulatory T cell and its mechanism of suppression. Nat Med 2000;6:782–9.

[122] Hanninen A, Harrison LC. Gamma delta T cells as mediators of mucosal tolerance: the autoimmune diabetes model. Immunol Rev 2000;173:109–19.

[123] Seo N, Tokura Y, Takigawa M, et al. Depletion of IL-10- and TGF-beta-producing regulatory

gamma delta T cells by administering a daunomycin-conjugated specific monoclonal antibody in early tumor lesions augments the activity of CTLs and NK cells. J Immunol 1999;163:242–9.

[124] Ke Y, Pearce K, Lake JP, et al. Gamma delta T lymphocytes regulate the induction and maintenance of oral tolerance. J Immunol 1997;158:3610–8.

[125] Seymour BW, Gershwin LJ, Coffman RL. Aerosol-induced immunoglobulin (Ig)-E unresponsiveness to ovalbumin does not require CD8 + or T cell receptor (TCR)-gamma/delta + T cells or interferon (IFN)-gamma in a murine model of allergen sensitization. J Exp Med 1998;187:721–31.

[126] Mauri C, Gray D, Mushtaq N, et al. Prevention of arthritis by interleukin 10-producing B cells. J Exp Med 2003;197:489–501.

[127] Akbari O, DeKruyff RH, Umetsu DT. Pulmonary dendritic cells producing IL-10 mediate tolerance induced by respiratory exposure to antigen. Nat Immunol 2001;2:725–31.

[128] Steinbrink K, Wolfl M, Jonuleit H, et al. Induction of tolerance by IL-10-treated dendritic cells. J Immunol 1997;159:4772–80.

[129] Morganti-Kossmann MC, Kossmann T, Brandes ME, et al. Autocrine and paracrine regulation of astrocyte function by transforming growth factor-beta. J Neuroimmunol 1992;39:163–73.

[130] Kao JY, Gong Y, Chen CM, et al. Tumor-derived TGF-beta reduces the efficacy of dendritic cell/tumor fusion vaccine. J Immunol 2003;170:3806–11.

[131] Rivas JM, Ullrich SE. Systemic suppression of delayed-type hypersensitivity by supernatants from UV-irradiated keratinocytes. An essential role for keratinocyte-derived IL-10. J Immunol 1992;149:3865–71.

[132] Lidstrom C, Matthiesen L, Berg G, et al. Cytokine secretion patterns of NK cells and macrophages in early human pregnancy decidua and blood: implications for suppressor macrophages in decidua. Am J Reprod Immunol 2003;50:444–52.

[133] Dowdell KC, Cua DJ, Kirtkman E, et al. NK cells regulate CD4 responses prior to antigen encounter. J Immunol 2003;171:234–9.

[134] Kitamura M, Suto T, Yokoo T, et al. Transforming growth factor-beta 1 is the predominant paracrine inhibitor of macrophage cytokine synthesis produced by glomerular mesangial cells. J Immunol 1996;156:2964–71.

[135] Weiner HL. Induction and mechanism of action of transforming growth factor-beta- secreting Th3 regulatory cells. Immunol Rev 2001;182:207–14.

[136] Jordan MS, Riley MP, von Boehmer H, et al. Anergy and suppression regulate CD4(+) T cell responses to a self peptide. Eur J Immunol 2000;30:136–44.

[137] Vermaelen KY, Carro-Muino I, Lambrecht BN, et al. Specific migratory dendritic cells rapidly transport antigen from the airways to the thoracic lymph nodes. J Exp Med 2001;193:51–60.

[138] Lambrecht BN, Pauwels RA, Fazekas De St Groth B. Induction of rapid T cell activation, division, and recirculation by intratracheal injection of dendritic cells in a TCR transgenic model. J Immunol 2000;164:2937–46.

[139] de Heer HJ, Hammad H, Soullie T, et al. Essential role of lung plasmacytoid dendritic cells in preventing asthmatic reactions to harmless inhaled antigen. J Exp Med 2004;200:89–98.

[140] Peek EJ, Richards DF, Faith A, et al. Interleukin-10-secreting "regulatory" T cells induced by glucocorticoids and beta2-agonists. Am J Respir Cell Mol Biol 2005;33:105–11.

[141] Karagiannidis C, Akdis M, Holopainen P, et al. Glucocorticoids upregulate FOXP3 expression and regulatory T cells in asthma. J Allergy Clin Immunol 2004;114:1425–33.

[142] Qin S, Cobbold SP, Pope H, et al. "Infectious" transplantation tolerance. Science 1993;259:974–7.

[143] Verhagen J, Akdis M, Traidl-Hoffmann C, et al. Absence of T-regulatory cell expression and function in atopic dermatitis skin. J Allergy Clin Immunol 2006;117:176–83.

[144] Thornton AM, Shevach EM. CD4 + CD25 + immunoregulatory T cells suppress polyclonal T cell activation in vitro by inhibiting interleukin 2 production. J Exp Med 1998;188:287–96.

[145] Nakamura K, Kitani A, Strober W. Cell contact-dependent immunosuppression by CD4(+) CD25(+) regulatory T cells is mediated by cell surface-bound transforming growth factor beta. J Exp Med 2001;194:629–44.

[146] Levings MK, Bachetta R, Schulz U, et al. The role of IL-10 and TGF-beta in the differentiation and effector function of T regulatory cells. Int Arch Allergy Appl Immunol 2002;129: 263–76.

[147] Itoh M, Takahashi T, Sakaguchi N, et al. Thymus and autoimmunity: production of CD25 + CD4 + naturally anergic and suppressive T cells as a key function of the thymus in maintaining immunologic self-tolerance. J Immunol 1999;162:5317–26.

[148] Fowell D, Mason D. Evidence that the T cell repertoire of normal rats contains cells with the potential to cause diabetes. Characterization of the CD4 + T cell subset that inhibits this autoimmune potential. J Exp Med 1993;177:627–36.

[149] Asano M, Toda M, Sakaguchi N, et al. Autoimmune disease as a consequence of developmental abnormality of a T cell subpopulation. J Exp Med 1996;184:387–96.

[150] Annunziato F, Cosmi L, Liotta F, et al. Phenotype, localization, and mechanism of suppression of CD4 + CD25 + human thymocytes. J Exp Med 2002;196:379–87.

[151] Takahashi T, Tagami T, Yamazaki S, et al. Immunologic self-tolerance maintained by CD25(+) CD4(+) regulatory T cells constitutively expressing cytotoxic T lymphocyte-associated antigen 4. J Exp Med 2000;192:303–10.

[152] Read S, Malmstrom V, Powrie F. Cytotoxic T lymphocyte-associated antigen 4 plays an essential role in the function of CD25(+)CD4(+) regulatory cells that control intestinal inflammation. J Exp Med 2000;192:295–302.

[153] Nishimura H, Nose M, Hiai H, et al. Development of lupus-like autoimmune diseases by disruption of the PD-1 gene encoding an ITIM motif-carrying immunoreceptor. Immunity 1999; 11:141–51.

[154] Carter L, Fouser LA, Jussif J, et al. PD-1:PD-L inhibitory pathway affects both CD4(+) and CD8(+) T cells and is overcome by IL-2. Eur J Immunol 2002;32:634–43.

[155] McHugh RS, Whitters MJ, Piccirillov CA. CD4(+)CD25(+) immunoregulatory T cells: gene expression analysis reveals a functional role for the glucocorticoid-induced TNF receptor. Immunity 2002;16:311–23.

[156] Shimizu J, Yamazaki S, Takahashi T, et al. Stimulation of CD25(+)CD4(+) regulatory T cells through GITR breaks immunological self-tolerance. Nat Immunol 2002;3:135–42.

[157] Nocentini G, Giunchi L, Ronchetti S, et al. A new member of the tumor necrosis factor/nerve growth factor receptor family inhibits T cell receptor-induced apoptosis. Proc Natl Acad Sci USA 1997;94:6216–21.

[158] Lehmann J, Huehn J, de la Rosa M, et al. Expression of the integrin alpha E beta 7 identifies unique subsets of CD25 + as well as CD25- regulatory T cells. Proc Natl Acad Sci USA 2002; 99:13031–6.

[159] Levings MK, Sangregorio R, Roncarolo MG. Human CD25(+)CD4(+) T regulatory cells suppress naive and memory T cell proliferation and can be expanded in vitro without loss of function. J Exp Med 2001;193:1295–302.

[160] Khattri R, Cox T, Yasayko SA, et al. An essential role for Scurfin in CD4 + CD25 + T regulatory cells. Nat Immunol 2003;4:337–42.

[161] Fontenot JD, Gavin MA, Rudensky AY. Foxp3 programs the development and function of CD4 + CD25 + regulatory T cells. Nat Immunol 2003;4:330–6.

[162] Kanangat S, Blair P, Reddy R, et al. Disease in the scurfy (sf) mouse is associated with overexpression of cytokine genes. Eur J Immunol 1996;26:161–5.

[163] Schubert LA, Jeffrey E, Zhang Y, et al. Scurfin (FOXP3) acts as a repressor of transcription and regulates T cell activation. J Biol Chem 2001;276:37672–9.

[164] Wildin RS, Ramsdell F, Peake J, et al. X-linked neonatal diabetes mellitus, enteropathy and endocrinopathy syndrome is the human equivalent of mouse scurfy. Nat Genet 2001;27:18–20.

[165] Walker LS, Chodos A, Eggena M, et al. Antigen-dependent proliferation of CD4 + CD25 + regulatory T cells in vivo. J Exp Med 2003;198:249–58.

[166] Sakaguchi S, Sakaguchi N. Organ-specific autoimmune disease induced in mice by elimination of T cell subsets. V. Neonatal administration of cyclosporin A causes autoimmune disease. J Immunol 1989;142:471–80.

[167] Sakaguchi S, Sakaguchi N, Asano M, et al. Immunologic self-tolerance maintained by activated T cells expressing IL-2 receptor alpha-chains (CD25). Breakdown of a single mechanism of self-tolerance causes various autoimmune diseases. J Immunol 1995;155:1151–64.

[168] Powrie F, Mauze S, Coffman RL. CD4 + T-cells in the regulation of inflammatory responses in the intestine. Res Immunol 1997;148:576–81.

[169] Salomon B, Lenschow DJ, Rhee L, et al. B7/CD28 costimulation is essential for the homeostasis of the CD4 + CD25 + immunoregulatory T cells that control autoimmune diabetes. Immunity 2000;12:431–40.

[170] Mottet C, Uhlig HH, Powrie F. Cutting edge: cure of colitis by CD4 + CD25 + regulatory T cells. J Immunol 2003;170:3939–43.

[171] Sutmuller RP, van Duivenvoorde LM, van Elsas A, et al. Synergism of cytotoxic T lymphocyte-associated antigen 4 blockade and depletion of CD25(+) regulatory T cells in antitumor therapy reveals alternative pathways for suppression of autoreactive cytotoxic T lymphocyte responses. J Exp Med 2001;194:823–32.

[172] Shimizu J, Yamazaki S, Sakaguchi S. Induction of tumor immunity by removing CD25 + CD4 + T cells: a common basis between tumor immunity and autoimmunity. J Immunol 1999; 163:5211–8.

[173] Jutel M, Watanabe T, Akdis M, et al. Immune regulation by histamine. Curr Opin Immunol 2002;14:735–40.

[174] Akdis CA, Blaser K. Histamine in the immune regulation of allergic inflammation. J Allergy Clin Immunol 2003;112:15–22.

[175] Del Valle J, Gantz I. Novel insights into histamine H2 receptor biology. Am J Physiol 1997; 273:G987–96.

[176] Mazzoni A, Young HA, Spitzer JH, et al. Histamine regulates cytokine production in maturing dendritic cells, resulting in altered T cell polarization. J Clin Invest 2001;108:1865–73.

[177] Osna N, Elliott K, Khan MM. Regulation of interleukin-10 secretion by histamine in TH2 cells and splenocytes. Int Immunopharmacol 2001;1:85–96.

[178] Kunzmann S, Mantel P-Y, Wohlfahrt J, et al. Histamine enhances TGF-beta1-mediated suppression of Th2 responses. FASEB J 2003;17:1089–95.

[179] Müller U, Hari Y, Berchtold E. Premedication with antihistamines may enhance efficacy of specific- allergen immunotherapy. J Allergy Clin Immunol 2001;107:81–6.

[180] Jutel M, Zak-Nejmark T, Wrzyyszcz M, et al. Histamine receptor expression on peripheral blood CD4 + lymphocytes is influenced by ultrarush bee venom immunotherapy. Allergy 1997;52(Suppl 37):88.

ELSEVIER
SAUNDERS

Immunol Allergy Clin N Am
26 (2006) 233–244

IMMUNOLOGY
AND ALLERGY
CLINICS
OF NORTH AMERICA

The Role of TGF-β in Allergic Inflammation

Carsten B. Schmidt-Weber, PhD*, Kurt Blaser, PhD

*Swiss Institute of Allergy and Asthma Research (SIAF), Obere Strasse 22,
CH-7270 Davos, Switzerland*

The transforming growth factor β (TGF-β) plays a dual role in allergic disease. It is important in suppressing T cells and also mediates repair responses that lead to unwanted remodeling of tissues [1]. Advances in the immunology of allergy indicate that allergens cause overreactions in the lymphocyte compartment because of the lack or decreased number of suppressive regulatory T cells (Tregs). TGF-β was shown to induce Tregs and participate directly in suppression of effector T cells (Teffs). Therefore, TGF-β may help return reactivity to allergens to normal subsymptomatic activity. Whether chronic inflammatory diseases such as asthma profit from TGF-β–mediated suppression of specific immune responses or whether TGF-β–mediated tissue remodeling aggravates diseases more than it helps control immune reactions is unclear. This article addresses these issues and future strategies in this field.

Immune responses observed in allergy, autoimmune diseases, and infectious diseases or transplantation share a combined effort of the innate and specific immune system to protect an organism from loss of function of chronically affected organs. The specific immune system, particularly the T cells, play a key role in the maintenance of peripheral tolerance against autologous, commensal, and environmental proteins such as proteins. The current understanding of this thymus-independent peripheral tolerance is that the commitment of antigen-naïve T cells to certain effector phenotypes such as T helper 1 (Th1) cells, Th2 cells, or Tregs can suppress Teffs [2]. Teffs are memory T cells and constitute the immunologic memory, thus affiliating an antigen specificity and quality from the response,

This work was supported by the Swiss National Foundation Grants Nr: 31-65436 and 32-100266 and 3100A0-100164, the Ehmann Foundation, the Saurer Foundation, Bonizzi-Theler Stiftung, and the Ernst-Göhner Stiftung, Zug.

* Corresponding author.

E-mail address: csweber@siaf.unizh.ch (C.B. Schmidt-Weber).

such as a certain cytokine profile, which is secreted on activation. To prevent the organism from damage, immunologic reactions are self-limited and Tregs are now recognized as key factors in silencing specific immune reactions. This fact is particularly important for those diseases that fail to recover and develop into chronic conditions. Recovery from inflammatory reactions must compensate cell lysis and lateral tissue damage to recover the function of the affected organ. A key cytokine in recovery responses is TGF-β1, which mediates suppression or Tregs generation and repair of damaged tissues.

Regulator and repair responses

The genes of the TGF-β family are key mediators in embryonic development and tissue repair and include three types of TGF-βs (TGF-β1, -β2, and -β3), in-

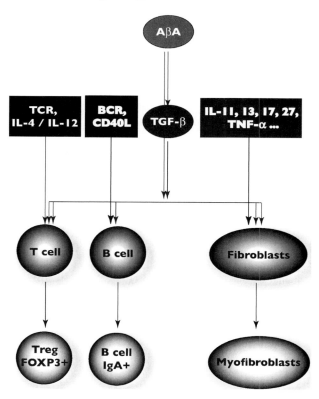

Fig. 1. Allergy relevant functions of activin βA. All of the depicted targets were described for TGF-β. Those on the left side of the circle represent negative side effects, whereas those on the right side may prevent allergic reactions.

hibins, activins, and various bone morphogenetic proteins (BMPs) and mullerian-inhibiting substances. Activin βA and TGF-β1 share functions in inflammatory reactions, including tissue repair and suppression [3,4]. They also share Smad2/3 and Smad4 as intracellular signaling targets of their receptors [5]. The overlap in function and signal transduction is also observed for the target genes induced by TGF-β and activin βA (Fig. 1), whereas BMP-1 differentially induces genes in osteoblasts [6]. Activin A has structural and functional homologies to TGF-β. Activin A itself is a homodimer of two βA subgroups, whereas activin AB consists of one βA and one βB subgroup [7]. A naturally occurring antagonist, inhibin α, also consists of one βA subunits, but differs in the additional inhibin α subgroup. Activin A is known to have a wide spectrum of functions, such as inducing apoptosis in several cell types, regulation of growth and development, and regulation of hemopoiesis [7]. Moreover, activin A has a promoting effect on proliferation and differentiation of human lung fibroblasts and on human airway smooth muscle cells, and therefore is considered as a critical cytokine in asthma [8–10]. Furthermore, human mast cells are potent sources of activin A in human asthma [8]. Whether activin βA also overlaps with TGF-β with respect to the induction of regulatory responses is unclear.

TGF-β and activin βAs in differentiation and suppression

The TGF-β superfamily members are involved in multiple cellular differentiation processes of embryogenesis and in the homeostasis of the mature organism. Activin βA and TGF-β are involved in the regulation of erythropoiesis [11,12] and mast cell differentiation and growth [13]. TGF-β controls growth of tissues such as epithelial cells, and fluid transport of epithelial barriers [14,15]. Activin stimulates proliferation of cells of various origins, including lung fibroblasts, keratinocytes, porcine thyroid cells, osteoblasts, and spermatogonial cells [4,16]. TGF-β was believed to be essential for the switch from IgM to IgA production [13]; however, recent data show that although reduced, IgA-secreting cells and IgA were still present in the systemic and mucosal compartments of mice that were engineered to lack the type II TGF-β receptor (TGF-βRII) in B cells. A significant reduction in antigen (Ag)-specific IgG2b and increased levels of IgG3 were observed in sera from these mice. Furthermore, Ag-specific IgA-secreting cells, serum IgA, and secretory IgA were undetectable in these mice, underlining that other factors such as IL-5 and IL-6 may be sufficient to switch IgA and that TGF-β is crucial for Ag-specific IgA responses [17]. TGF-β directly inhibits T-cell proliferation [18] and regulates lymphocyte homeostasis though preventing subsequent apoptosis of anergized cells [19,20].

The suppressive function of TGF-β in the control of peripheral tolerance is shown in transgenic animals that lack the TGF-βRII chain only on T cells, because these animals develop severe autoimmune diseases and uncontrolled T-cell differentiation [21–25]. The human CD25$^+$ subset of Tregs has been shown to express TGF-β [26], and current evidence suggests that TGF-β contributes to the reinduction of peripheral tolerance to allergens during allergen-specific immunotherapy [27–29]. Glucocorticoid treatment induces Tregs in vitro, increases IL-10 and FOXP3 expression in patients treated with inhaled or systemic glucocorticoids, and rescues TGF-β expression that is otherwise lower in patients who have untreated asthma compared with healthy individuals [17]. These data may indicate that TGF-β directly suppresses Teffs, but this concept conflicts with the observation that TGF-β is a soluble cytokine whereas T-cell suppression is a contact-dependent process. Treg suppression is independent of Smad3 and TGF-βRII because CD25$^+$ T cells of animals lacking these molecules still suppress their target cells [30,31]. In this context, one must consider that TGF-β is very hydrophobic and may therefore act in a surface-bound manner [32], and that TGF-β triggers multiple pathways that are Smad3-independent and differentially suppress T-cell activity [33].

Ag-specific activation, and probably also suppression, includes the generation of close cell contacts, creating an organized space with Ag-presenting cells and possibly with Tregs, providing a restricted space so that secreted cytokines such as IL-10 and TGF-β are focused on the target cell, as has been shown for interferon gamma [34]. We have recently shown that TGF-β receptors, specifically endoglin (CD105), are regulated through their expression on the cell surface. CD105 is a member of the TGF-β receptor family that plays an accessory role in the binding of TGF-β1 and -β3 to the receptor complex [35,36], but also binds activin-βA [36]. It is predominantly expressed on endothelial cells [35] but is also detected on various other hematopoietic cells [37–39], monocytes [40], and B-lineage cells [39,41,42]. Endoglin is a 95 kDa heavily glycosylated molecule that is present on the cell surface as covalently linked homodimers [43–45]. Mutations in the CD105 gene lead to hereditary hemorrhagic telangiectasia type 1, an autosomal dominant disorder associated with frequent nose bleeds and arteriovenous malformations [46–50]. Overexpression of CD105 was shown to inhibit several effects that are normally induced by TGF-β, such as downregulation of c-myc, stimulation of fibronectin synthesis, and cellular adhesion in a monocytic line [51]. Antisense oligonucleotides targeted at CD105 enhanced the suppressive activity of TGF-β in endothelial cells [52] but inhibited the TGF-β action in placental trophoblasts [53]. Thus, CD105 represents an accessory receptor that can negatively and positively modulate TGF-β responsiveness. CD105 is expressed on the surface by activated CD4$^+$ T cells and is actively regulated after T-cell receptor (TCR) engagement through post-translational means. Furthermore, CD105 acts as a regulatory receptor, counteracting TGF-β–mediated suppression [54]. It is also expressed on the surface of CD25$^+$ T cells. These data show that recognition of TGF-β is not a constitutive factor but is controlled by additional factors.

CD25$^+$ T cells of TGF-β–deficient mice can suppress CD25$^-$ cells in vitro, but do not protect recipient mice from colitis in the severe combined immuno deficiency (SCID) transfer model in vivo [55]. This observation can also mean that TGF-β is of secondary relevance for the actual suppression of Teffs and is more important for the expansion of Tregs through induction of Treg differentiation, as multiple and independent studies have suggested [56–60]. We hypothesized earlier that the ability of TGF-β to inhibit Th1 and Th2 differentiation through blocking T-BET or GATA-3 [24,61,62] may be of particular importance for Treg induction [1]. The lack of Th1 and Th2 decision signals during T-cell differentiation promotes the generation of Tregs [32] and is consistent with the fact that T-cell tolerance is only induced in the absence of danger signals in vivo [63]. Although TGF-β inhibits T-BET and GATA-3, it induces the expression of FOXP3, which is a transcription factor that promotes the generation of T cells with regulatory phenotype [56,64,65]. In fact, neutralization of IL-4 and IL-12 was found to be important in allowing FOXP3 mRNA expression [66]. We therefore hypothesize that the generation of Tregs represents a default pathway, requiring TCR activation as for any other T-cell differentiation, but in the absence of decision signals for Teffs. This model allows integration of several observations: (1) TGF-β induces FOXP3 mRNA and protein but not FOPX3-promoter constructs (unpublished results), (2) Tregs isolated from cord blood, characterized by a more uncommitted phenotype, show a more dramatic suppressive function than do Tregs from adult donors [67], (3) Tregs have been shown to be induced through engagement of TCRs in SCID transfer models, and (4) inhibitory receptors such as CD46 [68], CD200R [69], and CTLA-4 [70], and other inhibitory receptors [71] also convey an OFF signal that may guide activity away from Teff differentiation toward Treg induction.

The Treg-promoting capability of TGF-β is also supported by the ability of TGF-β to generate dendritic cells (DC) that promote tolerance in a major histocompatibility complex II–dependent way, as shown in an adoptive transfer model [72]. Specifically, immature DCs reportedly promote the generation of Tregs, and TGF-β prevents the maturation of DCs by keeping the expression of costimulatory molecules low [73,74].

TGF-β and activin βA in tissue remodeling

TGF-β and its close family member activin βA are known to induce expression of collagen and other extracellular matrix components [75–77]. Researchers have hypothesized that TGF-β requires an autocrine activin βA loop for effective collagen expression [78]. The deposition of matrix is required for tissue repair, but inflammatory responses represent a major complication in life-threatening conditions, particularly asthma and nephritis where the thickened basal membranes diminish gas or ion exchange. Myofibroblasts, which occur in areas of fibrosis and express the smooth muscle isoform α-actin (SMA) that is normally expressed constitutively only in smooth muscle cells, play a key role in this process. These cells represent a subpopulation of specialized fibroblasts that differentiate into this phenotype after induction by TGF-β or activin βA [78–80]. Follistatin, a naturally occurring antagonist of activin βA, was shown to inhibit not only activin βA–induced SMA expression but also TGF-β–induced SMA expression, whereas the activin βA–induced SMA expression was still intact in cells lacking the TGF-βRII [78]. Thus, TGF-β and activin βA act in concert to mediate cellular responses. We have shown that activin βA and TGF-β are in fact interdependent; TGF-β can induce activin βA and vice versa. However, in contrast to TGF-β, we show that activin βA is expressed in acute, immediate responses induced by allergens [81]. Thus, activin βA is an inflammatory cytokine produced by T cells and other sources, which may feed into the regulatory and chronic responses dominated by TGF-β.

The importance of T cells in fibrotic responses is also documented by the fact that antiparasitic reactions of the Th2 phenotype promote the fibrosing "walling-off" reaction. Among the Th2 cytokines, IL-13 seems to be an important factor in promoting fibrosis because transgene pulmonary overexpression of IL-13 results in airway and parenchymal fibrosis of the lung [82]. This effect of IL-13 was shown to be TGF-β–dependent because IL-13–induced fibrosis could be ameliorated using anti–TGF-β antagonists (soluble TGF-βR-Fc; [83]). In addition, IL-13 was shown to augment TGF-β–induced expression of tissue inhibitor of metalloproteinase (TIMP)-1 in fibroblasts [84]. Recent data show that IL-13 synergizes with IL-11 in allergic inflammation, fibrosis, hyaluronic acid accumulation, myofibroblast accumulation, alveolar remodeling, mucus metaplasia, and respiratory failure [85]. In addition to cytokine secretion, fibroblast–T cell contact seems to be relevant because engagement of the CD40 ligand (CD154) stimulates fibroblasts in synergy with IL-4/IL-13 [86,87]. Thus the potential role of T cells in matrix expression induction may be dependent on not only the production of TGF-β and activin βA but also the concomitant expression of interleukins such as IL-4, IL-13, IL-11, and IL-17 [88], and cell–cell contact, which lead to a persistent expression of matrix and, consequently airway remodeling.

TGF-β and activin βA good or bad for allergy?

The functions of TGF-β and activin βA are enormous and are reported in 1108 publications. However, they can be grouped under a homeostatic function, which covers the immunologic and tissue functions of these genes. Considering these systems, TGF-β seems to act in concert with other signals (Fig. 2): (1) Treg induction interacts with TCR, GATA-3, and T-bet signals, (2) B cells require B-cell–receptor engagement, and (3) fibroblasts and myofibroblasts develop pathogenicity through integration with signals, such as IL-13, IL-11, IL-17 [89], IL-22 [90,91], and TNF-α [92]. On the other hand, increasing evidence shows that mechanisms exist that keep remodeling under control (eg, expression of BMP-7 and Id2 [93] or IL-10 [94]). IL-10, which is also an effector cytokine for immune regulatory mechanisms, seems to play a key role in balanced remodeling. This balanced remodeling has been shown to be controlled by mechanical stress in osteoblasts [94]. Studies have shown the very interactive nature of TGF-β, which is also reflected by its very interactive and complex intracellular

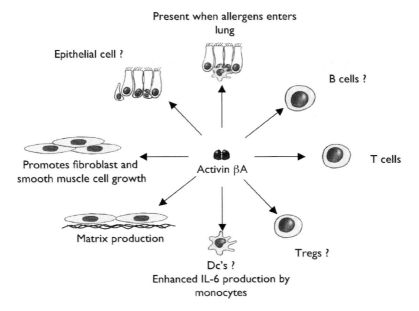

Present when allergens enters
lung

Epithelial cell ?

B cells ?

Promotes fibroblast and
smooth muscle cell growth

Activin βA

T cells

Matrix production

Dc's ?
Enhanced IL-6 production by
monocytes

Tregs ?

Fig. 2. Activin βA (AβA) induces TGF-β and also directly triggers similar signaling cascades.

signaling cascade [1]. Taken together, the pathogenicity of TGF-β seems to be mediated by accompanying factors, so whether TGF-β is good or bad for asthma cannot be determined without considering the context of TGF-β's environment.

Summary

The function of TGF-β was investigated under the focus of either tissue remodeling or immune regulation. TGF-β is currently considered a "recover" signal, comprising repair and regulation. As for the immune regulatory role of TGF-β, increasing evidence has shown that its remodeling capacity is controlled by additional signals that enhance or limit repair responses. These mechanisms may open new windows of therapeutic interventions and may allow selective control of airway remodeling components.

References

[1] Schmidt-Weber CB, Blaser K. Regulation and role of transforming growth factor-beta in immune tolerance induction and inflammation. Curr Opin Immunol 2004;16(6):709–16.
[2] Schmidt-Weber CB, Blaser K. The role of the FOXP3 transcription factor in the immune regulation of allergic asthma. Curr Allergy Asthma Rep 2005;5(5):356–61.

[3] Rosendahl A, Checchin D, Fehniger TE, et al. Activation of the TGF-beta/activin-Smad2 pathway during allergic airway inflammation. Am J Respir Cell Mol Biol 2001;25(1):60–8.

[4] Munz B, Hubner G, Tretter Y, et al. A novel role of activin in inflammation and repair. J Endocrinol 1999;161(2):187–93.

[5] Mak JC, Ho SP, Leung RY, et al. Elevated levels of transforming growth factor-beta(1) in serum of patients with stable bronchiectasis. Respir Med 2005;99(10):1223–8.

[6] de Jong DS, van Zoelen EJ, Bauerschmidt S, et al. Microarray analysis of bone morphogenetic protein, transforming growth factor beta, and activin early response genes during osteoblastic cell differentiation. J Bone Miner Res 2002;17(12):2119–29.

[7] Pangas SA, Woodruff TK. Activin signal transduction pathways. Trends Endocrinol Metab 2000;11(8):309–14.

[8] Cho SH, Yao Z, Wang SW, et al. Regulation of activin A expression in mast cells and asthma: its effect on the proliferation of human airway smooth muscle cells. J Immunol 2003;170(8):4045–52.

[9] Ohga E, Matsuse T, Teramoto S, et al. Effects of activin A on proliferation and differentiation of human lung fibroblasts. Biochem Biophys Res Commun 1996;228(2):391–6.

[10] Ohga E, Matsuse T, Teramoto S, et al. Activin receptors are expressed on human lung fibroblast and activin A facilitates fibroblast-mediated collagen gel contraction. Life Sci 2000;66(17):1603–13.

[11] Bohmer RM. IL-3-dependent early erythropoiesis is stimulated by autocrine transforming growth factor beta. Stem Cells 2004;22(2):216–24.

[12] Shiozaki M, Kosaka M, Eto Y. Activin A: a commitment factor in erythroid differentiation. Biochem Biophys Res Commun 1998;242(3):631–5.

[13] Funaba M, Ikeda T, Murakami M, et al. Transcriptional activation of mouse mast cell protease-7 by activin and transforming growth factor-beta is inhibited by microphthalmia-associated transcription factor. J Biol Chem 2003;278(52):52032–41.

[14] Clerici C, Matthay MA. Transforming growth factor-beta 1 regulates lung epithelial barrier function and fluid transport. Am J Physiol Lung Cell Mol Physiol 2003;285(6):L1190–1.

[15] Fjellbirkeland L, Cambier S, Broaddus VC, et al. Integrin alphavbeta8-mediated activation of transforming growth factor-beta inhibits human airway epithelial proliferation in intact bronchial tissue. Am J Pathol 2003;163(2):533–42.

[16] Ying SY, Zhang Z, Furst B, et al. Activins and activin receptors in cell growth. Proc Soc Exp Biol Med 1997;214(2):114–22.

[17] Borsutzky S, Cazac BB, Roes J, et al. TGF-beta receptor signaling is critical for mucosal IgA responses. J Immunol 2004;173(5):3305–9.

[18] Kunzmann S, Mantel PY, Wohlfahrt JG, et al. Histamine enhances TGF-beta mediated suppression of Th2 responses. FASEB J 2003;17(9):1089–95.

[19] Bommireddy R, Saxena V, Ormsby I, et al. TGF-beta 1 regulates lymphocyte homeostasis by preventing activation and subsequent apoptosis of peripheral lymphocytes. J Immunol 2003;170(9):4612–22.

[20] Schmidt-Weber CB, Blaser K. T-cell tolerance in allergic response. Allergy 2002;57(9):762–8.

[21] Gojova A, Brun V, Esposito B, et al. Specific abrogation of transforming growth factor-beta signaling in T cells alters atherosclerotic lesion size and composition in mice. Blood 2003;102(12):4052–8.

[22] Robertson AK, Rudling M, Zhou X, et al. Disruption of TGF-beta signaling in T cells accelerates atherosclerosis. J Clin Invest 2003;112(9):1342–50.

[23] Schramm C, Protschka M, Kohler HH, et al. Impairment of TGF-beta signaling in T cells increases susceptibility to experimental autoimmune hepatitis in mice. Am J Physiol Gastrointest Liver Physiol 2003;284(3):G525–35.

[24] Gorelik L, Fields PE, Flavell RA. Cutting edge: TGF-beta inhibits Th type 2 development through inhibition of GATA-3 expression. J Immunol 2000;165(9):4773–7.

[25] Gorelik L, Flavell RA. Immune-mediated eradication of tumors through the blockade of transforming growth factor-beta signaling in T cells. Nat Med 2001;7(10):1118–22.

[26] Levings MK, Sangregorio R, Sartirana C, et al. Human CD25(+)CD4(+) T suppressor cell clones

produce transforming growth factor beta, but not interleukin 10, and are distinct from type 1 T regulatory cells. J Exp Med 2002;196(10):1335–46.

[27] Jutel M, Akdis M, Budak F, et al. IL-10 and TGF-b cooperate in inducing peripheral T cell tolerance during specific immunotherapy with inhalant allergens and during natural allergen exposure. J Allergy Clin Immunol 2001;107(2):S90.

[28] Jutel M, Akdis M, Budak F, et al. IL-10 and TGF-beta cooperate in the regulatory T cell response to mucosal allergens in normal immunity and specific immunotherapy. Eur J Immunol 2003; 33(5):1205–14.

[29] Schmidt-Weber CB, Blaser K. Immunological mechanisms in specific immunotherapy. Springer Semin Immunopathol 2004;25(3–4):377–90.

[30] Piccirillo CA, Letterio JJ, Thornton AM, et al. CD4(+)CD25(+) regulatory T cells can mediate suppressor function in the absence of transforming growth factor beta1 production and responsiveness. J Exp Med 2002;196(2):237–46.

[31] Shevach EM. CD4 + CD25 + suppressor T cells: more questions than answers. Nat Rev Immunol 2002;2(6):389–400.

[32] Nakamura K, Kitani A, Strober W. Cell contact-dependent immunosuppression by CD4(+)CD25(+) regulatory T cells is mediated by cell surface-bound transforming growth factor beta. J Exp Med 2001;194(5):629–44.

[33] McKarns SC, Schwartz RH, Kaminski NE. Smad3 Is essential for TGF-beta1 to suppress IL-2 production and TCR-induced proliferation, but not IL-2-induced proliferation. J Immunol 2004; 172(7):4275–84.

[34] Maldonado RA, Irvine DJ, Schreiber R, et al. A role for the immunological synapse in lineage commitment of CD4 lymphocytes. Nature 2004;431(7008):527–32.

[35] Cheifetz S, Bellon T, Cales C, et al. Endoglin is a component of the transforming growth factor-beta receptor system in human endothelial cells. J Biol Chem 1992;267(27):19027–30.

[36] Barbara NP, Wrana JL, Letarte M. Endoglin is an accessory protein that interacts with the signaling receptor complex of multiple members of the transforming growth factor- beta super-family. J Biol Chem 1999;274(2):584–94.

[37] Quackenbush EJ, Letarte M. Identification of several cell surface proteins of non-T, non-B acute lymphoblastic leukemia by using monoclonal antibodies. J Immunol 1985;134(2):1276–85.

[38] Buhring HJ, Muller CA, Letarte M, et al. Endoglin is expressed on a subpopulation of immature erythroid cells of normal human bone marrow. Leukemia 1991;5(10):841–7.

[39] Rokhlin OW, Cohen MB, Kubagawa H, et al. Differential expression of endoglin on fetal and adult hematopoietic cells in human bone marrow. J Immunol 1995;154(9):4456–65.

[40] Lastres P, Bellon T, Cabanas C, et al. Regulated expression on human macrophages of endoglin, an Arg-Gly-Asp- containing surface antigen. Eur J Immunol 1992;22(2):393–7.

[41] Zhang H, Shaw AR, Mak A, et al. Endoglin is a component of the transforming growth factor (TGF)-beta receptor complex of human pre-B leukemic cells. J Immunol 1996;156(2):564–73.

[42] Dagdeviren A, Muftuoglu SF, Cakar AN, et al. Endoglin (CD 105) expression in human lymphoid organs and placenta. Ann Anat 1998;180(5):461–9.

[43] Gougos A, Letarte M. Primary structure of endoglin, an RGD-containing glycoprotein of human endothelial cells. J Biol Chem 1990;265(15):8361–4.

[44] Gougos A, Letarte M. Biochemical characterization of the 44G4 antigen from the HOON pre-B leukemic cell line. J Immunol 1988;141(6):1934–40.

[45] Altomonte M, Montagner R, Fonsatti E, et al. Expression and structural features of endoglin (CD105), a transforming growth factor beta1 and beta3 binding protein, in human melanoma. Br J Cancer 1996;74(10):1586–91.

[46] McAllister KA, Grogg KM, Johnson DW, et al. Endoglin, a TGF-beta binding protein of endothelial cells, is the gene for hereditary haemorrhagic telangiectasia type 1. Nat Genet 1994;8(4):345–51.

[47] Pece N, Vera S, Cymerman U, et al. Mutant endoglin in hereditary hemorrhagic telangiectasia type 1 is transiently expressed intracellularly and is not a dominant negative. J Clin Invest 1997; 100(10):2568–79.

[48] Shovlin CL, Letarte M. Hereditary haemorrhagic telangiectasia and pulmonary arteriovenous

malformations: issues in clinical management and review of pathogenic mechanisms. Thorax 1999;54(8):714–29.

[49] Pece-Barbara N, Cymerman U, Vera S, et al. Expression analysis of four endoglin missense mutations suggests that haploinsufficiency is the predominant mechanism for hereditary hemorrhagic telangiectasia type 1. Hum Mol Genet 1999;8(12):2171–81.

[50] Cymerman U, Vera S, Pece-Barbara N, et al. Identification of hereditary hemorrhagic telangiectasia type 1 in newborns by protein expression and mutation analysis of endoglin. Pediatr Res 2000;47(1):24–35.

[51] Lastres P, Letamendia A, Zhang H, et al. Endoglin modulates cellular responses to TGF-beta 1. J Cell Biol 1996;133(5):1109–21.

[52] Li C, Hampson IN, Hampson L, et al. CD105 antagonizes the inhibitory signaling of transforming growth factor beta1 on human vascular endothelial cells. FASEB J 2000;14(1):55–64.

[53] Caniggia I, Taylor CV, Ritchie JW, et al. Endoglin regulates trophoblast differentiation along the invasive pathway in human placental villous explants. Endocrinology 1997;138(11):4977–88.

[54] Schmidt-Weber CB, Letarte M, Kunzmann S, et al. TGF-{beta} signaling of human T cells is modulated by the ancillary TGF-{beta} receptor endoglin. Int Immunol 2005;17(7):921–30.

[55] Nakamura K, Kitani A, Fuss I, et al. TGF-beta 1 plays an important role in the mechanism of CD4 + CD25 + regulatory T cell activity in both humans and mice. J Immunol 2004;172(2): 834–42.

[56] Fantini MC, Becker C, Monteleone G, et al. Cutting edge: TGF-beta induces a regulatory phenotype in CD4 + CD25- T cells through Foxp3 induction and down-regulation of Smad7. J Immunol 2004;172(9):5149–53.

[57] Fu S, Zhang N, Yopp AC, et al. TGF-beta induces Foxp3 + T-regulatory cells from CD4 + CD25 - precursors. Am J Transplant 2004;4(10):1614–27.

[58] Huber S, Schramm C, Lehr HA, et al. Cutting edge: TGF-beta signaling is required for the in vivo expansion and immunosuppressive capacity of regulatory CD4 + CD25 + T cells. J Immunol 2004;173(11):6526–31.

[59] Jonuleit H, Schmitt E, Kakirman H, et al. Infectious tolerance: human CD25(+) regulatory T cells convey suppressor activity to conventional CD4(+) T helper cells. J Exp Med 2002;196(2):255–60.

[60] Verhasselt V, Vosters O, Beuneu C, et al. Induction of FOXP3-expressing regulatory CD4pos T cells by human mature autologous dendritic cells. Eur J Immunol 2004;34(3):762–72.

[61] Gorelik L, Constant S, Flavell RA. Mechanism of transforming growth factor beta-induced inhibition of T helper type 1 differentiation. J Exp Med 2002;195(11):1499–505.

[62] Chen CH, Seguin-Devaux C, Burke NA, et al. Transforming growth factor beta blocks Tec kinase phosphorylation, Ca2 + influx, and NFATc translocation causing inhibition of T cell differentiation. J Exp Med 2003;197(12):1689–99.

[63] Chen TC, Cobbold SP, Fairchild PJ, et al. Generation of anergic and regulatory T cells following prolonged exposure to a harmless antigen. J Immunol 2004;172(10):5900–7.

[64] Chen W, Jin W, Hardegen N, et al. Conversion of peripheral CD4 + CD25- naive T cells to CD4 + CD25 + regulatory T cells by TGF-beta induction of transcription factor Foxp3. J Exp Med 2003;198(12):1875–86.

[65] Peng Y, Laouar Y, Li MO, et al. TGF-beta regulates in vivo expansion of Foxp3-expressing CD4 + CD25 + regulatory T cells responsible for protection against diabetes. Proc Natl Acad Sci USA 2004;101(13):4572–7.

[66] Karagiannidis C, Akdis M, Holopainen P, et al. Glucocorticoids upregulate FOXP3 expression and regulatory T cells in asthma. J Allergy Clin Immunol 2004;114(6):1425–33.

[67] Godfrey WR, Spoden DJ, Ge YG, et al. Cord blood CD4(+)CD25(+)-derived T regulatory cell lines express FoxP3 protein and manifest potent suppressor function. Blood 2005;105(2):750–8.

[68] Kemper C, Chan AC, Green JM, et al. Activation of human CD4 + cells with CD3 and CD46 induces a T-regulatory cell 1 phenotype. Nature 2003;421(6921):388–92.

[69] Gorczynski RM, Lee L, Boudakov I. Augmented induction of CD4 + CD25 + Treg using monoclonal antibodies to CD200R. Transplantation 2005;79(4):488–91.

[70] Vasu C, Prabhakar BS, Holterman MJ. Targeted CTLA-4 engagement induces CD4 + CD25 +

CTLA-4high T regulatory cells with target (allo)antigen specificity. J Immunol 2004;173(4): 2866–76.

[71] Sinclair NR. Why so many coinhibitory receptors? Scand J Immunol 1999;50(1):10–3.

[72] Alard P, Clark SL, Kosiewicz MM. Deletion, but not anergy, is involved in TGF-beta-treated antigen-presenting cell-induced tolerance. Int Immunol 2003;15(8):945–53.

[73] Geissmann F, Revy P, Regnault A, et al. TGF-beta 1 prevents the noncognate maturation of human dendritic Langerhans cells. J Immunol 1999;162(8):4567–75.

[74] Roncarolo MG, Levings MK, Traversari C. Differentiation of T regulatory cells by immature dendritic cells. J Exp Med 2001;193(2):F5–9.

[75] Sugiyama M, Ichida T, Sato T, et al. Expression of activin A is increased in cirrhotic and fibrotic rat livers. Gastroenterology 1998;114(3):550–8.

[76] Kissin EY, Lemaire R, Korn JH, et al. Transforming growth factor beta induces fibroblast fibrillin-1 matrix formation. Arthritis Rheum 2002;46(11):3000–9.

[77] Jinnin M, Ihn H, Asano Y, et al. Tenascin-C upregulation by transforming growth factor-beta in human dermal fibroblasts involves Smad3, Sp1, and Ets1. Oncogene 2004;23(9):1656–67.

[78] Wada W, Kuwano H, Hasegawa Y, et al. The dependence of transforming growth factor-beta-induced collagen production on autocrine factor activin A in hepatic stellate cells. Endocrinology 2004;145(6):2753–9.

[79] Evans RA, Tian YC, Steadman R, et al. TGF-beta1-mediated fibroblast-myofibroblast terminal differentiation-the role of Smad proteins. Exp Cell Res 2003;282(2):90–100.

[80] Malmstrom J, Lindberg H, Lindberg C, et al. Transforming growth factor-beta 1 specifically induce proteins involved in the myofibroblast contractile apparatus. Mol Cell Proteomics 2004; 3(5):466–77.

[81] Karagiannidis C, Hense G, Martin C, et al. Activin A is an acute allergen-responsive cytokine and provides a link to TGF-beta-mediated airway remodeling in asthma. J Allergy Clin Immunol 2006;117(1):111–8.

[82] Zhu Z, Homer RJ, Wang Z, et al. Pulmonary expression of interleukin-13 causes inflammation, mucus hypersecretion, subepithelial fibrosis, physiologic abnormalities, and eotaxin production. J Clin Invest 1999;103(6):779–88.

[83] Lee CG, Homer RJ, Zhu Z, et al. Interleukin-13 induces tissue fibrosis by selectively stimulating and activating transforming growth factor beta(1). J Exp Med 2001;194(6):809–21.

[84] Zhou X, Trudeau JB, Schoonover KJ, et al. Interleukin-13 augments transforming growth factor-beta1-induced tissue inhibitor of metalloproteinase-1 expression in primary human airway fibroblasts. Am J Physiol Cell Physiol 2005;288(2):C435–42.

[85] Chen Q, Rabach L, Noble P, et al. IL-11 receptor alpha in the pathogenesis of IL-13-induced inflammation and remodeling. J Immunol 2005;174(4):2305–13.

[86] Atamas SP, Luzina IG, Dai H, et al. Synergy between CD40 ligation and IL-4 on fibroblast proliferation involves IL-4 receptor signaling. J Immunol 2002;168(3):1139–45.

[87] Kaufman J, Sime PJ, Phipps RP. Expression of CD154 (CD40 ligand) by human lung fibroblasts: differential regulation by IFN-gamma and IL-13, and implications for fibrosis. J Immunol 2004; 172(3):1862–71.

[88] Batra V, Musani AI, Hastie AT, et al. Bronchoalveolar lavage fluid concentrations of trans-forming growth factor (TGF)-beta1, TGF-beta2, interleukin (IL)-4 and IL-13 after segmental allergen challenge and their effects on alpha-smooth muscle actin and collagen III synthesis by primary human lung fibroblasts. Clin Exp Allergy 2004;34(3):437–44.

[89] Chakir J, Shannon J, Molet S, et al. Airway remodeling-associated mediators in moderate to severe asthma: effect of steroids on TGF-beta, IL-11, IL-17, and type I and type III collagen expression. J Allergy Clin Immunol 2003;111(6):1293–8.

[90] Andoh A, Zhang Z, Inatomi O, et al. Interleukin-22, a member of the IL-10 subfamily, induces inflammatory responses in colonic subepithelial myofibroblasts. Gastroenterology 2005;129(3): 969–84.

[91] Boniface K, Bernard FX, Garcia M, et al. IL-22 inhibits epidermal differentiation and induces proinflammatory gene expression and migration of human keratinocytes. J Immunol 2005; 174(6):3695–702.

[92] Theiss AL, Simmons JG, Jobin C, et al. Tumor necrosis factor alpha increases collagen accumulation and proliferation in intestinal myofibroblasts via TNF receptor 2. J Biol Chem 2005;280(43):36099–109.

[93] Izumi N, Mizuguchi S, Inagaki Y, et al. BMP-7 opposes TGF {beta}1-mediated collagen induction in mouse pulmonary myofibroblasts through Id2. Am J Physiol Lung Cell Mol Physiol 2006;290(1):L120–6.

[94] Yamamoto T, Eckes B, Krieg T. Effect of interleukin-10 on the gene expression of type I collagen, fibronectin, and decorin in human skin fibroblasts: differential regulation by transforming growth factor-beta and monocyte chemoattractant protein-1. Biochem Biophys Res Commun 2001;281(1):200–5.

ELSEVIER
SAUNDERS

Immunol Allergy Clin N Am
26 (2006) 245–259

IMMUNOLOGY
AND ALLERGY
CLINICS
OF NORTH AMERICA

Histamine Receptors in Immune Regulation and Allergen-Specific Immunotherapy

Marek Jutel, MD, PhD[a,b,*], Kurt Blaser, PhD[b],
Cezmi A. Akdis, MD, PhD[b]

[a]Department of Internal Medicine and Allergy, Wroclaw Medical University, Traugutta 57,
Wroclaw 50-417, Poland
[b]Swiss Institute of Allergy and Asthma Research (SIAF), Obere Strasse 22,
CH-7270 Davos, Switzerland

Histamine (2-[4-imidazole]-ethylamine) is a low-molecular-weight amine synthesized from L-histidine exclusively by histidine decarboxylase (HDC). It is produced by various cells throughout the body, including central nervous system neurons, gastric mucosa parietal cells, mast cells, basophils, and lymphocytes [1,2]. Since its discovery as a uterine stimulant more than 100 years ago, it has become one of the most intensely studied molecules in medicine. The name *histamine* was given after the Greek word for tissue, *histos,* when it was isolated first from liver and lung tissue and than from several other sites. Its smooth muscle stimulating and vasodepressor actions were demonstrated in the first experiments by Dale and Laidlaw [3], who found that the effects of histamine mimicked those occurring during anaphylaxis.

Histamine is involved in the regulation of many physiologic functions, including cell proliferation and differentiation, hematopoiesis, embryonic development, regeneration, and wound healing [2–6]. Within the central nervous system, it affects cognition and memory, the regulation of the cycle of sleeping and waking, and energy and endocrine homeostasis [4]. In human pathology, histamine triggers acute symptoms owing to its rapid activity on vascular endothelium and bronchial and smooth muscle cells, leading to the development of symptoms

The authors' laboratories are supported by Swiss National Foundation grants and Polish National Science Committee grant 1387/PO5/2000/19.

* Corresponding author. Department of Internal Medicine and Allergy, Wroclaw Medical University, Traugutta 57, Wroclaw 50-417, Poland.

E-mail address: mjutel@ak.am.wroc.pl (M. Jutel).

such as acute rhinitis, bronchospasm, cramping, diarrhea, or cutaneous wheal and flare responses. In addition to these effects on the immediate-type response, histamine significantly regulates the immune response and several chronic phase inflammatory events [1,2]. Consequently, the antihistamines should be viewed as systemic antiallergic agents and immune regulators. This article highlights the relevance of these findings for possible application of histamine signal in tolerance induction during therapeutic modalities such as allergen-specific immunotherapy (SIT).

Histamine receptors

The pleiotropic effects of histamine are triggered by activating on one or several histamine membrane receptors on different cells. Four subtypes of receptors (histamine receptor [HR] 1, HR2, HR3, and HR4) have been described (Table 1). All of these receptors belong to the G protein–coupled receptor family. They are heptahelical transmembrane molecules that transduce extracellular signal by using G proteins and intracellular second messenger systems [1,2]. The active and inactive states of HRs exist in equilibrium; however, it has been shown in recombinant systems that HRs can trigger downstream events in the absence of receptor occupancy by an agonist, which accounts for constitutive spontaneous receptor activity [5].

Histamine receptor agonists stimulate the active state in the receptor and inverse agonists, the inactive one. An agonist with a preferential affinity for the active state of the receptor stabilizes the receptor in its active conformation, lead-

Table 1
Histamine receptors, expression, coupled G proteins, and activated intracellular signals

Histamine receptors	Expression	Activated intracellular signals	G proteins
HR1	Nerve cells, airway and vascular smooth muscles, hepatocytes, chondrocytes, endothelial cells, epithelial cells, neutrophils, eosinophils, monocytes, dendritic cells, T and B cells	Ca^{++}, cGMP, phospholipase D, phospholipase A_2, NFκB	$G_{q/11}$
HR2	Nerve cells, airway and vascular smooth muscles, hepatocytes, chondrocytes, endothelial cells, epithelial cells, neutrophils, eosinophils, monocytes, dendritic cells, T and B cells	Adenylate cyclase, cAMP, c-Fos, c-Jun, PKC, p70S6K	$G\alpha_s$
HR3	Histaminergic neurons, eosinophils, dendritic cells, monocytes, low expression in peripheral tissues	Enhanced Ca^{++}, MAP kinase Inhibition of cAMP	$G_{i/o}$
HR4	High expression on bone marrow and peripheral hematopoietic cells, eosinophils, neutrophils, dendritic cells, T cells, basophils, mast cells; low expression in nerve cells, hepatocytes, peripheral tissues, spleen, thymus, lung, small intestine, colon and heart	Enhanced Ca^{+2}, Inhibition of cAMP	$G_{i/o}$

ing to continuous activation signal. An inverse agonist with a preferential affinity for the inactive state stabilizes the receptor in this conformation and consequently induces an inactive state, which is characterized by blocked signal transduction via the histamine receptor [5]. In reporter gene assays, constitutive HR1-mediated nuclear factor (NF)-κB activation has been shown to be inhibited by many of the clinically used H1 antihistamines, indicating that these agents are inverse HR1 agonists [5]. Constitutive activity has now been shown for all four histamine receptors [5].

Specific activation or blockade of histamine receptors showed that they differed in expression, signal transduction, or function and improved understanding of the role of histamine in physiology and disease mechanisms. Most positive effects of histamine are mediated by HR1, whereas HR2 is mostly involved in suppressive activities. The human $G_{q/11}$-coupled HR1 is encoded by a single exon gene located on the distal short arm of chromosome 3p25b and contains 487 amino acids. The HR1 is expressed in numerous cells, including airway and vascular smooth muscle cells, hepatocytes, chondrocytes, nerve cells, endothelial cells, dendritic cells, monocytes, neutrophils, and T and B cells [1,2]. Histamine binds to transmembrane domains 3 and 5. Activation of the HR1-coupled $G_{q/11}$ stimulates the inositol phospholipid signaling pathways, resulting in formation of inositol-1,4,5-triphosphate (IP_3) and diacylglycerol and an increase in intracellular calcium [6]. The rise in intracellular calcium accounts for nitric oxide production, liberation of arachidonic acid from phospholipids, and increased cyclic AMP (cAMP). The HR1 also activates phospholipase D and phospholipase A_2 and the transcription factor NF-κB through $G_{q/11}$ and $G_{\beta\gamma}$ upon agonist binding. Constitutive activation of NF-κB occurs only through $G_{\beta\gamma}$ [6]. The HR1 is responsible for the development of many symptoms of allergic disease. Targeted disruption of the H1-receptor gene in mice results in impairment of neurologic functions, such as memory, learning, locomotion, and nocioperception, and aggressive behavior. Immunologic abnormalities have also been described in HR1-deleted mice, with impairment of T- and B-cell responses [7]. Activation of HR1 is responsible for many symptoms of allergic disease.

In humans, the intronless gene encoding HR2 is located on chromosome 5. The human HR2 is a protein of 359 amino acids coupled to adenylate cyclase and phosphoinositide second messenger systems by separate GTP-dependent mechanisms including $G\alpha_s$ and induces activation of c-Fos, c-Jun, PKC, and p70S6 kinase [8]. Studies in different species and several human cells have demonstrated that inhibition of characteristic features of the cells by primarily cAMP formation dominates in HR2-dependent effects of histamine.

Human HR3 encoded by a gene that consists of four exons on chromosome 20 was demonstrated in 1987 and has recently been cloned [9]. HR3 was initially identified in the central and peripheral nervous system as a presynaptic receptor controlling the release of histamine and other neurotransmitters (dopamine, serotonin, noradrenaline, GABA, and acetylcholine). HR3 signal transduction involves $G_{i/o}$ of G proteins, leading to inhibition of cAMP and accumulation of Ca^{++} and activation of the mitogen-activated protein kinase (MAPK) pathway.

R-α-methylhistamine and imetit are agonists of HR3, whereas thioperamide and clobenpropit are antagonists. The control of mast cells by histamine acting on HR3 involves neuropeptide-containing nerves and might be related to a local neuron–mast cell feedback loop controlling neurogenic inflammation. Dysregulation of this feedback loop may lead to excessive inflammatory responses and suggests a novel therapeutic approach by using HR3 agonists. Probably more than one HR3 subtype exists, which differ in central nervous system localization and signaling pathways.

Human HR4 is encoded by a gene containing three exons separated by two large introns located in chromosome 18q11.2. It has 37% to 43% homology to HR3 (58% in the transmembrane region). HR4 is functionally coupled to G protein $G_{i/o}$, inhibiting forskolin-induced cAMP formation like HR3 [10]. HR4 shows high expression in bone marrow and peripheral hematopoietic cells, neutrophils, eosinophils and T cells, basophils, and mast cells, and moderate expression in spleen, thymus, lung, small intestine, colon, and heart [11]. Until now, relatively little has been known about the biologic function of HR4. It seems to be involved in immune regulatory functions including chemotaxis and cytokine secretion [1,2].

Histamine receptors form dimers and even oligomers, which allows cooperation between the histamine receptors and other G protein–coupled receptors; therefore, the effects of histamine upon receptor stimulation can be complex.

Synthesis and metabolism of histamine

The classical cellular sources of histamine are mast cells and basophils, gastric enterochromaffinlike cells, platelets, and histaminergic neurons. Interestingly, cells in the immune system, which do not store histamine, show high HDC activity and are capable of producing high amounts of histamine, which is secreted immediately after synthesis [12]. These cells include platelets, monocytes/macrophages, dendritic cells, neutrophils, and T and B lymphocytes.

Histamine is synthesized by decarboxylation of histidine by L-HDC, which is dependent on the cofactor pyridoxal-5′-phosphate [13]. Mast cells and basophils are the major source of granule-stored histamine, where it is closely associated with the anionic proteoglycans and chondroitin-4-sulfate. Histamine is released when these cells degranulate in response to various immunologic and nonimmunologic stimuli. In addition, several myeloid and lymphoid cell types (dendritic cells and T cells), which do not store histamine, show high HDC activity and are capable of producing high amounts of histamine [12]. HDC activity is modulated by cytokines, such as interleukin-1 (IL-1), IL-3, IL-12, IL-18, granulocyte-macrophage colony-stimulating factor (GM-CSF), macrophage-colony stimulating factor, tumor necrosis factor-α (TNF-α), and calcium ionophore, in vitro [14]. HDC activity has been demonstrated in vivo in conditions such as lipopolysaccharide (LPS) stimulation, infection, inflammation, and graft rejection [6]. The generation of HDC-deficient mice provided histamine-free systems to study the role of endogenous histamine in a broad range of normal and disease processes. These mice show decreased numbers of mast cells and significantly reduced granule content, which suggests that histamine might affect the synthesis of mast cell granule proteins [10]. IgE binding to the FcERI on IL-3–dependent mouse bone marrow–derived mast cells induces the expression of HDC through a signaling pathway distinct from that operating during antigen-stimulated $Fc\varphi RI$ activation [15]. More than 97% of the histamine is metabolized in two major pathways before excretion [16]. Histamine N-methyltransferase metabolizes the majority of histamine to N-methylhistamine, which is further metabolized to the primary urinary metabolite M-methylimidazole acetic acid by monoamine oxidase. Diamine oxidase metabolizes 15% to 30% of histamine to imidazole acetic acid.

Histamine signal in chronic inflammatory responses

A chronic inflammatory response is one of the hallmarks of allergic diseases. Over the course of pollen season, there may be a tenfold increase in the number of nasal epithelial submucosal mast cells. Histamine released from these cells may not only induce acute allergic symptoms but also be crucial for sustaining this response into a chronic phase, because increasing evidence suggests that it influences several immune/inflammatory and effector functions [2].

Histamine contributes to the progression of allergic-inflammatory responses by enhancement of the secretion of proinflammatory cytokines, such as IL-1α, IL-1β, and IL-6, as well as chemokines such as RANTES or IL-8, in several cell types and local tissues [17–20]. Histamine induces the CC chemokines, mono-cyte chemotactic proteins 1 and 3, RANTES, and eotaxin in explant cultures of human nasal mucosa via HR1, suggesting a prolonged inflammatory cycle in allergic rhinitis between the cells that release histamine and their enhanced migration to nasal mucosa. Endothelial cells express functional HR1 and HR2, and increased adhesion molecule expression such as ICAM-1, VCAM-1, and P-selectin has been demonstrated by histamine infusion via HR1 [21–23]. Histamine regulates the expression of its own receptors on endothelial cells and influences the overall inflammatory reaction [24].

Histamine regulates granulocyte accumulation to tissues in distinct ways. Allergen-induced accumulation of eosinophils in the skin, nose, and airways is potently inhibited by H1 antihistamines [25]. The effect of histamine on eosino-phil migration may differ according to the dose. High doses inhibit eosinophil chemotaxis via HR2, whereas low doses enhance eosinophil chemotaxis via HR1 [26]. Recently, it has been shown that the histamine receptor responsible for the selective recruitment of eosinophils is HR4 [27]. Histamine possesses all of the properties of a classical leukocyte chemoattractant (ie, agonist-induced actin polymerization, mobilization of intracellular calcium, alteration in cell shape, and upregulation of adhesion molecule expression). The eosinophil chemoattractive ability of histamine is weak when compared with the potent CCR3-binding chemokines, eotaxin and eotaxin-2 [26–29]. Nevertheless, histamine upon activation of the HR4 induces enhanced migration of eosinophils toward eotaxin and eotaxin-2 [28]. The potential of histamine alone to act as an eosinophil chemoattractant in vivo might be augmented by other factors, such as growth factors or cytokines like IL-5, the cytokines specific for the differentiation, activation, and survival of eosinophils [27]. Triggering of HR4 also induces chemotaxis of mast cells [30]. Experiments in mice showed that mast cells from wild-type and HR3-deleted mice migrated in response to histamine, whereas mast cells from the HR4-deleted mice did not. Chemotaxis of eosinophils and mast cells via histamine is triggered mainly through the HR4. The HR4-mediated chronic inflammatory effects of histamine may be aborted by administration of HR4 antagonists, and combination therapies with the HR1 antagonists are a promising approach.

Histamine inhibits neutrophil chemotaxis owing to HR2 triggering, which is mimicked by impromidine (HR2 agonist) but not by betahistine (HR1 agonist). In addition, histamine inhibits neutrophil activation, superoxide formation, and degranulation via HR2 [31]. Downregulation of NF-κB, which acts as a potent transcription factor in initiating inflammation, may represent a possible mechanism for H1 antihistamines to inhibit inflammatory cell accumulation [32]. Low concentrations of H1 antihistamines, cetirizine, and azelastine have been demonstrated to downregulate NF-κB expression in parallel with inhibition of pro-inflammatory cytokines [33]. A recent study with HDC-deficient and mast cell–deficient mice demonstrated that histamine mainly derived from non–mast cells had an essential role in angiogenesis and the generation of inflammatory granulation [34]. Pretreatment of the nasal mucosa and conjunctivae with topical H1 antihistamines has been shown to downregulate inflammation locally after an allergen challenge [35]. Decreased macrophage production of IL-6, as well as decreased expression of CD86 and decreased IL-8 production in dendritic cells, was shown [36,37].

These findings open a new therapeutic window for antihistamines as systemic antiallergic agents. Although the use of H1 antihistamine in persistent asthma is currently not recommended, some recent evidence might lead to a re-evaluation of this approach. Histamine has been found in the airways of asthma patients even during asymptomatic periods [38,39]. An increased number of degranulated mast cells and basophils has been detected in biopsies of asthmatic airways long after an acute asthma attack [40]. The level of histamine in bronchoalveolar lavage fluid (BALF) has been found to correlate with the severity of asthma and airway hyperresponsiveness [41].

Inhaled and intravenous histamine causes bronchoconstriction as one of the first recognized properties, which is inhibited by H1 antihistamines. As a manifestation of airway hyperresponsiveness, asthmatic individuals are more sensitive to the bronchoconstrictor effect of histamine than are normal individuals. In addition, in vitro studies have shown increased histamine release in basophils and mast cells obtained from asthmatic subjects when compared with cells obtained from persons without asthma [38]. In lavage fluid of patients treated with

H1 antihistamines, decreased levels of proinflammatory cytokines and mediators (eg, histamine, leukotrienes, prostaglandin), cell adhesion molecules (eg, intercellular adhesion molecules and vascular cell adhesion molecules), cells (eg, eosinophils and neutrophils), and plasma exudation along with a reduced symptom score have been found [42].

The potential efficacy of H1 antihistamines in asthma has been investigated intensively [42]. Inhalation, intravenous, or oral administration of clemastine or chlorpheniramine induces significant bronchodilatation, whereas second-generation H1 antihistamines induce only a limited increase of FEV1 (5% to 10% over baseline) with recommended doses [43,44]. There is variable effect on allergen challenge or exercise-induced bronchospasm. Only terfenadine given in three times the recommended dose inhibited early and late bronchoconstrictor responses [44]. Terfenadine, cetirizine, and loratadine in two to five times the usual dose appeared to improve symptoms in patients with mild seasonal or perennial asthma, but did not block the development of bronchial hyperresponsiveness in seasonal pollen asthma nor show apparent benefit in patients with more severe asthma [43,44]. In patients with concurrent symptoms of allergic rhinitis and asthma, treatment with H1 antihistamine results in a significant decrease in symptoms of rhinitis and asthma, a decrease in the use of beta-2 agonists, and some improvement of airway function [45]. Montelukast sodium, a leukotriene receptor antagonist, showed a similar effect as desloratadine [45].

The mechanisms of the beneficial effect of HR1 antihistamines in asthma have been investigated in a mice model. Fexofenadine was found to suppress allergic immune/inflammatory responses in sensitized mice [46]. Treatment with fexofenadine diminished the Th2-like response that typically follows sensitization and challenge with allergen. Decreased secretion of IL-4 and IL-5, prevention of the allergen-specific IgE increase, reduced eosinophilia in lung tissue and BALF, as well as normalization of airway response to metacholine was observed.

In an adoptive transfer model, it was demonstrated that the target mechanism was T cell mediated. Lung T cells from sensitized mice when transferred to naïve recipient mice triggered airway hyperresponsiveness and allergic inflammatory features after allergen challenge. In contrast, naïve mice that received T cells from sensitized mice treated before with fexofenadine showed no such responses to allergen challenge [46]. The inability of T cells from HR1 antihistamine–treated allergen-sensitized mice to transfer allergic sensitivity to naïve recipients resulted from an alteration in the cytokine production profile of the transferred cells.

Consistently, histamine-induced concentration-dependent release of IL-6 and β-glucuronidase from macrophages isolated from human lung parenchyma was inhibited by fexofenadine but not by ranitidine, an H2 receptor antagonist [47]. Long-term treatment with H1 antihistamines can alter disease progression in patients with respiratory allergy associated with tissue damage/remodeling mediated by macrophage and Th2 cell activation. Treatment with cetirizine over period of 18 months delayed the onset of asthma in some young children with atopic dermatitis [48]. Although H1 antihistamines clearly show weaker anti-inflammatory effects than corticosteroids, they may subtly affect the immune response by modulating the balance among Th1, Th2, and T regulatory cells and suppressing the accumulation of inflammatory cells.

Although previous studies have suggested a basal tone of smooth muscle mediated by histamine binding to HR1, constitutive intrinsic activity of HR1 without any occupation by histamine could be more relevant. Histamine also induces proliferation of cultured airway smooth muscle cells [49].

A difference in histamine response between species has been reported, indicating a role for HR2-mediated bronchodilatation in the cat, rat, rabbit, sheep, and horse [50]. In humans, H2 antihistamines such as cimetidine and ranitidine do not cause bronchoconstriction in normal or asthmatic individuals [51]. Although there is no direct evidence that it has a role in disease pathogenesis, HR2-mediated gastric secretion is impaired in asthma [52]. Histamine may have an important role in modulation of the cytokine network in the lung via HR2, HR3, and HR4, which are expressed in distinct cells and cell subsets. Apparently, owing to the same signal transduction patterns, β2-adrenergic receptors may function similar to HR2 in humans. The role of histamine and other redundant G protein–coupled receptors in regulation of the immune/inflammatory pathways in the lung will be the focus of future studies.

Histamine signal in the regulation of immune response

Antigen-presenting cells

Dendritic cells are often located near various histamine sources such as connective tissue mast cells. They are potent antigen-presenting and cytokine-producing cells; therefore, histamine may effectively influence the immune response through dendritic cells. These professional antigen-presenting cells mature from monocytic and lymphoid precursors and acquire DC1 and DC2 phenotypes, which, in turn, facilitate the development of Th1 and Th2 cells, respectively. Endogenous histamine is actively synthesized during cytokine-induced dendritic cell differentiation, which acts in autocrine and paracrine fashion and modifies dendritic cell markers [53]. Histamine actively participates in the functions and activity of dendritic cell precursors as well as their immature and mature forms (Fig. 1). Immature and mature dendritic cells express all four histamine receptors; however, a comparison of their levels of expression has not yet been performed. In the differentiation process of DC1 from monocytes, HR1 and HR3 act as positive stimulants that increase antigen presentation capacity and proinflammatory cytokine production and Th1 priming activity. In contrast, HR2 acts as a suppressive molecule for antigen presentation capacity, enhances IL-10 production, and induces IL-10–producing T cells or Th2 cells [54,55].

In monocytes stimulated with Toll-like receptor–triggering bacterial products, histamine inhibits the production of proinflammatory IL-1–like activity, TNF-α, IL-12, and IL-18, but enhances IL-10 secretion through HR2 stimulation [17,55]. Histamine also downregulates CD14 expression via H2 receptors on

HR1 blocks humoral immunity, induces cellular immunity
HR2 blocks cellular immunity
HR1-deficient mice show increased specific IgE,
HR2-deficient mice show suppressed specific IgE

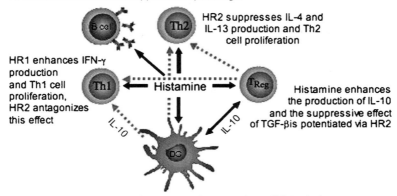

HR2 suppresses IL-4 and IL-13 production and Th2 cell proliferation

HR1 enhances IFN-γ production and Th1 cell proliferation, HR2 antagonizes this effect

Histamine enhances the production of IL-10 and the suppressive effect of TGF-βis potentiated via HR2

HR1 increases antigen-presenting capacity and Th1 priming.
HR2 induces IL-10 production, suppresses antigen-presentation and aids development of IL-10-secreting T cells

Fig. 1. Histamine regulates monocyte, dendritic cell (DC), T cell, and B cell functions. Monocytes and DCs express all four histamine receptors. Activation of HR1 and HR3 triggers proinflammatory events and increases antigen-presenting cell capacity. HR2 has a suppressive role on monocytes and monocyte-derived DCs. Th1 cells show predominant, but not exclusive, expression of HR1, whereas Th2 cells show upregulation of HR2. Histamine induces increased proliferation and IFN-γ production in Th1 cells. Th2 cells express predominant HR2, which acts as the negative regulator of proliferation, IL-4, and IL-13 production. Histamine enhances Th1-type responses by triggering the HR1, whereas both Th1- and Th2-type responses are negatively regulated by HR2, showing an essential role in immune regulation for this receptor. Distinct effects of histamine suggest roles of HR1 and HR2 on T cells for autoimmunity and peripheral tolerance, respectively. Histamine also modulates antibody production. Histamine directly affects B-cell antibody production as a co-stimulatory receptor on B cells. HR1 predominantly expressed on Th1 cells may block humoral immune responses by enhancing Th1-type cytokine IFN-γ. In contrast, HR2 enhances humoral immune responses. Allergen-specific IgE production is differentially regulated in HR1- and HR2-deficient mice. HR1-deleted mice show increased allergen-specific IgE production, whereas HR2-deleted mice show suppressed IgE production. Histamine regulates the functions of antigen-presenting cells and T cells. The controlled release of histamine from effector cells of allergy induces IL-10 in dendritic cells (DCs) and suppresses Th1 and Th2 responses through HR2. HR1-deficient mice show increased specific IgE, whereas HR2-deficient mice show suppressed specific IgE production from B cells. IL-10 affects the maturation of DCs to IL-10–producing types, which may further contribute to T regulatory cell generation. DCs express all known histamine receptors. HR1 and HR3 induce proinflammatory activity and increased antigen-presentation capacity; in contrast, HR2 has a suppressive role in DCs. Th1 cells show predominant expression of HR1, whereas Th2 cells show a higher expression of HR2. HR1 induces increased proliferation and IFN-γ production in Th1 cells. HR2 acts as a negative regulator of proliferation, IL-4, and IL-13 production in Th2 cells. HR2 negatively regulates Th1 and Th2 responses, induces IL-10 production, and potentiates the suppressive effect of TGF-β (*solid line*: activation; *dotted line*: suppression).

human monocytes [56]. The inhibitory effect of histamine via H2 receptor appears through the regulation of ICAM-1 and B7.1 expression, leading to the reduction of innate immune response stimulated by LPS [57].

Histamine induces intracellular Ca^{++} flux, actin polymerization, and chemotaxis in immature dendritic cells owing to stimulation of HR1 and HR3 subtypes. Maturation of dendritic cells results in loss of these responses. In maturing dendritic cells, histamine dose dependently enhances intracellular cAMP levels and stimulates IL-10 secretion while inhibiting production of IL-12 via HR2 [16]. Interestingly, although human monocyte-derived dendritic cells (MoDC) have both histamine H1 and H2 receptors and can induce CD86 expression by histamine, human epidermal Langerhans cells express neither H1 nor H2 receptors [58].

T cells and antibody isotypes

Histamine has been shown to intervene in the Th1, Th2, and T regulatory cell balance and, consequently, antibody formation. Differential patterns of histamine receptor expression on Th1 and Th2 cells determine reciprocal T-cell responses following histamine stimulation (Fig. 1) [59]. Th1 cells show predominant, but not exclusive, expression of HR1, whereas Th2 cells show increased expression of HR2. Histamine enhances Th1-type responses by triggering the HR1, whereas both Th1- and Th2-type responses are negatively regulated by HR2 owing to activation of different biochemical intracellular signals [59]. In mice, deletion of HR1 results in suppression of IFN-γ and dominant secretion of Th2 cytokines (IL-4 and IL-13). HR2-deleted mice show upregulation of Th1 and Th2 cytokines. *Bphs*, a non–major histocompatibility complex-linked gene involved in the susceptibility to many autoimmune diseases, has been identified as the HR1 gene in mice. HR1-deleted mice showed delayed disease onset and decreased disease severity when immunized to develop experimental allergic encephalomyelitis [60]. Histamine stimulation induces IL-10 secretion through HR2 [1,2]. Increased IL-10 production in dendritic cells and T cells may account for an important regulatory mechanism in the control of inflammatory functions through histamine. Various cytokines regulate the production of histamine and its receptor expression. IL-3 stimulation significantly increases HR1 expression on Th1 cells but not on Th2 cells [59].

In mice, histamine enhances anti-IgM–induced proliferation of B cells, which is abolished in HR1-deleted mice. In HR1-deleted mice, antibody production against a T cell–independent antigen, TNP-Ficoll, is decreased [7], suggesting an important role of HR1 signaling in responses triggered from B-cell receptors. Antibody responses to T cell–dependent antigens like ovalbumin (OVA) show a different pattern [7]. HR1-deleted mice produced high OVA-specific IgG1 and IgE in comparison with wild-type mice. In contrast, HR2-deleted mice showed decreased serum levels of OVA-specific IgE in comparison with wild-type mice and HR1-deficient mice. Although T cells of HR2-deficient mice secreted increased IL-4 and IL-13, OVA-specific IgE was suppressed in the presence of highly increased IFN-γ. These findings suggest that HR1 and the related Th1 response may have a dominant role in the suppression of humoral immune response.

The relevance of histamine signal during allergen-specific immunotherapy

The rationale for the use of H1 antihistamines during SIT is diverse and may include the reduction of side effects, which may develop immediately after shots of vaccine, and providing help in the long-term induction of allergen tolerance induced by vaccination. Pretreatment with antihistamines was proposed as early as the 1980s as an effective approach to reduce the side effects of allergen immunotherapy [61]. Several studies have confirmed that administration of high doses of second-generation H1 antihistamines before vaccine shots of insect venom or grass pollen is effective in reducing local allergic reactions and generalized symptoms of urticaria and angioedema [62–64]. Unfortunately, this modality is much less effective in the reduction of more severe systemic symptoms [62–64].

The effect of pretreatment with terfenadine on the long-term protection from honeybee stings during rush immunotherapy with honeybee venom was analyzed in a double-blind, placebo-controlled trial [65]. After an average of 3 years, 41 patients were re-exposed to honeybee stings. Surprisingly, none of 20 patients who had been given HR1 antihistamine premedication had a systemic allergic reaction to the re-exposure by either a field sting or a sting challenge, whereas 6 of 21 given placebo did have a reaction. This highly significant difference suggests that H1 antihistamine premedication during the initial dose increase phase may have enhanced the long-term efficacy of immunotherapy and indicates a positive role for histamine in immune regulation during SIT [66]. Similarly, the ETAC (Early Treatment of the Atopic Child) study, a double-blind, placebo-controlled trial, was performed to determine the preventative effect of cetirizine on the development of asthma. The ETAC included 830 children with atopic dermatitis aged 12 to 24 months and showed that treatment with cetirizine reduced the relative risk of developing asthma for children sensitized to grass pollen or house dust mites [67]. These findings indicate the immunoregulatory and anti-inflammatory effects of H1 antihistamines. The underlying mechanisms are not fully elucidated. On one hand, treatment with HR1 antagonists also results in HR2 predominance. Moreover, the expression of HR1 on T lymphocytes is strongly reduced during ultrarush immunotherapy, which may lead to a dominant expression of HR2.

Peripheral T-cell tolerance characterized by immune deviation to regulatory/suppressor T cells represents a key event in the control of specific immune response during SIT [68]. Although multiple suppressor factors including contact dependent or independent mechanisms might be involved, IL-10 and TGF-β predominantly produced by allergen-specific T cells have an essential role [69,70]. Histamine interferes with the peripheral tolerance induced during SIT in several pathways. It induces the production of IL-10 by dendritic cells [54]. In addition, histamine induces IL-10 production by Th2 cells [71]. Furthermore, histamine enhances the suppressive activity of TGF-β on T cells [72]. All three of these effects are mediated via HR2, which is relatively highly expressed on Th2 cells and suppresses IL-4 and IL-13 production and T-cell proliferation. These findings suggest that HR2 may represent an essential receptor that participates in peripheral tolerance or active suppression of inflammatory/immune responses. Although the selective activation of HR2 might be a more promising approach as compared with the use of H1 antihistamines, thus far, it has not been investigated in vivo.

Selective HR2 antagonists have attracted interest because of their potential immune response–modifying activity [73]. Most data suggest that cimetidine has a stimulatory effect on the immune system, possibly by blocking the receptors on subsets of T lymphocytes and inhibiting HR2-induced immune suppression. Cimetidine has also been used successfully to restore immune functions in patients with malignant disorders, hypogammaglobulinemia, and AIDS-related complexes.

References

[1] Akdis CA, Blaser K. Histamine in the immune regulation of allergic inflammation. J Allergy Clin Immunol 2003;112:15–22.
[2] Jutel M, Watanabe T, Akdis M, et al. Immune regulation by histamine. Curr Opin Immunol 2002;14:735–40.
[3] Dale HH, Laidlaw PP. The physiological action of beta-imidazolylethylamine. J Physiol 1910; 41:318–44.
[4] Haas HPP. The role of histamine and the tuberomamillary nucleus in the nervous system. Rev Neurosci 2003;4:121–30.
[5] Leurs R, Church MK, Taglialatela M. H1-antihistamines: inverse agonism, anti-inflammatory actions and cardiac effects. Clin Exp Allergy 2002;32:489–98.
[6] Leurs R, Smit MJ, Timmerman H. Molecular and pharmacological aspects of histamine receptors. Pharmacol Ther 1995;66:413–63.
[7] Banu Y, Watanabe T. Augmentation of antigen receptor-mediated responses by histamine H1 receptor signaling. J Exp Med 1999;189:673–82.
[8] Del Valle J, Gantz I. Novel insights into histamine H2 receptor biology. Am J Physiol 1997;273: G987–96.
[9] Lovenberg TW, Roland BL, Wilson SJ, et al. Cloning and functional expression of the human histamine H3 receptor. Mol Pharmacol 1999;55:1101–7.
[10] Ohtsu H, Tanaka S, Terui T, et al. Mice lacking histidine decarboxylase exhibit abnormal mast cells. FEBS Lett 2001;502:53–6.
[11] Nakamura K, Kitani A, Strober W. Cell contact-dependent immunosuppression by CD4(+)CD25(+) regulatory T cells is mediated by cell surface-bound transforming growth factor beta. J Exp Med 2001;194:629–44.
[12] Kubo Y, Nakano H. Regulation of histamine in mouse CD4+ and CD8+ lymphocytes. Inflamm Res 1999;48:149–53.
[13] Endo Y. Simultaneous induction of histidine and ornithine decarboxylases and changes in their product amines following the injection of Escherichia coli lipopolysaccharide into mice. Biochem Pharmacol 1982;31:1643–7.

[14] Yoshimoto T, Tsutsui H, Tominaga K, et al. IL-18, although antiallergic when administered with IL-12, stimulates IL-4 and histamine release by basophils. Proc Natl Acad Sci USA 1999; 96:13962–6.

[15] Tanaka S, Takasu Y, Mikura S, et al. Antigen-independent induction of histamine synthesis by immunoglobulin E in mouse bone marrow-derived mast cells. J Exp Med 2002;196:229–35.

[16] Abe Y, Ogino S, Irifune M, et al. Histamine content, synthesis and degradation in human nasal mucosa. Clin Exp Allergy 1993;23:132–6.

[17] Vannier E, Dinarello CA. Histamine enhances interleukin (IL)-1-induced IL-1 gene expression and protein synthesis via H2 receptors in peripheral blood mononuclear cells: comparison with IL-1 receptor antagonist. J Clin Invest 1993;92:281–7.

[18] Meretey K, Falus A, Taga T, et al. Histamine influences the expression of the interleukin-6 receptor on human lymphoid, monocytoid and hepatoma cell lines. Agents Actions 1991;33: 189–91.

[19] Jeannin P, Delneste Y, Gosset P, et al. Histamine induces interleukin-8 secretion by endothelial cells. Blood 1994;84:2229–33.

[20] Bayram H, Devalia JL, Khair OA, et al. Effect of loratadine on nitrogen dioxide-induced changes in electrical resistance and release of inflammatory mediators from cultured human bronchial epithelial cells. J Allergy Clin Immunol 1999;104:93–9.

[21] Lo WW, Fan TP. Histamine stimulates inositol phosphate accumulation via the H1-receptor in cultured human endothelial cells. Biochem Biophys Res Commun 1987;148:47–53.

[22] Kubes P, Kanwar S. Histamine induces leukocyte rolling in post-capillary venules: a P-selectin-mediated event. J Immunol 1994;152:3570–7.

[23] Yamaki K, Thorlacius H, Xie X, et al. Characteristics of histamine-induced leukocyte rolling in the undisturbed microcirculation of the rat mesentery. Br J Pharmacol 1998;123:390–9.

[24] Schaefer U, Schmitz V, Schneider A, et al. Histamine induced homologous and heterologous regulation of histamine receptor subtype mRNA expression in cultured endothelial cells. Shock 1999;12:309–15.

[25] Fadel R, Herpin-Richard N, Rihoux JP, et al. Inhibitory effect of cetirizine 2HCl on eosinophil migration in vivo. Clin Allergy 1987;17:373–9.

[26] Clark RA, Sandler JA, Gallin JI, et al. Histamine modulation of eosinophil migration. J Immunol 1977;118:137–45.

[27] O'Reilly M, Alpert R, Jenkinson S, et al. Identification of a histamine H4 receptor on human eosinophils: role in eosinophil chemotaxis. J Recept Signal Transduct Res 2002;22:431–48.

[28] Buckland KF, Williams TJ, Conroy DM. Histamine induces cytoskeletal changes in human eosinophils via the H(4) receptor. Br J Pharmacol 2003;140:1117–27.

[29] Ling P, Ngo K, Nguyen S, et al. Histamine H4 receptor mediates eosinophil chemotaxis with cell shape change and adhesion molecule upregulation. Br J Pharmacol 2004;142:161–71.

[30] Gantz I, Schaffer M, Del Valle J. Molecular cloning of a gene encoding the histamine H2 receptor. Proc Natl Acad Sci USA 1991;88:429–33.

[31] Seligmann BE, Fletcher MP, Gallin JI. Histamine modulation of human neutrophil oxidative metabolism, locomotion, degranulation, and membrane potential changes. J Immunol 1983;130: 1902–9.

[32] Oda T, Morikawa N, Saito Y, et al. Molecular cloning and characterization of a novel type of histamine receptor preferentially expressed in leukocytes. J Biol Chem 2000;275:36781–6.

[33] Yoneda K, Yamamoto T, Ueta E, et al. Suppression by azelastine hydrochloride of NF-kappa B activation involved in generation of cytokines and nitric oxide. Jpn J Pharmacol 1997;73: 145–53.

[34] Ghosh AK, Hirasawa N, Ohtsu H, et al. Defective angiogenesis in the inflammatory granulation tissue in histidine decarboxylase–deficient mice but not in mast cell–deficient mice. J Exp Med 2002;195:973–82.

[35] Simons FER. Antihistamines. In: Adkinson Jr NF, Yunginger JW, Busse WW, et al, editors. Middleton's allergy: principles & practice. Philadelphia: Mosby; 2003. p. 834–69.

[36] Paolieri F, Battifora M, Riccio AM. Terfenadine and fexofenadine reduce in vitro ICAM-1 expression on human continuous cell lines. Ann Allergy Asthma Immunol 1988;81:601–7.

[37] Caron G, Delneste Y, Roelandts E. Histamine induces CD86 expression and chemokine production by human immature dendritic cells. J Immunol 2001;166:6000–6.

[38] Casolaro V, Gale D. Functional comparisons of cells obtained from peripheral blood, lung parenchyma, and bronchoalveolar lavage in asthmatics. Am Rev Respir Dis 1989;139:1375–82.

[39] Wenzel SE, Fowler AA, Schwartz LB. Activation of pulmonary mast cells by bronchoalveolar allergen challenge: in vivo release of histamine and tryptase in atopic subjects with and without asthma. Am Rev Respir Dis 1988;137:1002–8.

[40] Crimi E, Chiaramondia M, Milanese M. Increase of mast cell numbers in mucosa after the late-phase asthmatic response to allergen. Am Rev Respir Dis 1991;144:1282–6.

[41] Nakamura T, Itadani H, Hidaka Y, et al. Molecular cloning and characterization of a new human histamine receptor, HH4R. Biochem Biophys Res Commun 2000;279:615–20.

[42] Milligan G, Bond R, Lee M. Inverse agonism: pharmacological curiosity or potential therapeutic strategy? Trends Pharmacol Sci 1995;16:10–3.

[43] Malick A, Grant JA. Antihistamines in the treatment of asthma. Allergy 1997;52:55–66.

[44] Town GI, Holgate ST. Comparison of the effect of loratadine on the airway and skin responses to histamine, methacholine, and allergen in subjects with asthma. J Allergy Clin Immunol 1990;86: 886–93.

[45] Baena-Cagnani CE, Berger WE, Du-Buske LM. Comparative effects of desloratadine versus montelukast on asthma symptoms and use of beta 2-agonists in patients with seasonal allergic rhinitis and asthma. Int Arch Allergy Immunol 2003;130:307–13.

[46] Gelfand EW, ZH C, Takeda K, et al. Fexofenadine modulates T-cell function, preventing allergen-induced airway inflammation and hyperresponsiveness. J Allergy Clin Immunol 2002; 110:85–95.

[47] Triggiani M, Gentile M, Secondo A, et al. Histamine induces exocytosis and IL-6 production from human lung macrophages through interaction with H1 receptors. J Immunol 2001;166: 4083–91.

[48] Warner JO. A double-blind, randomized, placebo-controlled trial of cetirizine in preventing the onset of asthma in children with atopic dermatitis: 18 months' treatment and 18 months' posttreatment followup. J Allergy Clin Immunol 2001;108:929–37.

[49] Panettieri RA, Yadvish PA, Kelly AM, et al. Histamine stimulates proliferation of airway smooth muscle and induces c-fos expression. Am J Physiol 1990;259:L365–71.

[50] Chand N, Eyre P. Classification and biological distribution of histamine receptor subtypes. Agents Actions 1975;5:277–95.

[51] Thomson NC, Kerr JW. Effect of inhaled H1 and H2 receptor antagonist in normal and asthmatic subjects. Thorax 1980;35:428–34.

[52] Gonzales H, Ahmed T. Suppression of gastric H2-receptor-mediated function in patients with bronchial asthma and ragweed allergy. Chest 1986;89:491–6.

[53] Szeberenyi JB, Pallinger E, Zsinko M, et al. Inhibition of effects of endogenously synthesized histamine disturbs in vitro human dendritic cell differentiation. Immunol Lett 2001;76:175–82.

[54] Mazzoni A, Young HA, Spitzer JH, et al. Histamine regulates cytokine production in maturing dendritic cells, resulting in altered T cell polarization. J Clin Invest 2001;108:1865–73.

[55] van der Pouw Kraan TC, Snijders A, Boeije LC, et al. Histamine inhibits the production of interleukin-12 through interaction with H2 receptors. J Clin Invest 1998;102:1866–73.

[56] Takahashi HK, Morichika T, Iwagaki H, et al. Histamine downregulates CD14 expression via H2 receptors on human monocytes. Clin Immunol 2003;108:274–81.

[57] Morichika T, Takahashi HK, Iwagaki H, et al. Histamine inhibits lipopolysaccharide-induced tumor necrosis factor-alpha production in an intercellular adhesion molecule-1- and B7.1-dependent manner. J Pharmacol Exp Ther 2003;304:624–33.

[58] Ohtani T, Aiba S, Mizuashi M, et al. H1 and H2 histamine receptors are absent on Langerhans cells and present on dermal dendritic cells. J Invest Dermatol 2003;121:1073–9.

[59] Jutel M, Watanabe T, Klunker S, et al. Histamine regulates T-cell and antibody responses by differential expression of H1 and H2 receptors. Nature 2001;413:420–5.

[60] Ma RZ, Gao J, Meeker ND, et al. Identification of Bphs, an autoimmune disease locus, as histamine receptor H1. Science 2002;297:620–3.

[61] Jarisch R, Goetz M, Aberer W, et al. Reduction of side effects of specific immunotherapy by premedication with antihistamines and reduction of maximal dosage to 50 000 SQ-U/mL. Arbeiten aus dem Paul-Ehrlich Institut 1988;82:163–75.

[62] Berchtold E, Maibach R, Muller UR. Reduction of side effects from rush-immunotherapy with honeybee venom by pretreatment with terfenadine. Clin Exp Allergy 1992;22:59–65.

[63] Nielsen L, Johnsen CR, Mosbech H, et al. Antihistamine premedication in specific cluster immunotherapy: a double blind placebo-controlled study. J Allergy Clin Immunol 1996;97: 1207–13.

[64] Reimers A, Hari Y, Muller UR. Reduction of side effects from ultra-rush immunotherapy with honeybee venom by pretreatment with fexofenadine: a double-blind, placebo controlled trial. Allergy 2000;55:484–8.

[65] Muller U, Hari Y, Berchtold E. Premedication with antihistamines may enhance efficacy of specific-allergen immunotherapy. J Allergy Clin Immunol 2001;107:81–6.

[66] Jutel M, Zak-Nejmark T, Wrzyyszcz M, et al. Histamine receptor expression on peripheral blood CD4+ lymphocytes is influenced by ultrarush bee venom immunotherapy. Allergy 1997; 52(Suppl. 37):88.

[67] Diepgen TL. Long-term treatment with cetirizine of infants with atopic dermatitis: a multi-country, double-blind, randomized, placebo-controlled trial (the ETAC trial) over 18 months. Pediatr Allergy Immunol 2002;13:278–86.

[68] Akdis CA, Blaser K, Akdis M. Genes of tolerance. Allergy 2004;59:897–913.

[69] Akdis CA, Blesken T, Akdis M, et al. Role of IL-10 in specific immunotherapy. J Clin Invest 1998;102:98–106.

[70] Jutel M, Akdis M, Budak F, et al. IL-10 and TGF-beta cooperate in the regulatory T cell response to mucosal allergens in normal immunity and specific immunotherapy. Eur J Immunol 2003;33: 1205–14.

[71] Osna N, Elliott K, Khan MM. Regulation of interleukin-10 secretion by histamine in Th2 cells and splenocytes. Int Immunopharmacol 2001;1:85–96.

[72] Kunzmann S, Mantel P-Y, Wohlfahrt J, et al. Histamine enhances TGF-beta-1-mediated suppression of Th2 responses. FASEB J 2003;17:1089–95.

[73] Gifford R, Schmidke J. Cimetidine-induced augmentation of human lymphocyte blastogenesis: comparison with levamisole in mitogen stimulation. Surg Forum 1979;30:113–5.

ELSEVIER
SAUNDERS

Immunol Allergy Clin N Am
26 (2006) 261–281

IMMUNOLOGY
AND ALLERGY
CLINICS
OF NORTH AMERICA

Strategies for Recombinant Allergen Vaccines and Fruitful Results from First Clinical Studies

Oliver Cromwell, PhD*, Helmut Fiebig, PhD,
Roland Suck, PhD, Helga Kahlert, PhD, Andreas Nandy, PhD,
Jens Kettner, PhD, Annemie Narkus, MD

*Research and Development, Allergopharma Joachim Ganzer KG, Hermann-Koerner-Strasse 52,
D-21465, Reinbek, Germany*

The prevalence of allergic airway disease attributable to inhalant allergens such as pollen has been increasing steadily. A European-based survey of allergic rhinitis published in 2004 reported a prevalence of 23%, with values as high as 29% in some countries [1]. The only potentially curative and specific treatment for IgE-mediated type I allergy is allergen-specific immunotherapy, a causal therapy based on administration of the disease-eliciting allergens or derivatives thereof with the objective of reducing allergic symptoms. Once a prescribed dose or a maximum tolerated dose has been achieved, this dose can be administered repeatedly at intervals until it is deemed to have been therapeutically effective. The treatment has been shown to be particularly beneficial in allergic rhinitis, mild and moderate asthma, and insect venom hypersensitivity.

Whole aqueous extracts of natural allergen source materials such as pollens, mites, molds, and animal epithelia are the basis for therapeutic preparations that are currently used in clinical practice. The extracts are standardized in terms of total allergenic activity, or potency, and possibly the concentration of one individual major allergen, whereas product consistency is assessed in terms of protein and allergen profiles determined by various techniques including electrophoresis and immunoblotting. An extract may contain numerous proteins only some of

* Corresponding author.
  E-mail address: oliver.cromwell@allergopharma.de (O. Cromwell).

which are allergens. The composition is determined to a large extent by the quality of the raw material and the method of extraction and purification. Raw materials are provided by certified suppliers and produced under controlled conditions. Nevertheless, there are differences. For example, the allergen content of mold cultures is highly dependent on the time and conditions of culture; climatic factors or pollution can influence the allergenicity of pollen; and, while some manufacturers use whole cultures of house dust mites, including the nutrient medium and fecal particles, others use purified mite bodies. In addition, many extracts derived from natural materials contain endotoxin [2].

There is clearly considerable scope for improving allergen vaccines to obtain more precisely defined preparations that are the basis for achieving improved quality and consistency, which, in turn, can lead to enhanced clinical efficacy with respect to diagnosis and treatment. The use of recombinant DNA technology seems to provide a realistic means of achieving such improvements. Furthermore, the technology provides the possibility to create allergen derivatives with reduced IgE reactivity, that is, hypoallergenic molecules that have a reduced risk for inducing undesirable allergic reactions during the course of immunotherapy but retain their therapeutic activity.

Recombinant allergens

Many hundreds of allergens have been identified, and, often, several allergens originate from one source. For example, more than 20 allergens have been characterized from the house dust mites *Dermatophagoides pteronyssinus* and *D farinae*, more than 20 have been identified as coming from *Aspergillus fumigatus*, and *Ambrosia artemisiaefolia* (short ragweed) is a source of nine different allergens. Although numerous allergens have been cloned for research purposes, only a few have been developed to the stage at which they can be used in clinical studies.

Once an allergen source has been identified, mRNA is isolated and used as a template to synthesize cDNA. IgE immunoscreening of cDNA libraries can then be used to select cDNA encoding allergens that most closely resemble their natural counterparts. Allergen-specific monoclonal antibodies can also be used. Alternatively, DNA-based screening techniques may be used, such as polymerase chain reaction (PCR) amplification, which relies on the use of oligonucleotide primers designed based on known amino acid sequence data for the allergen. Phage surface display technology has also been used to great advantage to identify a number of allergens. A physical linkage between the gene product and its cDNA facilitates isolation of the specific cDNA from large libraries [3,4].

The next step is to insert the cDNA into a suitable vector (viral, plasmid DNA), which enables it to be expressed and produced in a suitable host organism. Bacterial host organisms, such as *Escherichia coli,* produce the recombinant proteins without posttranslational modification, and, in many cases, it is possible to obtain the allergens with reactivity comparable with the native form. When correct folding and posttranslational modifications, including glycosylation, become an issue, a eukaryotic expression system such as the yeast *Pichia pastoris*, Baculovirus in host insect cells, and various plants including the tobacco plant *Nicotiana benthamiana* [5] and barley [6] may be used. Nevertheless, these systems do not necessarily introduce glycosylation that is comparable with that of

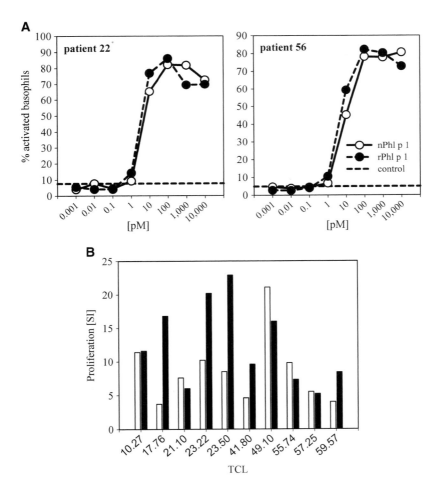

Fig. 1. Comparison of natural glycosylated and recombinant nonglycosylated Phl p 1. (*A*) Peripheral blood mononuclear cells from grass pollen–allergic subjects were incubated with various concentrations of the allergens or the diluent solution. Basophil activation was measured by fluorescence activated flow cytometry in terms of expression of the surface marker CD203c. (*B*) Lymphocyte proliferation, expressed as a stimulation index (SI), was determined in terms of ³H-thymidine incorporation by T-cell lines (TCL) derived from grass pollen–allergic subjects. White bars denote natural glycosylated Phl p 1; black bars denote nonglycosylated recombinant Phl p 1.

the natural glycoprotein. One example of this is the expression of the house dust mite allergen Der p 1 in *Pichia pastoris*, which results in inappropriate hyper-glycosylation [7].

Following a fermentation process and the induction of gene expression, the heterologous recombinant protein is recovered from the cell culture and purified using appropriate chromatographic methods. Optimal production conditions must be determined for each protein to ensure that correct and reproducible secondary and tertiary structures are achieved. Once these are established, the use of contemporary technology enables pure protein to be produced with consistent pharmaceutical quality [8,9].

The so-called "wild-type" recombinant allergens exhibiting IgE reactivity comparable with that of the natural allergen are particularly suitable for diagnostic applications and may also substitute for natural allergens used in specific immunotherapy. The success of the latter is dependent primarily on the T-cell reactivity and immunogenicity of the protein. The allergen Phl p 1 from timothy grass is naturally glycosylated, but the presence of the carbohydrate moiety does not seem to be important for IgE reactivity. When compared for their ability to activate peripheral blood basophils and T-cell lines from grass pollen–allergic subjects, the purified natural molecule and a recombinant nonglyco-sylated form obtained by expression in *E coli* gave essentially identical results (Fig. 1).

Characterization and quality of recombinant allergens

The production of recombinant proteins depends initially on the creation of a master cell bank incorporating a DNA construct including the expression vector together with the cDNA encoding the protein. This cell bank is the starting point for all routine production batches. Each production run starts with an aliquot of cells derived from the one cell bank, ensuring that the identical protein is always produced.

Quality control of the recombinant proteins is undertaken using an array of analytical methods. Identity is confirmed by reactivity with specific antibodies on immunoblot, peptide fingerprinting, and N-terminal amino acid analysis. Purity is determined by sodium dodecyl sulfate (SDS) polyacrylamide gel electrophoresis (PAGE) and native PAGE [10], both in conjunction with protein staining; by size exclusion high-performance liquid chromatography (HPLC); and by reverse phase HPLC, taking account of peak symmetry. Allergen concentration is expressed in terms of absolute protein concentration determined from the UV absorption at 280 nm and the specific extinction coefficient of the particular protein, and confirmed as appropriate by specific antibody immunoassays and integrated HPLC peak areas. It is important to be able to determine the potency, and, with natural allergen equivalents, this can best be achieved by measuring IgE-binding activity in an inhibition immunoassay. The use of such a potency measure in preparations for immunotherapy assumes a relationship between IgE reactivity and antigenicity. This measurement is clearly not appropriate for recombinant allergen derivatives that have been specifically designed to achieve a hypoallergenic character while conserving or even enhancing antigenic activity. In such cases, IgE reactivity provides little more than an indication of batch consistency. It will be necessary to establish new definitions of potency, possibly based on determination of antigenicity, but it is likely that no one method will be generally applicable.

Levels of possible contaminants, including endotoxin and host cell proteins, are also measured. Endotoxin (lipopolysaccharide) is derived from the outer membrane of gram-negative bacteria and can be detected in many allergen extracts [2]. This contaminant is a potential problem for recombinant allergens expressed in gram-negative bacteria such as *E coli*, but the chromatographic purification steps for the protein can be designed to ensure that it is rendered effectively free of contamination.

Only some of the previously described techniques can be applied in the routine quality control of allergen extracts. Furthermore, interpretation is made difficult because of the complexity of the preparations, the one exception being the specific allergen immunoassays. Consequently, the levels of characterization and standardization that can be achieved for recombinant preparations are far superior to that for allergen extracts.

Further methods can be used to confirm aspects of protein structure, identity, and potency, but, in many cases, these methods are suitable for use in development of the proteins and not in routine quality control. Techniques include circular dichroism spectroscopy to determine secondary structure; mass spectroscopy for measurement of molecular mass; basophil activation, measured in terms of expression of the activation marker CD203c [11], and basophil histamine release to assess potency; and T-cell reactivity determined using allergen-specific T-cell lines or clones to confirm immunoreactivity.

In contrast to pure recombinant proteins, allergen extracts may contain many irrelevant proteins and other macromolecules from the source material. Furthermore, relevant allergens may be instable and prone to degradation in the complex extract, particularly if proteases are present. A possibility exists that extracts may be contaminated with unrelated allergens. One particular example that has been reported is the contamination of a dog dander extract with house dust mite allergens, which gave rise to false-positive skin test results [12]. In animal-derived extracts, such as cat and dog dander or poultry feathers and meat, there is a theoretical risk of viral contamination, although this risk can be excluded by the use of accredited material from certified suppliers.

The subject of effective therapeutic and diagnostic allergen concentrations has attracted a great deal of attention. The acceptable safe dose for an allergen extract may be dictated by the contribution of one or two allergens to the extract's biologic potency, defined in terms of IgE reactivity. Some other allergens may be present in relatively small amounts that render them ineffective for diagnosis or therapy. Working with pure recombinant molecules provides the opportunity to formulate preparations in which all of the components are consistently present in effective concentrations.

Hypoallergenic variants of recombinant allergens

The idea of hypoallergenic allergen derivatives is not new, and, indeed, several successful products derived by chemical modification of the extracts are on the European market. The most commonly used methods of chemical modification involve treatment with formaldehyde and glutaraldehyde using an approach first adopted in the development of vaccines against tetanus and diphtheria. The resulting intra- and intermolecular cross-linking changes the three-dimensional structures of the proteins and consequently the IgE-binding epitopes, resulting in so-called "allergoids." The reduced IgE reactivity can be demonstrated using in vitro techniques, such as RAST inhibition and basophil activation, and in vivo methods including skin testing and nasal provocation [13]. The immunogenicity of the preparations can be demonstrated by the ability to activate allergen-specific T cells and induce allergen-specific IgG-antibody responses [14–16]. The advantage of such preparations is that they have a reduced risk for inducing IgE-mediated side reactions and allow a maximum therapeutic dose to be achieved in a relatively short course of injections when compared with the native allergen [16,17]. The experience with these hypoallergenic preparations suggests that it should be possible to combine the benefits of the hypoallergenic nature with the advantages offered by recombinant proteins.

Recombinant DNA technology provides the opportunity to use genetic engineering techniques to create such hypoallergenic variants. Detailed information concerning IgE-binding epitopes, T-cell epitopes, and three-dimensional structure can help in the design of such molecules. The advantages of this approach are that the new molecules can be precisely defined and the design features validated in respect to the specific immunotherapeutic application [18,19].

Hypoallergenic allergen variants can be created by various production methods. One approach is chemical modification. The methods used to produce allergoids, that is, formaldehyde and glutaraldehyde treatment, can be applied to recombinant allergens, but a disadvantage is that the end product cannot be defined in molecular terms. Conjugation with particular unrelated chemical entities may influence IgE reactivity. The coupling of an average of four 22-base CpG-oligonucleotide sequences per molecule of the major ragweed allergen Amb a 1, for example, resulted in a threefold increase in the concentration of allergen required to achieve 50% inhibition in an IgE ELISA and a similar 30-fold increase for the basophil histamine release assay [20]. In a second approach, peptides represent continuous, discontinuous, or portions of T- or B-cell epitopes expressed or synthesized singly or in combination to create a new molecular form. Peptide mixtures derived by proteolytic digestion of allergen extracts were considered for immunotherapy more than 20 years ago but were dismissed because of the problems of consistent production and standardization. The availability of detailed information on protein structure now allows a designer approach. In the major cat allergen, Fel d 1, a mixture of overlapping 16 to 17 amino acid peptides spanning most of the sequence of both of the two chains was selected on the basis of T-cell reactivity and the ability to bind to MHC molecules [21]. The peptide mixture was shown to be effective in modifying surrogate markers of allergy, including cutaneous responses to allergen challenge and ex vivo parameters of T-cell activation [22,23]. An alternative strategy is to combine several T-cell determinants to form a large hybrid peptide, as has been achieved for the two major allergens of Japanese cedar [24]. In this case, the hybrid failed to bind allergen-specific IgE and was substantially more effective in inducing T-cell proliferation than a mixture of the individual peptides.

A third approach involves fragmentation of the allergen so that the correct molecular folding of the intact molecule is lost, as are conformational IgE-binding epitopes. This method has been used successfully in the birch pollen allergen Bet v 1, which can be expressed as two hypoallergenic fragments [25]. In a fourth approach, recombinant oligomers are produced by linking several copies of a gene in sequence (homomer) or several different genes in sequence (heteromer). A trimeric form of Bet v 1 has been shown to be hypoallergenic [26]. A construct of the group 5 and 6 allergens of *Phleum pratense* has been shown to have partial hypoallergenic properties [27]. On the other hand, Phl p 2–Phl p 6, Phl p 6–Phl p 2, and Phl p 5–Phl p 1 hybrids appear to retain the IgE reactivity of the individual allergens while immunogenicity is enhanced [28]. These results clearly indicate that oligomerization, per se, does not ensure hypoallergenic properties, and it must be concluded that the success of the technique is allergen dependent.

A fifth strategy involves producing variants through mutations introduced by site-directed mutagenesis either directly in IgE-binding epitopes to compromise their activity, or at sites outside the epitopes in positions such that they influence the conformation of the molecule and thereby IgE-binding activity. Substituting single amino acids can have dramatic effects on the overall structure. Disulfide bonds can be destroyed by replacing one or more cysteine residues, resulting in degeneration of tertiary structure and conformational changes, an approach used successfully to produce variants of Der p/f 2 with reduced IgE reactivity [29,30]. Alteration of the surface charge in antigenic regions, such as by substituting aspartic acid (negative charge) for alanine (nonpolar) or vice versa, may modify folding and the ability to react with antibody. The deletion of short sequences can also be used to good effect providing that T-cell epitopes are left undisturbed [31]. PCR amplification in conjunction with oligonucleotide primers may give rise to allergen variants with little or no IgE-binding activity as a result of chance mutations. Various variants of Bet v 1 have been characterized [32]. The isoform Bet v 1a was identified based on high IgE reactivity, whereas the Bet v 1d isoform, which differed by seven amino acid residues, was found to have little IgE reactivity. Cutaneous reactivity was 100-fold lower, and a conjunctival provocation was negative in 48 patients tested, whereas 38 of these patients reacted to the Bet v 1a molecule [33]. Both isoforms show good T-cell reactivity, although failure in both cases to stimulate a number of T-cell clones indicates that some T-cell epitopes are compromised.

A sixth strategy for creating hypoallergenic variants involves gene rearrangement to produce modified protein sequences. This rearrangement may be achieved by a random approach using "gene shuffling," also referred to as molecular breeding, which gives rise to a large number of new sequences and necessitates screening to identify candidate molecules [19,34]. Alternatively, a gene may be cut at preselected points and reassembled before expression to create a "mosaic" protein [35]. The latter approach can be extended by mixing gene fragments from various allergens.

Selection of allergens for a therapeutic vaccine

In addition to the advantages in quality, the expectation is that recombinant allergens or their hypoallergenic derivatives will be better than allergen extracts in terms of the degree of therapeutic benefit they can confer and the specificity of the diagnosis.

In many cases, it will not be realistic to represent all allergens from a particular source; therefore, it will be important to identify the most important allergens that contribute to sensitization and symptoms. Grass pollen, for example, has 11 different allergens that have been identified and characterized in detail, some of which are known to occur as several different isoforms. Only some of these allergens have major general importance, being associated with a high prevalence of sensitization in the grass pollen–allergic population and together accounting for a large part of the specific IgE response directed against the whole pollen extract. The group 1 and 5 allergens are strong candidates for inclusion in a therapeutic vaccine. More than 90% of grass pollen–allergic subjects react to group 1 allergens and as many as 85% to group 5 [36,37]. There are two isoallergens of the timothy grass pollen allergen Phl p 5, the principal difference being that two 14/15 amino acid sequences are missing from the N-terminal half of Phl p 5b when compared with Phl p 5a. The molecules show extensive homology. Although there is a high degree of IgE antibody cross-reactivity, the immunologic differences in terms of T-cell reactivity may justify the inclusion of both isoallergens in a vaccine. The allergens Phl p 2 and Phl p 6 show prevalences of sensitization in the range of 40% to 60% and 60% to 70%, respectively, and are classified as major allergens. Although as many as 80% of grass pollen–sensitized subjects may have IgE antibodies directed to the group 4 allergen, the concentrations are relatively low compared with those specific for Phl p 1 and 5, as is specific skin test reactivity. Further allergens including Phl p 7, 10, 11, and 12 are classified as minor allergens and are not strong contenders for inclusion in a vaccine. The prevalence of sensitization to the calcium-binding protein designated Phl p 7 is about 10% [38], and subjects reacting to Phl p 10 (cytochrome c) are seldom found [36]. Both Phl p 11 (profilin) and Phl p 13 are glycosylated, and a substantial part of the IgE reactivity appears to involve cross-reactive carbohydrate determinants.

It seems reasonable to conclude that any preparation for grass pollen–specific immunotherapy must include the group 1 and group 5 allergens. These allergens may be supplemented by other relatively important allergens, such as group 2 and 6 and possibly group 4. A study conducted using two purified natural allergens of *Phleum pratense*, subsequently identified as Phl p 5 and Phl p 6, found that they were significantly less effective clinically than a partially purified whole allergen extract, and one can speculate that this result might have been attributable to the lack of Phl p 1 [39,40].

Similar considerations will have to be applied in preparations for house dust mites. Although more than 20 allergen groups have been identified in association with *D pteronyssinus* and *D farinae*, the group 1 and 2 allergens, which were the first to be identified, are apparently the most important and account for a large proportion of the specific IgE response directed against the mite extracts.

In other instances, there is a real prospect that one allergen or allergen derivative will suffice to achieve a substantial improvement in clinical symptoms (eg, cat [Fel d 1] and birch [Bet v 1] allergens), the rationale being that one major allergen dominates and accounts for most or all of the specific IgE response directed against the one sensitizing agent.

One concept that has been propagated is patient-tailored immunotherapy [41]. The availability of pure recombinant allergens will make it possible to perform component-resolved diagnosis and to produce IgE reactivity profiles for individual patients. Furthermore, the information will help to elucidate the role played by cross-reacting allergens in clinically relevant sensitizations. With this information, it would be possible to define a vaccine to match an individual's sensitization profile. One day this may become a reality; the more immediate prospect is the introduction of standard combinations of allergens from one source, or in some cases single allergens, to provide immunotherapy for the sensitizations most frequently implicated in allergic disease.

Recombinant hypoallergenic variants of birch pollen allergen Bet v 1

The IgE-binding reactivity of allergens such as Bet v 1 from birch pollen is dependent on their three-dimensional structure. Cleaving the cDNA and expressing the two parts separately results in two allergen fragments (amino acid residues 1–73 and 74–159) showing only minimal allergenicity and a random coil conformation [25]. The cleavage point was chosen to prevent compromising any of the recognized T-cell epitopes. Three-dimensional mapping of the Bet v 1 molecule revealed that the IgE-binding structure involved residues 9 to 22 and 104 to 123, regions that are segregated between the two fragments, resulting in the loss of IgE-antibody binding activity. It has been proposed that a similar approach could be used for the grass pollen allergen Phl p 6 [42], but experience has shown that the approach is not generally applicable.

The birch pollen protein has also been used as a model system to investigate the potential of oligomerization to influence IgE reactivity. Linking three copies of the Bet v 1 cDNA in sequence and expression in *E coli* resulted in a trimeric form of the protein. IgE reactivity was reduced as judged by histamine release and skin testing, but circular dichroism spectroscopy showed that the secondary structure was essentially the same as monomeric Bet v 1 [26]. Basophil activation measured in terms of CD203c expression indicated that the trimer was less hypoallergenic than the fragments [43]. The reasons for the hypoallergenic nature have not been elucidated, but steric hindrance of the IgE-binding sites seems a likely explanation. The general utility of this approach has not been confirmed.

The hypoallergenic nature of these preparations was investigated in two studies involving skin prick and intradermal testing. When skin prick testing was performed at concentrations of 100 μg/mL in birch pollen–allergic subjects who had not received specific immunotherapy, 18 of 23 and 15 of 23 failed to react to the fragment mixture and the trimer, respectively [44]. All subjects reacted to unmodified Bet v 1, but groups of nonatopic individuals and atopic individuals without birch pollen sensitivity showed negative test results to all preparations. A similar result emerged from intradermal testing. Eight of 23 and 13 of 23 of the birch pollen–allergic subjects failed to react to 1 μg/mL concentrations of the fragment mixture and the trimer, respectively. Clear dose-response effects were seen with each of the allergen derivatives. The second study produced similar results [45]; however, there was a large intersubject variation in the endpoint of the intradermal tests. Analysis of the ratios of the endpoint concentrations of Bet v 1 to each of the derivatives showed that although the derivatives were hypoallergenic in all birch pollen–allergic subjects, the degree of hypoallergenicity varied. The two Bet v 1 fragments were tested separately, and both were shown to be hypoallergenic in nature. Subjects proved to be more sensitive to all preparations when tested during the *Fagales* pollen season, suggesting that natural exposure to this tree pollen primed the subjects' response to the birch pollen allergen.

The first study of allergen-specific immunotherapy with recombinant preparations investigated the clinical effects, immunologic activity, and tolerance of a mixture of the two Bet v 1 fragments and the Bet v 1 trimer in comparison with placebo. The recombinant preparations were adsorbed to aluminium hydroxide suspensions at concentrations of 100 μg/mL, and immunotherapy was planned with a course of eight preseasonal injections of increasing concentrations from 1 to 80 μg of total protein, with further injections up until the beginning of the pollen season. Subjects were assessed at baseline, after treatment, during and after the pollen season, and after 12 months [46].

Results from 71 patients from one of the three study centers showed that both active preparations induced Bet v 1–specific IgG1, IgG2, and IgG4 antibody responses as well as an IgA response. Responses to the trimer were stronger, and this preparation also induced IgM antibodies, indicating its good immunogenic properties. The serum antibodies were shown to be able to inhibit allergen-induced histamine release in vitro from basophils of birch pollen–allergic subjects. Sera from the trimer-treated subjects were more effective, reflecting the higher IgG antibody titers. It was possible to show a correlation between IgG1 antibody titers and an improvement in clinical symptoms, as judged by a ten-point interval scale, as well as a reduction in skin test reactivity to Bet v 1. Measurement of Bet v 1–specific IgE responses showed a threefold increase in the placebo group owing to seasonal pollen exposure, whereas the responses in the two treatment groups were blunted.

Nasal lavage fluids were collected from a randomly selected subgroup of 23 subjects at the end of the birch pollen season following the course of immunotherapy and again 12 months after the time point at which treatment had commenced [47]. Bet v 1–specific lavage fluid IgG1 levels were significantly raised at the end of the pollen season in subjects who had received the active preparations (10 trimer; 3 fragment mixture) when compared with placebo subjects. Higher levels of IgG2 and IgG4 were also detected as in serum, but these differences were not significant. There were also no apparent differences in IgA levels. There were correlations between the various IgG subgroup concentrations in serum and lavage fluid. At the end of the birch pollen season, there was a correlation between nasal IgG4 and reduced specific nasal sensitivity. Perhaps not surprisingly, the nasal antibody levels mirrored those in serum. The reduced nasal sensitivity may be accounted for by the inhibitory effect of the antibodies on basophil and mast cell mediator release as demonstrated for the serum antibodies in vitro.

Investigations of cytokine responses conducted in one of the other two study centers showed that treatment with trimer resulted in significant reductions in interleukin-5 (IL-5) and IL-13 producing cells when compared pre- and posttreatment, which was indicative of a suppression of the Th2 response [48]. There were also trends for decreased numbers of IL-4 producing cells and increased numbers of IL-12 producing cells, but the differences were not significant, most likely because of the small number of subjects (8 trimer, 10 fragment mixture, and 8 placebo). The results from measurements of immunologic parameters provide an encouraging basis for pursuing the development of hypoallergenic derivatives, but emphasis must be placed on the generation of data to provide evidence of clinical efficacy.

An alternative strategy for developing a hypoallergenic derivative came from the observation that recombinant Bet v 1 can be induced to adopt a stable random coil structure that can be clearly distinguished from the secondary structure of the native molecule by circular dichroism spectroscopy. This folding variant, designated Bet v 1-FV, exhibits hypoallergenic properties as judged by immunoassay inhibition tests and basophil activation [43,49]. The first clinical trial to test this derivative began in 2003. Subjects with birch pollen rhinitis were included in an open randomized comparative study of recombinant Bet v 1-FV and a natural birch pollen extract, both adsorbed to aluminum hydroxide. Treatment was administered over a period of 4 months before the birch pollen season, with injections given at weekly intervals. The maximum dose of Bet v 1-FV was 80μg, fourfold higher than the Bet v 1 content of the natural allergen preparation. Preliminary results following the first year's treatment indicate that the combined

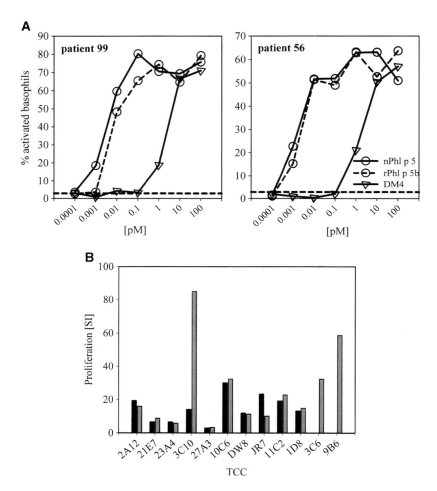

Fig. 2. Comparison of the natural timothy grass pollen allergen Phl p 5 with recombinant Phl p 5b and the genetically engineered derivative DM4. (*A*) Peripheral blood mononuclear cells from grass pollen–allergic subjects were incubated with various concentrations of the proteins or the diluent solution. Basophil activation was measured by fluorescence activated flow cytometry in terms of expression of the surface marker CD203c. (*B*) Lymphocyte proliferation, expressed as a stimulation index (SI), was determined in terms of ^{3}H-thymidine incorporation by T-cell clones (TCC) derived from nine grass pollen–allergic subjects and showed specificity for five distinct T-cell epitopes distributed throughout the protein. Cells were stimulated with rPhl p 5b (*black bars*) and rPhl p 5 variant DM4 (*gray bars*).

symptom-medication score for subjects receiving the recombinant preparation is favorably less than that for subjects receiving the natural pollen extract. The scores for both groups are superior to those of a reference group with only antisymptomatic treatment (parallel control group). Improvements in specific nasal sensitivity, as judged by a nasal provocation test, have been seen in both study groups, and the immunogenic activity of the recombinant preparation is confirmed by its ability to induce strong IgG1 and IgG4 antibody responses. Safety data indicate that the preparations are comparable with respect to the occurrence of adverse events. Again, the results are encouraging for further development of the hypoallergenic preparation, but final data on clinical efficacy will be important.

Recombinant hypoallergenic variants of grass pollen allergens

Information on both T cell and IgE-binding epitopes was used as a basis for designing mutants of group 5 allergens from timothy grass and rye grass pollen [31,50]. Various candidate derivatives were produced. Although partial reduction in IgE reactivity could be achieved through introduction of point mutations, more dramatic results were obtained by creating small deletions in the molecule. Two deletions, one of 20 amino acid residues and one of 25, were introduced at sites outside five distinct T-cell epitope regions and resulted in a variant (designated DM4) with substantially reduced IgE-binding activity, skin test reactivity, and histamine-releasing activity while largely retaining T-cell reactivity (Fig. 2). Larger deletions or deletions at other sites often resulted in hypoallergenic molecules but invariably considerable loss of T-cell reactivity [31].

The DM4 mutant was subsequently tested in a group of 22 grass pollen–allergic subjects, 19 of whom reacted with at least one concentration of natural or recombinant Phl p 5b, which served as reference preparations [51]. The wheal responses to recombinant Phl p 5b were smaller than those to the natural molecule but not significantly. In contrast, the wheal response to DM4 was significantly smaller than that to the two reference preparations (Fig. 3). The measurement of IgE reactivity to each of the proteins supported these results, and, in the majority of cases, serum IgE failed to bind to the DM4.

The DM4 variant of Phl p 5b is seen as a potential candidate for a thera-peutic vaccine for grass pollen–specific immunotherapy, but before planning any clinical studies, it will be necessary to develop derivatives of other grass pollen allergens to create a mixture that can account for all of the major causes of sensitization.

Recombinant grass pollen allergens

The grass *Phleum pratense* is a member of the subfamily Pooideae, which, in turn, belongs to the family Poaceae. It shows substantial cross-reactivity with

274 CROMWELL et al

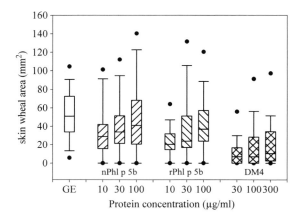

Fig. 3. Comparison of median skin test wheal responses to the natural timothy grass pollen allergen Phl p 5b with those to recombinant Phl p 5b and the genetically engineered derivative DM4. A grass pollen extract (GE) and three concentrations of each of the test proteins were skin prick tested in triplicate on the volar forearms of 22 grass pollen–allergic subjects using a random scheme. Boxes show the 25th and 75th percentiles; bars show the fifth and 95th percentiles; and dots show the outliers.

other members of the subfamily [36]; therefore, it can be considered representative of grasses found in temperate regions. Separate aluminum hydroxide adsorbates of the recombinant allergens Phl p 1, Phl p 2, Phl p 5a, Phl p 5b, and Phl p 6 were prepared and mixed together to create a therapeutic vaccine, with approximately equimolar amounts of the individual allergens. This mixture of allergens accounts for a substantial proportion of the specific IgE sensitization developed against grass pollen; therefore, it is realistic to expect that it could be effective against a substantial part of the symptoms.

A double-blind, placebo-controlled clinical trial was undertaken with 62 grass pollen–allergic patients sustaining rhinoconjunctivitis with or without asthma [52]. The recombinant allergen adsorbate was administered in subcutaneous injections of increasing concentrations at 7-day intervals before the pollen season in 2002, starting with 0.02 µg of total protein, followed by 0.16 µg and then doubling to 40 µg of total protein (0.8 mL). The maximum dose contained 10 µg of Phlp1, 5 µg of Phlp 2, 10 µg of Phlp 5a, 10 µg of Phlp 5b, and 5 µg of Phlp 6. Maintenance injections were continued until after the subsequent pollen season with a 50% reduction during each pollen season. The median cumulative dose was 490 µg of total protein, corresponding to 122.5 µg each of Phl p 1, Phl p 5a, and Phl p 5b, and 61.25 µg of Phl p 2 and Phl p 6.

A symptom-medication score was the primary outcome measure to assess efficacy. Subjects kept diaries for 3 months over each pollen season to record the nature and severity of eye, nose, and chest symptoms and the type and dose of any medication. The intensity of symptoms was documented as follows: 0 = no symptoms, 1 = mild symptoms, 2 = moderate symptoms, 3 = severe symptoms. The same rescue medication was available to all subjects, and use was scored taking into account pharmacokinetic and pharmacodynamic characteristics. A per protocol analysis included 24 active treatment and 25 placebo patients. A combined symptom-medication score adopted as the primary endpoint showed a 39% improvement in the active treatment group when compared with the placebo group ($P = .0\,44$). Symptoms alone improved by 37% ($P = .015$), and the use of symptomatic medication decreased by 36.5% in a comparison with the placebo group.

A validated rhinitis quality of life questionnaire was a secondary endpoint [53]. Questionnaires were completed every 2 weeks during the pollen season, and the questionnaire following the maximum pollen count was used for analysis. Benefits were registered for subjects on active treatment during the first pollen season. The per protocol evaluation during the second pollen season showed even greater differences between active and placebo treatment with an overall significant benefit ($P = .024$), providing further evidence of clinical efficacy. Significant effects were seen in five of seven domains tested (Fig. 4). The level of clinically relevant improvement for individual subjects was considered to be 0.5, and the mean between group differences that were judged statistically significant were all considerably in excess of this figure. Conjunctival provocation tests were performed before therapy (inclusion criterion) and at the end of the study using a standardized six-grass allergen extract. The concentration was increased in half-log steps starting with 5 biologic units (BU)/mL until a positive reaction was obtained or a maximum concentration of 5000 BU/mL (0.18μg of group 5 allergen/drop) was reached. A favorable trend was observed ($P = .081$),

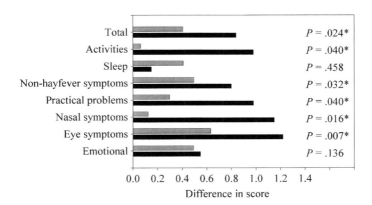

Fig. 4. Rhinitis quality of life questionnaire for subjects undergoing immunotherapy with a mixture of five recombinant *Phleum pratense* pollen allergens. Bars show differences between active and placebo treatment groups in pollen seasons during the first and second years of the study, 2002 (*gray*) and 2003 (*black*), respectively. Questionnaires completed immediately following the maximum pollen count were used for analysis. Mann-Whitney U-test results and *P* values for the 2003 season are shown. (*From* Jutel M, Jaeger L, Suck R, et al. Allergen-specific immunotherapy with recombinant grass pollen allergens. J Allergy Clin Immunol 2005:116(3);611; with permission from the American Academy of Allergy, Asthma, and Immunology.)

with an increase in the threshold dose in favor of treatment with the active preparation. The failure to achieve a significant result was most likely attributable to the small numbers of patients.

Active treatment induced highly significant increases in IgG1 and IgG4 grass pollen–specific antibody concentrations together with a significant decrease in

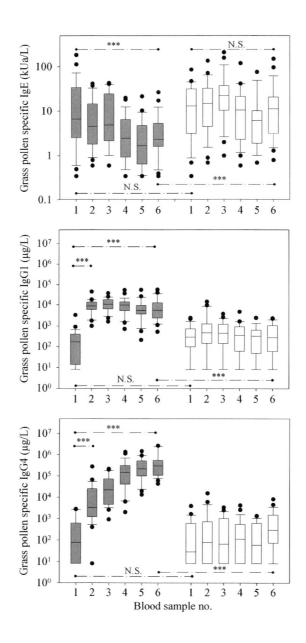

IgE (Fig. 5). IgG1 increased approximately 60-fold, peaking during the first 12 months of the study. IgG4 showed a continuing upward trend, achieving an approximately 4000-fold increase by the end of treatment. Specific IgE levels were not significantly different between groups at the beginning of the study, but thereafter the active treatment group showed a downward trend with values significantly less than baseline. Four subjects in each group had no Phl p 5a/b–specific IgE before the study but reacted to Phl p 1 and other grass pollen allergens. None of these subjects developed Phl p 5a/b IgE antibodies during the study, although the four subjects receiving active treatment developed strong IgG4 and IgG1 Phl p 5a/b responses consistent with induction of a protective immune response. This observation obviously needs to be substantiated. It will also be of interest to look at the prophylactic effects of the treatment in guarding against the development of new sensitizations.

Treatment-related adverse events were seen in association with 78 injections (10.7%) in the active treatment group and 44 injections (5.9%) in the placebo group. Local reactions involving erythema and swelling near the injection site, with or without pruritus, accounted for nearly all of these events. Single systemic reactions were seen in seven active treatment and two placebo subjects, the former including general urticaria (2 cases), local urticaria (2 cases), dyspnea (1 case), rhinoconjunctivitis (1 case), and asthma (1 case) 2 days following the injection. All of these subjects continued treatment without further problems, and it was concluded that the preparation showed a favorable safety profile when compared with findings from other immunotherapy studies.

Potential benefits of recombinant allergens for specific immunotherapy

Recombinant DNA technology has delivered the prospect of a new generation of preparations for allergen-specific immunotherapy. The first clinical studies with recombinant allergens have yielded encouraging results, suggesting that there is a good chance that such preparations will become available for use in the

Fig. 5. Grass pollen–specific IgE, IgG1, and IgG4 antibody concentrations in blood from subjects undergoing immunotherapy with a mixture of five recombinant *Phleum pratense* pollen allergens. Median values are shown with 25th/75th and 10th/90th percentiles represented by boxes and error bars, respectively, and outliers by points. Gray bars denote the active group and white bars the placebo group. Time points: 1, before immunotherapy, 1/2002–2/2002; 2, after initial dosage increase and before pollen season, 4/2002–5/2002; 3, after the pollen season, 7/2002–9/2002; 4, after 12 months, 1/2003–3/2003; 5, before the pollen season, 4/2003–5/2003; 6, at the end of the study, 8/2003–9/2003. ***$P < .001$; NS, nonsignificant. (*From* Jutel M, Jaeger L, Suck R, et al. Allergen-specific immunotherapy with recombinant grass pollen allergens. J Allergy Clin Immunol 2005:116(3);611; with permission from the American Academy of Allergy, Asthma, and Immunology.)

routine management of allergic disease. Some of the advantages and benefits that may be achieved with these preparations can be summarized as follows:

- Although a large proportion of the proteins and other molecules in an allergen extract may have no relevance to allergy, recombinant preparations include only allergens or allergen derivatives.
- The proteins can be produced in high purity to exacting pharmaceutical standards.
- There is no risk that unrelated allergens, infectious agents, or irritants can contaminate a preparation.
- Different allergens stemming from the same source (eg, grass pollen) can be mixed together in appropriate amounts (possibly equimolar concentrations) to achieve an optimal therapeutic formulation in contrast to the composition of native allergen extracts, which is determined largely by the raw material from which they are derived.
- Standardization, product consistency, and declaration of the concentrations of the active pharmaceutical ingredients are easily achieved.
- The technology provides the means for producing precisely defined hypoallergenic derivatives that may make it possible to achieve an enhanced benefit-risk ratio.

References

[1] Bauchau V, Durham SR. Prevalence and rate of diagnosis of allergic rhinitis in Europe. Eur Resp J 2004;24(5):758–64.
[2] Trivedi B, Valerio C, Slater JE. Endotoxin content of standardized allergen vaccines. J Allergy Clin Immunol 2003;111(4):777–83.
[3] Crameri R, Jaussi R, Menz G, et al. Display of expression products of cDNA libraries on phage surfaces: a versatile screening for selective isolation of genes by specific gene-product/ligand interaction. Eur J Biochem 1994;226:53–8.
[4] Crameri R. Recombinant *Aspergillus fumigatus* allergens: from the nucleotide sequences to clinical applications. Int Arch Allergy Immunol 1998;115(2):99–114.
[5] Wagner B, Fuchs H, Adhami F, et al. Plant virus expression systems for transient production of recombinant allergens in *Nicotiana benthamiana*. Methods 2004;32(3):227–34.
[6] Horvath H, Huang J, Wong O, et al. The production of recombinant proteins in transgenic barley grains. Proc Natl Acad Sci USA 2000;97(4):1914–9.
[7] Jacquet A, Magi M, Petry H, et al. High-level expression of recombinant house dust mite allergen Der p 1 in *Pichia pastoris*. Clin Exp Allergy 2002;32(7):1048–53.
[8] Cromwell O, Suck R, Kahlert H, et al. Transition of recombinant allergens from bench to clinical application. Methods 2004;32(3):300–12.
[9] Batard T, Didierlaurent A, Chabre H, et al. Characterization of wild-type recombinant Bet v 1a as a candidate vaccine against birch pollen allergy. Int Arch Allergy Immunol 2005; 136(3):239–49.
[10] Suck R, Petersen A, Weber B, et al. Analytical and preparative native polyacrylamide gel electrophoresis: investigation of the recombinant and natural major grass pollen allergen Phl p 2. Electrophoresis 2004;25:14–9.
[11] Kahlert H, Cromwell O, Fiebig H. Measurement of basophil-activating capacity of grass

pollen allergens, allergoids and hypoallergenic recombinant derivatives by flow cytometry using anti-CD203c. Clin Exp Allergy 2003;33(9):1266–72.

[12] van der Veen MJ, Mulder M, Witteman AM, et al. False-positive skin prick test responses to commercially available dog dander extracts caused by contamination with house dust mite (*Dermatophagoides pteronyssinus*) allergens. J Allergy Clin Immunol 1996;98(6 Pt 1): 1028–34.

[13] Maasch HJ, Marsh DG. Standardized extracts: modified allergens—allergoids. Clin Rev Allergy 1987;5(1):89–106.

[14] Kahlert H, Stüwe HT, Cromwell O, et al. Reactivity of T cells with grass pollen allergen extract and allergoid. Int Arch Allergy Immunol 1999;120:146–57.

[15] Kahlert H, Grage-Griebenow E, Stüwe HT, et al. T cell reactivity with allergoids: influence of the type of APC. J Immunol 2000;165:1807–15.

[16] Corrigan C, Kettner J, Doemer C, et al. Efficacy and safety of preseasonal-specific immunotherapy with an aluminum-adsorbed six-grass pollen allergoid. Allergy 2005;60(6):801–7.

[17] Akdis CA, Blaser K. Regulation of specific immune responses by chemical and structural modifications of allergens. Int Arch Allergy Immunol 2000;121:261–9.

[18] Bhalla PL, Singh MB. Engineered allergens for immunotherapy. Curr Opin Allergy Clin Immunol 2004;4(6):569–73.

[19] Ferreira F, Wallner M, Breiteneder H, et al. Genetic engineering of allergens: future therapeutic products. Int Arch Allergy Immunol 2002;128(3):171–8.

[20] Tighe H, Takabayashi K, Schwartz D, et al. Conjugation of immunostimulatory DNA to the short ragweed allergen Amb a 1 enhances its immunogenicity and reduces its allergenicity. J Allergy Clin Immunol 2000;106(1):124–34.

[21] Haselden BM, Kay AB, Larche M. Immunoglobulin E-independent major histocompatibility complex-restricted T cell peptide epitope-induced late asthmatic reactions. J Exp Med 1999; 189(12):1885–94.

[22] Kay AB, Larche M. Allergen immunotherapy with cat allergen peptides. Springer Semin Immunopathol 2004;25(3–4):391–9.

[23] Verhoef A, Alexander C, Kay AB, et al. T cell epitope immunotherapy induces a CD4+ T cell population with regulatory activity. PLoS Med 2005;2(3):e78.

[24] Hirahara K, Tatsuta T, Takatori T, et al. Preclinical evaluation of an immunotherapeutic peptide comprising 7 T-cell determinants of Cry j 1 and Cry j 2, the major Japanese cedar pollen allergens. J Allergy Clin Immunol 2001;108(1):94–100.

[25] Vrtala S, Hirtenlehner K, Vangelista L, et al. Conversion of the major birch pollen allergen, Bet v 1, into two nonanaphylactic T cell epitope-containing fragments: candidates for a novel form of specific immunotherapy. J Clin Invest 1997;99(7):1673–81.

[26] Vrtala S, Hirtenlehner K, Susani M, et al. Genetic engineering of a hypoallergenic trimer of the major birch pollen allergen, Bet v 1. FASEB J 2001;15(11):2045–7.

[27] Fiebig H, Suck R, Kahlert H, et al. Immunologische Eigenschaften von rekombinanten Allergenen. In: Ring J, Darsow U, editors. Allergie 2000: Probleme, Strategien und praktische Konsequenzen. München: Dustri-Verlag; 2001. p. 75–82.

[28] Linhart B, Hartl A, Jahn-Schmid B, et al. A hybrid molecule resembling the epitope spectrum of grass pollen for allergy vaccination. J Allergy Clin Immunol 2005;115(5):1010–6.

[29] Linhart B, Jahn-Schmid B, Verdino P, et al. Combination vaccines for the treatment of grass pollen allergy consisting of genetically engineered hybrid molecules with increased immunogenecity. FASEB J 2002;16:1301–3.

[30] Takai T, Yokota T, Yasue M, et al. Engineering of the major house dust mite allergen Der f 2 for allergen-specific immunotherapy. Nat Biotechnol 1997;15(8):754–8.

[31] Schramm G, Kahlert H, Suck R, et al. "Allergen engineering": Variants of the timothy grass pollen allergen Phl p 5b with reduced IgE-binding capacity but conserved T cell reactivity. J Immunol 1999;162(4):2406–14.

[32] Ferreira F, Hirtenlehner K, Jilek A, et al. Dissection of immunoglobulin E and T lymphocyte reactivity of isoforms of the major birch pollen allergen bet v 1: potential use of hypoallergenic isoforms for immunotherapy. J Exp Med 1996;183(2):599–609.

[33] Arquint O, Helbling A, Crameri R, et al. Reduced in vivo allergenicity of Bet v 1d isoform, a natural component of birch pollen. J Allergy Clin Immunol 1999;104(6):1239–43.

[34] Punnonen J. Molecular breeding of allergy vaccines and antiallergic cytokines. Int Arch Allergy Immunol 2000;121(3):173–82.

[35] Linhart B, Valenta R. Vaccine engineering improved by hybrid technology. Int Arch Allergy Immunol 2004;134(4):324–31.

[36] Andersson K, Lidholm J. Characteristics and immunobiology of grass pollen allergens. Int Arch Allergy Immunol 2003;130(2):87–107.

[37] Suphioglu C. What are the important allergens in grass pollen that are linked to human allergic disease? Clin Exp Allergy 2000;30(10):1335–41.

[38] Rossi RE, Monasterolo G, Monasterolo S. Measurement of IgE antibodies against purified grass-pollen allergens (Phl p 1, 2, 3, 4, 5, 6, 7, 11, and 12) in sera of patients allergic to grass pollen. Allergy 2001;56(12):1180–5.

[39] Osterballe O. Immunotherapy in hay fever with two major allergens 19, 25 and partially purified extract of timothy grass pollen: a controlled double-blind study. In vivo variables, season I. Allergy 1980;35:473–89.

[40] Osterballe O, Lowenstein H, Prahl P, et al. Immunotherapy in hay fever with two major allergens 19, 25 and partially purified extract of timothy grass pollen: a controlled double-blind study. In vitro variables, season I. Allergy 1981;36:183–99.

[41] Valenta R, Lidholm J, Niederberger V, et al. The recombinant allergen-based concept of component-resolved diagnostics and immunotherapy (CRD and CRIT). Clin Exp Allergy 1999; 29(7):896–904.

[42] Vrtala S, Focke M, Sperr W, et al. Recombinant hypoallergenic fragments of the major Timothy grass pollen allergen, Phl p 6, for immunotherapy. J Allergy Clin Immunol 2001; 107(2):S257.

[43] Kahlert H, Weber B, Cromwell O, et al. Evaluation of the allergenicity of hypoallergenic recombinant derivatives of Bet v 1 using basophil activation by CD203c expression measurement. In: Marone G, editor. Clinical immunology and allergy in medicine. Naples: JGC Editions; 2003. p. 735–40.

[44] van Hage-Hamsten M, Kronqvist M, Zetterström O, et al. Skin test evaluation of genetically engineered hypoallergenic derivatives of the major birch pollen allergen, Bet v 1: results obtained with a mix of two recombinant Bet v 1 fragments and recombinant Bet v 1 trimer in a Swedish population before the birch pollen season. J Allergy Clin Immunol 1999; 104(5):969–77.

[45] Pauli G, Purohit A, Oster JP, et al. Comparison of genetically engineered hypoallergenic rBet v 1 derivatives with rBet v 1 wild-type by skin prick and intradermal testing: results obtained in a French population. Clin Exp Allergy 2000;30(8):1076–84.

[46] Niederberger V, Horak F, Vrtala S, et al. Vaccination with genetically engineered allergens prevents progression of allergic disease. Proc Natl Acad Sci USA 2004;101(Suppl.2): 14677–82.

[47] Reisinger J, Horak F, Pauli G, et al. Allergen-specific nasal IgG antibodies induced by vaccination with genetically modified allergens are associated with reduced nasal allergen sensitivity. J Allergy Clin Immunol 2005;116(2):347–54.

[48] Gafvelin G, Thunberg S, Kronqvist M, et al. Cytokine and antibody responses in birch-pollen-allergic patients treated with genetically modified derivatives of the major birch pollen allergen Bet v 1. Int Arch Allergy Immunol 2005;138(1):59–66.

[49] Weber B, Slamal H, Suck R. Size exclusion chromatography as a tool for quality control of recombinant allergens and hypoallergenic variants. J Biochem Biophys Meth 2003;56(1–3): 219–32.

[50] Swoboda I, de Weerd N, Bhalla PL, et al. Mutants of the major rye grass pollen allergen, Lol p 5, with reduced IgE-binding capacity: candidates for grass pollen-specific immunotherapy. Eur J Immunol 2002;32(1):270–80.

[51] Lepp U, Eberhardt F, Schramm G, et al. Approaches based on mutated or modified recombinant

grass pollen allergens: in vivo evaluation of the constructs. Arb Paul Ehrlich Inst Bundesamt Sera Impfstoffe Frankf A M 2003;94:188–91.

[52] Jutel M, Jaeger L, Suck R, et al. Allergen-specific immunotherapy with recombinant grass pollen allergens. J Allergy Clin Immunol 2005;116(3):608–13.

[53] Juniper EF, Guyatt GH. Development and testing of a new measure of health status for clinical trials in rhinoconjunctivitis. Clin Exp Allergy 1991;21(1):77–83.

ELSEVIER
SAUNDERS

Immunol Allergy Clin N Am
26 (2006) 283–306

IMMUNOLOGY
AND ALLERGY
CLINICS
OF NORTH AMERICA

Novel Ways for Immune Intervention in Immunotherapy: Mucosal Allergy Vaccines

Laurent Mascarell, PhD, Laurence Van Overtvelt, PhD, Philippe Moingeon, PhD*

Research and Development, Stallergènes SA, 6 Rue Alexis de Tocqueville, Antony Cedex 92160, France

Subcutaneous immunotherapy (SCIT) has been investigated for almost a century [1,2] and is currently used to treat allergies to insect venom, house dust mites (HDMs), grass and tree pollens, and animal epithelia [3–8]. Currently, allergen-specific immunotherapy is considered the only curative treatment for type I allergies because of its capacity to reorient inappropriate humoral and cellular immune responses. Although SCIT is considered a reference therapy, it requires multiple injections and can be associated with severe side effects, including anaphylactic shock. Thus, safer and noninvasive mucosal routes, including nasal, oral, and sublingual routes of administration, are considered an alternative to SCIT.

A rationale for administering immunotherapy through the mucosal route is that the immune system in aerodigestive mucosae is poised to induce immune tolerance rather than immunostimulation when exposed to antigens and allergens from the environment [9,10]. Mucosal tolerance is believed to be a consequence of either anergy (after the depletion of responsive cells) or the induction of suppressive mechanisms mediated by regulatory T lymphocytes [11]. In light of a better understanding of immune mechanisms associated with successful antiallergic treatments, new strategies can be implemented to improve mucosal allergy vaccines. The latter may rely on modified or unmodified recombinant

* Corresponding author.
E-mail address: pmoingeon@stallergenes.fr (P. Moingeon).

Table 1
Comparison between systemic and mucosal routes for allergy vaccination

Route of immunization	Allergens	Comments	References
Subcutaneous immunotherapy (SCIT)	Pollens (ragweed, birch, grasses, *Parietaria*, olive), dust mites, cat dander, venoms Used as natural biologic extracts, allergoids, recombinant protein (Bet v 1, Phl p 1, 2, 5, 6), purified natural allergen (Amb a1) or peptides (Fel d 1, PLA A2), associated with an adjuvant (eg, CaPO4, alum, monophosphoryl lipid A [MPL])	Clinical efficacy: SCIT with house dust mites (HDM) or pollen (grass and tree) extracts reduces asthma and rhinoconjunctivitis symptoms and antiallergic drug intake. SCIT decreases allergen-specific skin, nose, and eye sensitivity after natural allergen exposure or challenge. SCIT with hypoallergenic Bet v 1 forms (peptide fragment and trimer) inhibits immediate-type allergic reactions. Patients treated with Fel d 1 peptides experience a decrease in skin reactivity concomitantly with a decrease in Th1/Th2 responses and an induction of circulating IL10–producing regulatory T (Treg) cells. Immunotherapy with peptides from PLA A2 (a major bee venom allergen) induces tolerance after allergen and bee sting challenge in allergic patients. Immune mechanisms: Antibody responses: During SCIT (grass, ragweed and birch pollens), an improvement in symptoms is often associated with an increase in allergen-specific IgG (mostly IgG4) and a reduction of specific IgE antibodies. IgG4 inhibit binding of allergen-IgE complexes to inflammatory cells, thereby preventing histamine release. SCIT with recombinant grass pollen allergens (hypoallergenic Bet v 1 or a mixture of five allergens) improves rhinitis symptoms while up-regulating IgG (1, 2, and 4) antibodies. MPL associated with grass pollen allergens increases the production of specific IgG1 and IgG4 antibodies.	[3–8,24] [118–120] [17,22,24,80,81, 121,122]

Cellular responses:

SCIT prevents migration and activation of inflammatory cells (mast cells, eosinophils, basophils, neutrophils) within target organs (skin, nose, lung). After successful SCIT, the level of inflammatory mediators (histamine, kinins, PGD2, myeloperoxidase) is reduced. [18,19,25–30]

SCIT reorients allergen-specific T-cell responses in atopic patients from a Th2 to Th1 pattern. A correlation is often established between successful SCIT and an increase in the Th1/Th2 cytokine balance. In certain studies, the increase of the Th1/Th2 ratio is not observed at the beginning of the treatment, but only during high-dose maintenance therapy. The shift from Th2 to Th1 responses is sometimes noticeable mostly within the target organ (eg, nasal mucosa, skin). Successful SCIT with recombinant hypoallergenic Bet v 1 (peptide fragments and trimer) is associated with a reduced production of IL-4, IL-5, and IL-13 by allergen-specific T cells, whereas IFN-γ and IL-12 production is increased. SCIT for wasp venom, HDM, cat, and grass or birch pollen allergies induces allergen-specific regulatory cells (CD4+ CD25+ or Type 1 regulatory cells [Tr1]) in the blood. [19,33–37,123]

[23,119,124–126]

Clinical efficacy:

LNIT with HDM or pollen (tree and grass) allergens in natural or allergoid forms reduces symptoms/medication scores in patients with allergic rhinitis. Allergoids are better-tolerated than aqueous extracts when used intranasally but the therapeutic benefit is lower. Macronized powder forms of pollens (eg, *Parietaria*, birch, grass) or mites have been used, leading to improved clinical efficacy and long-lasting protective effects in patients who have rhinitis. [41–47,50]

Local nasal immunotherapy (LNIT)

Pollens (ragweed, grasses, *Parietaria*), dust mites
Used as natural biologic extracts, allergoids, macronized powder forms, without any adjuvant

(continued on next page)

Table 1 (*continued*)

Route of immunization	Allergens	Comments	References
Local nasal immunotherapy (LNIT)		Immune mechanisms: Antibody responses: A rise in IgA, IgE, and IgG antibodies is observed during LNIT with aqueous or chemically modified (allergoid) pollens (ragweed and grass). No significant immunologic change is induced in LNIT with macronized powder pollen extracts (eg, *Parietaria*).	[41–47,50]
		Cellular responses: Successful LNIT to *Parietaria* significantly reduces inflammatory infiltration and intercellular adhesion molecule (ICAM-1) expression on nasal epithelial cells after allergen challenge. No change in soluble eosinophil cationic protein is detected.	[48]
		In preclinical models, nasal administration of recombinant Ves v 5 before sensitization with wasp venom reduces Th2 polarization (humoral and cellular responses) in association with an increase in TGF-β and IL-10 mRNA in spleen cells. In another study, immunologic tolerance was achieved after intranasal immunization with ovalbumin (OVA) as a consequence of induction of anergy and stimulation of OVA-specific CD4 + regulatory T cells.	[51,52]
Oral immunotherapy (OIT)	Grass and birch pollens Used as natural biologic extract in aqueous, freeze-dried, powder forms, tablets, enterosoluble capsules, without any adjuvant	Clinical efficacy: OIT using low or high doses of grass pollen does not improve skin and nasal reactivity to allergens. In contrast, OIT with birch pollen extracts reduces asthma/rhinitis symptoms in adults and children. Oral tolerance induction with myelin basic protein or collagen-derived peptides in	[10,55–57,60–62]

multiple sclerosis or rheumatoid arthritis, respectively, leads to some level of clinical improvement.

Immune mechanisms:

Antibody responses:

No changes in specific IgE and IgG have been detected in OIT with grass pollen allergen extracts. OIT with birch pollen extracts decreases specific IgE and up-regulates IgG antibodies. [55–57,60–62,127]

Cellular responses:

OIT with grass pollen does not change histamine secretion by basophils. [56]

Numerous studies in murine models show that CD4+ Treg cells are involved in oral tolerance induction.

These Treg cells include Th3 cells synthesizing TGF-β and/or IL-10, Tr1 cells producing IL-10, and CD4+ CD25+ T cells. [11]

Clinical efficacy:

SLIT to HDM or pollens is safe and improves symptoms (asthma, rhinitis) and quality-of-life in adults and children. Current protocols use the sublingual–swallow procedure (rather than the sublingual–spit, which is less efficacious). After a 4- to 6-week titration phase, the maximal dose is administered several times a week over years. Doses of allergens used for SLIT are at least 50 fold higher than for SCIT. High doses of *Parietaria judaica* extracts given to allergy prone children reduce rhinitis symptoms and skin reactivity after the second year of SLIT treatment. In adults, preseasonal rush SLIT against *P judaica* decreases clinical symptoms. Side effects for SLIT include oral itching, swelling and abdominal pain. [69,70,86,128]

Sublingual immunotherapy (SLIT)

Venoms, pollens (ragweed, birch, grasses, *Parietaria*, olive), dust mites

Used as natural biologic extracts, allergoids without any adjuvant

(continued on next page)

Table 1 (*continued*)

Route of immunization	Allergens	Comments	References
Sublingual immunotherapy		Immune mechanisms: Antibody responses: SLIT enhances allergen-specific IgG4 production in many studies, whereas IgE is often unaltered. In a few studies, a dose-dependent induction of allergen-specific IgA is observed.	[68,69,71,129]
		Cellular responses: SLIT with grass pollen or HDM down-regulates ICAM-1 expression in epithelial cells. Preseasonal rush SLIT using *Parietaria* in patients who have asthma reduces recruitment of neutrophils and eosinophils and ICAM-1 expression in the nose after allergen provocation. In children allergic to olive pollen, SLIT reduces rhinitis and skin reactivity in parallel with seric eosinophil cationic protein (ECP) during the peak season. SLIT against grass pollen or HDM decreases nasal secretion of ECP and tryptase in children.	[72,75,82–86]
		In several studies, SLIT had no impact on the Th1/Th2 balance. Children who have asthma treated with *Dermatophagoides pteronyssinus* extracts exhibited a decrease in seric IL-13 and T-cell proliferation.	[87–89]
		A pilot study indicated that peripheral blood mononuclear cells from patients treated with HDM-SLIT produce high levels of IL-10.	[90]

allergens or derived peptides associated with new vectors and adjuvant molecules to enhance allergen-specific regulatory T-cell responses.

Immune tolerance after subcutaneous allergen-specific immunotherapy

After the pioneer studies by Noon [1] almost a century ago, allergen-specific SCIT was established based on clinical efficacy as a reference for curative treatment of allergies [3–8]. Venom SCIT is a very effective treatment in patients allergic to Vespula or honeybees. SCIT is also efficacious in treating rhinoconjunctivitis and asthma associated with grass and tree pollens, dust mites (eg, *Dermatophagoides pteronyssinus, D farinae, Lepidoglyphus destructor*), cat dander, and *Cladosporium* or Alternaria [3]. SCIT reduces immediate (ie, linked to the release of inflammatory mediators such as histamine or prostaglandin D2) and late phase (ie, linked to the activation of mast cells and eosinophils) allergen-induced symptoms in target organs (Table 1) [4,12–16].

Successful SCIT is often associated with a decrease in the sera of allergen-specific IgE antibody production concomitant with an up-regulation of IgGs, particularly IgG1 and IgG4s, some of which may exhibit a potential blocking activity (see Table 1) [17]. Such an altered IgE/IgG4 antibody balance contributes to the reduction of IgE-mediated histamine release by basophils and antigen presentation to T cells [18–21]. Researchers have suggested that during SCIT, the affinity of IgE antibodies for allergens is potentially decreased, whereas the affinity of allergen-specific IgG4 antibodies seems enhanced [22]. A limited number of studies have also documented an increase in seric IgA antibodies [23,24]. Successful SCIT also inhibits the recruitment and activation of proinflammatory cells, such as mast cells, basophils, and eosinophils in the skin, nose, eye, and bronchial mucosae, as shown after provocation or natural exposure to allergens (see Table 1) [18,19,25–30].

In the current view of the immune system (Fig. 1), CD4+ T lymphocytes play a critical role in controlling the various immune effector mechanisms contributing to allergic inflammation [31]. That allergic patients mount allergen-specific CD4+ T-cell responses of the T helper 2 (Th2) type (ie, associated with the secretion of interleukin (IL)-4, IL-5, and IL-13 cytokines [13,32]) is well established. Successful SCIT redirects those allergen-specific Th2 responses toward the Th1 type [33–37], with an increased production of IL-12 and interferon (IFN)-γ within the blood and target organs, such as the nasal mucosa or the skin (see Table 1). More recently, research established that SCIT also stimulates allergen-specific subsets of CD4+ regulatory T cells capable of down-regulating Th1 and Th2 responses through the production of IL-10 or transforming growth factor (TGF)-β and cell-to-cell contact (see Table 1) [31].

Taken together, SCIT is widely agreed to be effective in curing allergic rhinoconjunctivitis and preventing progression to asthma. However, repeated injections are needed over several years in the course of SCIT, which makes this treatment cumbersome, particularly for children. In addition, a major drawback

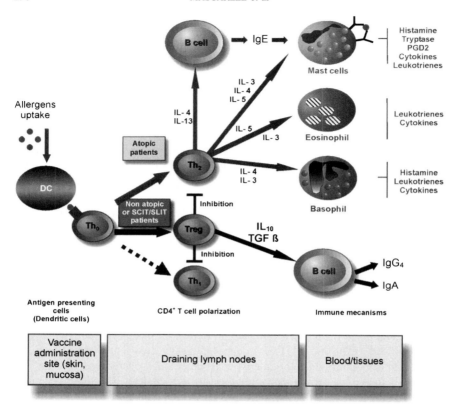

Fig. 1. Cellular and humoral mechanisms of allergen-specific immunotherapy. After allergen capture at the administration site, dendritic cells mature and migrate to draining lymph nodes where they stimulate naïve T cells (Th0). Depending on the cytokine milieu, Th0 cells can differentiate into various CD4$^+$ T helper cells producing distinct patterns of cytokines. Such CD4$^+$ T helper cells stimulated after allergen exposure or desensitization with the vaccine are critical in controlling antibody production and isotype switching, and recruitment and activation of proinflammatory cells (eg, mast cells, eosinophils, basophils). The purpose of allergen-specific immunotherapy is to restore immune tolerance by shifting T-cell responses from Th2 to Th1 regulatory T cells.

is the risk for serious systemic reactions such as anaphylaxis, which is infrequent but can be lethal [38]. Therefore, alternative vaccination strategies through the nasal, oral, or sublingual mucosal routes are being investigated.

Tolerance induction by mucosal immunotherapy

Intranasal immunotherapy

Local nasal immunotherapy (LNIT) has been evaluated in clinical trials for almost 3 decades with some encouraging results in terms of safety and efficacy (see Table 1) [39]. For example, LNIT with either aqueous extracts or chemically modified allergens (allergoids) elicited a marked reduction in symptoms and medication scores in patients who had allergic rhinitis to ragweed and grass pollens [40–42]. In general, chemically modified allergens were better-tolerated than aqueous extracts, although a lower therapeutic benefit was sometimes observed with the former [41,42]. Several studies have shown clinical efficacy of LNIT in patients who have allergic rhinitis to various pollens (eg, *Parietaria*, birch, grass) or mites when using allergens in a macronized powder form [43–47]. Medication and symptoms scores were improved and a long-lasting protective effect was observed, most particularly with regard to nasal symptoms [48]. In contrast, no significant clinical efficacy of LNIT could be shown in the second year after treatment with an allergoid grass vaccine [49]. Adverse reactions during LNIT are infrequent and generally restricted to the upper respiratory tract.

No clear immunologic changes correlating with vaccine efficacy have been noted in LNIT clinical trials [41–47,50]. Immune mechanisms underlying LNIT-induced tolerance have been investigated in mice. In such preclinical models, T-cell anergy, a decrease in Th2 responses, and an induction of TGF-β– and IL-10–producing regulatory T cells have been proposed to be potential mechanisms for tolerance induction through the nasal route [51,52]. Biodistribution studies of radiolabeled *Parietaria judaica* allergen (Par j 1) have been conducted in humans after intranasal administration. Such studies showed that most of the allergen is swallowed and absorbed through the gastrointestinal tract in volunteers who had allergies and those who did not, leading to a plasmatic peak 1 hour after administration [53,54]. A fraction of the allergen seems to persist up for to 24 hours in the nasal cavity in healthy volunteers but not in patients who are allergic. The rapid local clearance of the allergen observed in volunteers who were allergic likely involves IgE-mediated capture mechanisms.

Altogether, LNIT represents a safe and efficient treatment against grass pollen rhinitis. However, it requires particular technical skills, and controlling the exact dose administered is not trivial. Thus, these limitations have hampered its broad use in allergen-specific immunotherapy.

Oral immunotherapy

Oral immunotherapy (OIT) was investigated in the early 1980s in allergic patients [55–57]. Several studies were conducted in adults and children using an orally administered grass pollen extract, either as an aqueous solution, a powder, or enterosoluble tablets [55,56]. Although such oral grass pollen vaccines were well tolerated, no major impact was observed on symptom and medication scores or on skin or nasal reactivity (see Table 1). In addition, no significant alteration of seric allergen-specific IgG or IgE levels was found in patients undergoing OIT compared with those of patients undergoing therapy with placebo [55–57]. In parallel studies, immunotherapy using high doses of allergen formulated as enterosoluble grass pollen capsules also lacked any therapeutic effect [58,59]. In contrast, oral immunotherapy with high doses of encapsulated birch pollen extracts showed some clinical efficacy in adults and children who were allergic [58,59]. When compared with the placebo group, patients undergoing birch pollen OIT showed an increase in seric-specific IgG antibody levels, associated with a reduction in seasonal IgE levels [60–62]. Encouraging clinical efficacy data were also obtained for OIT in patients allergic to either *Dermatophagoides* sp, *Artemisia*, or ragweed pollen [63–65].

OIT has also been extensively evaluated as a potential treatment for non-allergic inflammatory or autoimmune diseases [9,10]. Because tolerance break-down of the intestinal immune system is known to cause inflammatory disorders, such as celiac or Crohn's disease, OIT is being considered in these patholo-gies [66]. Also, oral tolerance has shown some efficacy in preclinical models of autoimmune encephalomyelitis, arthritis, type I diabetes, thyroiditis, uveitis, ath-erosclerosis, and cerebrovascular stroke [9]. Using peptide vaccines, OIT was evaluated in patients who had rheumatoid arthritis, diabetes, or multiple sclerosis [10,11], with only a limited clinical benefit observed [10,11].

Regarding immunologic mechanisms involved during OIT, high doses of antigen administered orally are believed to promote T-cell depletion or anergy [11]. Alternatively, low-dose antigen tolerance is likely mediated through active suppressive mechanisms involving regulatory T cells. In all circumstances, in-creasing evidence suggests that dendritic cells play a crucial role in the regulation of mucosal immunity and tolerance as a consequence of their capacity to direct the fate of T cells. The level of costimulatory molecules and the cytokine milieu influence the degree of antigen-presenting cell (APC) maturation and activation, leading to systemic or suppressive T-cell responses [67]. Several studies focusing on $CD4^+$ regulatory T cells have shown that such cells are critical in the induction of oral tolerance [11]. Regulatory T cells induced during OIT are highly hetero-geneous and include Th3 cells (producing TGF-β or IL-10), Tr1 cells (producing IL-10), and $CD4^+$ $CD25^+$ cells, which mediate their regulatory function through cytokine secretion or cell contact–dependent mechanisms involving the cytotoxic T-lymphocyte associated antigen-4 (CTLA-4) or programmed death-1 (PD-1) mole-cules [11].

Although oral tolerance induction has been successful in several animal models, its clinical efficacy has not been firmly established in humans. Thus, a purely oral route of administration is not recommended as a routine approach in allergic immunotherapy.

Sublingual immunotherapy

More than a decade ago, SLIT was investigated in patients with allergies [68–75]. During sublingual immunization, the allergen extract is held under the tongue for at least 1 to 2 minutes to allow capture by oral Langerhans-like dendritic cells (LLDCs) before being swallowed. Wilson and colleagues [70] conducted a meta-analysis encompassing 22 randomized clinical studies evaluat-ing SLIT in 979 patients who had allergic rhinitis to HDMs, pollens (from grass, *Parietaria*, olive, ragweed, *Cupressus*), or cat dander. They concluded that

SLIT significantly reduces symptoms and medication requirements [70]. For example, high-dose SLIT has beneficial effects on nasal symptoms during the peak pollen season in patients who have severe seasonal allergic rhinitis, even if 2 years of treatment are required [76]. The safety and efficacy profile of SLIT has been confirmed in children, including those younger than 5 years [77]. In adults and children who had rhinitis, long-term clinical benefits in the form of prevention of new sensitizations or asthma were observed after SLIT [70]. A comparison of SCIT and SLIT regimens performed in a clinical trial in adult patients allergic to birch pollen showed no statistical difference in terms of efficacy between the two routes when high-dose SLIT regimens were used [78].

Biologic mechanisms underlying SLIT are being clarified [79]. As shown for the subcutaneous route, the IgE/IgG4 ratio is decreased in several clinically effective SLIT studies. SLIT most particularly increases allergen-specific IgG4 levels compared with placebo, as shown with house dust mites (HDM) and *Parietaria*/grass pollen vaccines [68,69,71]. Allergen-specific IgG (and possibly IgA) antibodies induced during SLIT are believed to compete with IgEs for binding to the allergen, thus preventing basophil or mastocyte degranulation (see Table 1) [24,80,81]. Within target organs (eg, eye or nose), SLIT reduces the recruitment of inflammatory cells induced by allergen challenge [75,82–85]. SLIT with grass pollen or HDM extracts also decreases the release of inflammatory mediators such as tryptase or eosinophil cationic protein in sputum or nasal secretions [82,84]. The expression of the *intercellular adhesion molecule 1* (*ICAM-1*), is also down-regulated on epithelial cells after SLIT [83,85]. Similarly, rush SLIT to *Parietaria* reduces the recruitment of neutrophils and eosinophils to the nasal mucosa, and the expression of the ICAM-1 molecule [86]. The impact of SLIT on allergen-specific T-cell polarization is still poorly documented. Although several SLIT studies have shown no impact on T-cell responses [87,88], successful sublingual immunotherapy in patients allergic to HDMs reduces the production of the Th2 cytokine IL-13 and the proliferation of peripheral blood mononuclear cells [89,90]. In a recent preliminary report, SLIT was found to stimulate IL-10–producing T cells in the peripheral blood of patients allergic HDMs, although no functional test was used to confirm that those cells were bona fide regulatory T cells [91].

Biodistribution studies in humans showed that no direct plasmatic absorption of allergens occurs through the sublingual mucosa [53,92]. Radiolabeled Par j 1 administered sublingually was detected in the plasma only after ingestion, with a peak between 1 and 2 hours after administration, implying absorption through the gut mucosa. Radiolabeled allergens persisted for up to 20 hours at the mucosal surface after SLIT, suggesting that allergen capture by Langerhans cells can occur during this time frame. The sublingual mucosa contains many LLDCs expressing constitutively high-affinity receptors for IgE (FcεRI), which are believed to play a crucial role in tolerance induction during desensitization [93]. Cross-linking of IgE receptors on LLDCs induces TGF-β and IL-10 cytokine production and the synthesis of indoleamine 2,3-dioxygenase (IDO), a tryptophan-catabolizing enzyme regulating T-cell proliferation [94,95]. After allergen capture in the sub-

Table 2
Vector systems and adjuvants for tolerance induction with mucosal allergy vaccines

	Comments	References
Immunodulators		
Whole bacteria		
Lactococcus lactis, Lactobacillus plantarum, Lactobacillus casei	In mice, mucosal administration of commensal bacteria adapted to the intestine such as *Lactococcus lactis* or *Lactobacillus plantarum* together with recombinant Bet v 1 induces IgG2a antibodies and IFN-γ production in mice sensitized to the allergen. A mutant of *Lactobacillus plantarum* altered in the teichoic acid biosynthesis pathway exhibits a superior protective capacity in a murine colitis model, as a consequence of enhanced production of IL-10. *Lactobacillus casei* reduces CD8+ T-cell–mediated skin inflammation controlled by specific CD4+ Treg cells.	[100–103]
Heat-killed *Mycobacterium vaccae*	Heat-killed *Mycobacterium vaccae* induces Treg cells secreting IL-10 and TGF-β, conferring protection against airway inflammation in mice. Some efficacy in children who have atopic dermatitis has also been observed after intradermal administration.	[104,105]
Natural/synthetic bacterial products		
Toxins and derivatives (CT, LT, CTB, LTB)	Genetically detoxified CT and LT (or B subunits) without ADP ribosyl transferase activity retain a strong mucosal adjuvanticity (ie, induction of seric and mucosal neutralizing IgA). Mice vaccinated with influenza virus hemagglutinin concomitantly with LTB or genetically detoxified LT develop strong and protective antigen-specific IgG and IgA responses. The antigen/allergen can be mixed, fused, or chemically conjugated with the toxin moiety.	[106,130,131]
Lipid A analogs (OM-174, monophosphoryl lipid A (MPL), RC 529)	Lipid A derivatives are powerful Th1 adjuvants when administered through a systemic route. OM-174 promotes DC migration to lymphoid organs and their maturation. Mucosal administration (nasal, oral) of antigen of interest with MPL or RC 529 induces seric and local IgA and Th1 responses (IgG2a and CTL). Grass pollen allergens combined with MPL induce a strong production of specific IgG1 and IgG4 antibodies through the subcutaneous route. MPL is being tested in humans as an adjuvant for the sublingual route.	[132–134]
CpG	Synthetic oligonucleotides containing CpG motifs (CpG ODN) are potent Th1 adjuvants. Mucosal delivery of CpG ODN together with proteins promotes systemic (IgG2a and CTLs) and mucosal (IgA and CTLs) responses. Intradermal immunization with Amb a 1 fused to CpG oligonucleotides prevents allergen-induced hyperresponsiveness in mice. A conjugate Amb a1-cpG vaccine is being tested in ragweed allergic humans through the subcutaneous route.	[135,136]

Synthetic muramyldipeptides (MDP)	MDP-Lys (L18) induces mucosal immune responses protecting against a lethal viral challenge (using Sendai virus or rotavirus).	[137]
Bacterial subunits	The purified protein derivative (PPD) from *Mycobacterium tuberculosis* can induce IL-10-producing T cells in humans. The filamentous hemagglutinin (FHA) from *Bordetella pertussis* can induce Tr1 cells *in vivo* in mice.	[138,139]
Cytokines		
IL-1, IL-12, IL-15, IL-18, GM-CSF, IFN-γ/β	Combinations of cytokines (mainly IL-1 + IL-12, IL-18, and GM-CSF) with an HIV-env peptide induce mucosal protection, with specific CTLs and IgG1 and IgA antibodies. IFN-γ/β is a strong mucosal adjuvant against influenza virus. DNA vaccines expressing cytokine genes also induce efficient mucosal immune responses. Coimmunization with plasmid-expressing influenza hemagglutinin with the IL-15 gene generates protective cytotoxic T-lymphocyte responses.	[107,108] [140,141]
Small synthetic molecules	In murine models, imidazoquinolines (ligands for TLR7), dihydroxyvitamin D₃ plus glucocorticoids, calcineurin inhibitors (cyclosporin A, FK 506), rapamycin, and mycophenolate mofetil can enhance regulatory T-cell responses.	[142]
Vectors/delivery systems **Particulate formulations** Liposomes, virosomes	Lipid-based vehicles such as liposomes can incorporate functional viral envelope proteins (leading to Virosomes). Mucosal administration of such particulate formulations increases IgG and neutralizing IgA antibodies. Nasal administration of plasmid DNA complexes formulated with cationic lipids induces specific secretory IgA antibodies in the vaginal and rectal mucosae and seric IgG and IgA antibodies. Intranasal immunization with the antigen formulated in liposomes together with immunopotentiators (eg, LPS, MPL, LTB) induces strong systemic and mucosal responses (with IgG and IGA in the lung and nose).	[111,143–145]
ISCOMs (structured complex of saponins and lipids)	These complexes are spherical structures (30–100 nm diameter) comprising the saponin-adjuvant Quil A, cholesterol, and phospholipids mixed with the antigen of interest. ISCOMs exhibit a strong systemic and mucosal adjuvant activity. ISCOMs particles target the endosomal and cytosolic compartments, thus leading to class I and class II presentation of antigens for T cell stimulation. Nasal administration of influenza virus submits formulated as ISCOMs induce protective immune responses.	[109,146]
Poly (D,L-lactide-co-glycolic) acid (PLGA)	PLGA can be used to present the antigen within nano- or microparticles to target antigen-presenting cells.	[147]

(continued on next page)

Table 2 (continued)

	Comments	References
Virus-like particles (VLPs)		
From human papilloma viruses, Norwalk virus, porcine parvovirus	After spontaneous assembly of capsid proteins, VLPs are formed that can stimulate humoral and cellular immune responses. Oral or nasal administration of recombinant hepatitis E virus (HEV) or Norwalk VLPs induce specific mucosal antibody responses in animals and humans. Oral vaccination with recombinant HEV-VLPs expressing B-cell epitopes induces specific IgG and IgA antibody secretion. Oral administration of DNA vaccines encapsulated in VLPs stimulates mucosal and systemic responses. Other potential VLP delivery systems include the porcine parvovirus VLP (PPV-VLP) and human papilloma virus VLPs, which specifically target immature DCs.	[112,113,148–151]
DC-targeting vectors		
Bacterial molecules (OmpA, CyaA, STxB)	Antigens coupled to the OmpA from *Klebsiella pneumoniae* (kpOmpA) target CD11$^+$ c mucosal (e.g. nasal) DCs through Toll-like receptor 2. The CyaA from *Bordetella pertussis* binds specifically to CD11b/CD18 α2 integrins expressed on DCs and delivers its catalytic domain into the cytosol together with antigen epitopes, leading to presentation to the class I and class II MHC pathways. The STxB also targets DCs, and antigens fused to this vector are delivered into the class I presentation pathway, leading to specific Th1-polarized T-cell responses and strong humoral responses. These vectors (CyaA, STxB) have not been evaluated for their capacity to elicit mucosal immune responses.	[114–117]
Anti-DEC205 antibodies	Anti-DEC-205 antibodies coupled to ovalbumin (OVA) target the antigen to DCs and induce strong OVA-specific T-cell responses in mice when administered together with anti-CD40 antibodies.	[152]

Abbreviations: CT, cholera toxin; CTB, B subunits of CT; CTL, cytotoxic T lymphocyte; CyaA, adenylate cyclase; DC, dendritic cell; GM-CSF, granulocyte-macrophage colony-stimulating factor; ICAM-1, intercellular adhesion molecule 1; ISCOMs, immunostimulating complexes; LT, heat-labile enterotoxin; LTB, B subunits of LT; OmpA, outer membrane protein A; STxB, B subunit of Shiga toxin.

lingual mucosa, LLDCs rapidly migrate to proximal-draining lymph nodes of the cervical/submaxillary chain [96]. The latter represents a TGF-β–rich environment that likely favors the activation of B cells expressing "blocking IgG" antibodies (IgG2b in mice) and the induction of suppressive T cells [97].

Because of its well-established safety profile, with more than 500 million doses administered to humans, SLIT is currently considered a valid alternative to SCIT [78].

Novel mucosal vector systems and adjuvants

In SCIT, mineral adjuvant molecules (eg, calcium phosphate, aluminum hydroxide) are used as part of allergy vaccines [73]. No such adjuvants are currently used during mucosal immunotherapy, implying that the dose of allergens should be increased. For example, it is well-documented that up to 50 to 100 fold more allergen is needed in SLIT to reach a level of efficacy similar to SCIT [73]. Specialized Langerhans cells in mucosae are prone to elicit regulatory T cells, favoring the development of allergen-specific IgG or IgA antibodies instead of IgE responses through IL-10 and TGF-β cytokine production. Capitalizing on the better understanding of immune mechanisms associated with immune tolerance, more efficacious mucosal vaccines can be rationally designed, particularly adjuvants/formulations that better target mucosal Langerhans cells, to improve stimulation of allergen-specific regulatory T cells. Schematically, antigen presentation platforms that can be used to improve mucosal tolerance include (1) immunopotentiators (ie, synthetic or biologic adjuvant molecules modulating immune responses by providing cosignals to immune cells) and (2) vector systems (targeting the antigen/allergen to APCs within the mucosa).

Immunopotentiators

Using appropriate immunopotentiators together with antigens/allergens may be necessary to redirect T-lymphocyte polarization from Th2 to regulatory T-cell responses. Several adjuvants are currently available from the vaccine industry that could lead to more efficient mucosal and systemic immune responses after administration at mucosal surfaces. Some are explored as novel approaches to potentiate antigen-specific Th1 or regulatory T-cell responses. For example, the Th1 adjuvant monophosphoryl lipid A has been used successfully through the subcutaneous route as part of grass pollen vaccines [98,99] and is currently being tested in humans through the sublingual route. In preclinical models, living or heat-killed bacteria (eg, *Lactobacillus plantarum, Lactococcus lactis, Mycobacterium vaccae*) showed some benefits as adjuvants in murine models of asthma (Table 2) [100–105]. Other potential mucosal adjuvants include bacterial toxins, such as cholera toxin and the closely related *Escherichia coli* heat-labile enterotoxin or their nontoxic derivatives (genetically detoxified or B subunits).

These bacterial toxins can be coadministered as a mix, conjugated, or fused with soluble antigens (see Table 2) [106]. A combination of cytokines mimicking signals induced by bacterial toxins can be used instead [107,108]. Triggering Toll-like receptors by lipid A or synthetic muramyl dipeptide analogs is also effective in inducing systemic and mucosal responses (see Table 2). Immuno-suppressive drugs (eg, glucocorticoids with vitamin D_3) also represent potential regulatory T-cell adjuvants for allergy immunotherapy because they are powerful inducers of IL-10 through immune cells (see Table 2).

Mucosal vector systems

Selected formulations can be used to present allergens in a particulate form, thereby targeting antigen-presenting cells (eg, Langerhans cells) with phagocytic activity. They may be used in association with immunopotentiators to further increase immune responses (see Table 2). These formulations include liposomes, virosomes, or immunostimulating complexes [109]. Ideal mucosal vectors should protect the allergens in the vaccine (mostly proteins or glycoproteins) from degradation by local proteases while targeting mucosal inductive sites or antigen-presenting cells.

Several vector systems to express antigen/allergen at mucosal surfaces have been tested. Using naked plasmid DNA or DNA absorbed on microparticles, markedly enhanced systemic and mucosal immune responses have been obtained [110,111]. Nonreplicating virus-like particles (VLPs) generated by the sponta-neous assembly of viral capsid proteins also represent an attractive alternative for expressing either the whole antigen/allergen, or selected T- or B-cell epitopes within a particulate vector system [112,113]. As an advantage for mucosal ap-plication, VLPs are often derived from viruses for which mucosae represent a natural route of transmission (see Table 2). Genetically detoxified or nontoxic bacterial products, such as the adenylate cyclase from *Bordetella pertussis,* the outer membrane protein A (OmpA) from *Klebsiella pneumoniae*, or the Shiga toxin B subunit, can be conjugated to antigens/allergens to target antigen-presenting cells (see Table 2) [114–116]. Delivering epitopes of interest through these vectors generates specific protective cytotoxic T lymphocytes and sys-temic antibody responses [114–116]. Nasal administration of OmpA induces mucosal immune responses [117]. Collectively, several vector systems are avail-able to target antigens/allergens to mucosal Langerhans cells. Although such vec-tors were initially designed and tested to elicit effector immune responses of the Th1 and Th2 types, none of these potential mucosal vectors has been estab-lished as a means to enhance antigen-specific regulatory T cells.

Summary

Building on the success of SCIT in curing allergic disease, improved allergy vaccines that rely on mucosal routes of administration are needed. To varying degrees, desensitization through the oral, nasal, and sublingual routes has shown some efficacy. The development of allergy vaccines has almost exclusively been based on natural or modified allergen extracts. A second generation will consist of vaccines based on recombinant proteins. In this regard, a major interest exists in developing hypoallergenic forms of recombinant allergens capable of inducing IgGs and stimulating T cells while exhibiting reduced IgE-binding capacity. Although this approach is definitively promising for vaccines administered parenterally, a more appropriate strategy for mucosal immunization, particularly for sublingual immunotherapy, is perhaps to rely on recombinant allergens presented in the most native form to allow IgE-mediated targeting and capture of allergens by mucosal Langerhans cells [93]. A better understanding of immune mechanisms involved in the induction and maintenance of antigen-specific immune tolerance provides opportunities for the design and development of improved mucosal vaccines. An emergent working hypothesis is that allergy vaccines should induce allergen-specific regulatory T lymphocytes capable of producing suppressive cytokines (eg, IL-10, TGF-β). Developing a new generation of safer and more efficient allergy vaccines administered through nonparenteral routes implies the need for adjuvants or vector systems specifically selected to enhance tolerance at mucosal surfaces. Identifying allergen presentation systems suitable for mucosal application will help develop more efficient allergy vaccines while simplifying immunization schemes.

Acknowledgments

The authors wish to thank Danielle Michel for excellent secretarial assistance and Patrick Buchoux for helping prepare the figure.

References

[1] Noon L. Prophylactic inoculation against hay fever. Lancet 1911;2:1572–3.
[2] Freeman J. Further observations on the treatment of hay fever by hypodermic inoculations of pollen vaccine. Lancet 1911;2:814–7.
[3] Bousquet J, Lockey R, Malling HJ. Allergen immunotherapy: therapeutic vaccines for allergic diseases. A WHO position paper. J Allergy Clin Immunol 1998;102:558–62.
[4] Larche M. Specific immunotherapy. Br Med Bull 2000;56:1019–36.
[5] Gehlhar K, Schlaak M, Becker W, et al. Monitoring allergen immunotherapy of pollen-allergic patients: the ratio of allergen-specific IgG4 to IgG1 correlates with clinical outcome. Clin Exp Allergy 1999;29:497–506.
[6] Michils A, Mairesse M, Ledent C, et al. Modified antigenic reactivity of anti-phospholipase A2 IgG antibodies in patients allergic to bee venom: conversion with immunotherapy and relation to subclass expression. J Allergy Clin Immunol 1998;102:118–26.
[7] Pichler CE, Helbling A, Pichler WJ. Three years of specific immunotherapy with house-dust-mite extracts in patients with rhinitis and asthma: significant improvement of allergen-specific parameters and of nonspecific bronchial hyperreactivity. Allergy 2001;56:301–6.
[8] Moller C, Dreborg S, Ferdousi HA, et al. Pollen immunotherapy reduces the development of

asthma in children with seasonal rhinoconjunctivitis (the PAT-study). J Allergy Clin Immunol 2002;109:251–6.

[9] Mowat AM, Parker LA, Beacock-Sharp H, et al. Oral tolerance: overview and historical perspectives. Ann N Y Acad Sci 2004;1029:1–8.

[10] Mayer L, Shao L. Therapeutic potential of oral tolerance. Nat Rev Immunol 2004;4:407–19.

[11] Faria AM, Weiner HL. Oral tolerance. Immunol Rev 2005;206:232–59.

[12] Akdis CA, Blaser K. Mechanisms of allergen-specific immunotherapy. Allergy 2000;55: 522–30.

[13] Durham SR, Till SJ. Immunologic changes associated with allergen immunotherapy. J Allergy Clin Immunol 1998;102:157–64.

[14] Till SJ, Francis JN, Nouri-Aria K, et al. Mechanisms of immunotherapy. J Allergy Clin Immunol 2004;113:1025–34 [quiz 35].

[15] Ebner C. Systemic immune response to specific immunotherapy. Clin Exp Allergy 1998;28: 781–3.

[16] Garcia NM, Lynch NR, Di Prisco MC, et al. Nonspecific changes in immunotherapy with house dust extract. J Investig Allergol Clin Immunol 1995;5:18–24.

[17] Wachholz PA, Durham SR. Induction of 'blocking' IgG antibodies during immunotherapy. Clin Exp Allergy 2003;33:1171–4.

[18] Iliopoulos O, Proud D, Adkinson Jr NF, et al. Effects of immunotherapy on the early, late, and rechallenge nasal reaction to provocation with allergen: changes in inflammatory mediators and cells. J Allergy Clin Immunol 1991;87:855–66.

[19] Durham SR, Ying S, Varney VA, et al. Grass pollen immunotherapy inhibits allergen-induced infiltration of CD4 + T lymphocytes and eosinophils in the nasal mucosa and increases the number of cells expressing messenger RNA for interferon-gamma. J Allergy Clin Immunol 1996;97:1356–65.

[20] van Neerven RJ, Wikborg T, Lund G, et al. Blocking antibodies induced by specific allergy vaccination prevent the activation of CD4 + T cells by inhibiting serum-IgE-facilitated allergen presentation. J Immunol 1999;163:2944–52.

[21] van Neerven RJ, Arvidsson M, Ipsen H, et al. A double-blind, placebo-controlled birch allergy vaccination study: inhibition of CD23-mediated serum-immunoglobulin E-facilitated allergen presentation. Clin Exp Allergy 2004;34:420–8.

[22] Pierson-Mullany LK, Jackola D, Blumenthal M, et al. Altered allergen binding capacities of Amb a 1-specific IgE and IgG4 from ragweed-sensitive patients receiving immunotherapy. Ann Allergy Asthma Immunol 2000;84:241–3.

[23] Jutel M, Akdis M, Budak F, et al. IL-10 and TGF-beta cooperate in the regulatory T cell response to mucosal allergens in normal immunity and specific immunotherapy. Eur J Immunol 2003;33:1205–14.

[24] Niederberger V, Horak F, Vrtala S, et al. Vaccination with genetically engineered allergens prevents progression of allergic disease. Proc Natl Acad Sci USA 2004;101(Suppl 2): 14677–82.

[25] Hakansson L, Heinrich C, Rak S, et al. Priming of eosinophil adhesion in patients with birch pollen allergy during pollen season: effect of immunotherapy. J Allergy Clin Immunol 1997;99: 551–62.

[26] Durham SR, Varney VA, Gaga M, et al. Grass pollen immunotherapy decreases the number of mast cells in the skin. Clin Exp Allergy 1999;29:1490–6.

[27] Monteseirin J, Bonilla I, Camacho J, et al. Elevated secretion of myeloperoxidase by neutrophils from asthmatic patients: the effect of immunotherapy. J Allergy Clin Immunol 2001;107: 623–6.

[28] Wilson DR, Irani AM, Walker SM, et al. Grass pollen immunotherapy inhibits seasonal increases in basophils and eosinophils in the nasal epithelium. Clin Exp Allergy 2001;31: 1705–13.

[29] Furin MJ, Norman PS, Creticos PS, et al. Immunotherapy decreases antigen-induced eosinophil cell migration into the nasal cavity. J Allergy Clin Immunol 1991;88:27–32.

[30] Wilson DR, Nouri-Aria KT, Walker SM, et al. Grass pollen immunotherapy: symptomatic

improvement correlates with reductions in eosinophils and IL-5 mRNA expression in the nasal mucosa during the pollen season. J Allergy Clin Immunol 2001;107:971–6.

[31] Robinson DS, Larche M, Durham SR. Tregs and allergic disease. J Clin Invest 2004;114: 1389–97.

[32] El Biaze M, Boniface S, Koscher V, et al. T cell activation, from atopy to asthma: more a paradox than a paradigm. Allergy 2003;58:844–53.

[33] Mavroleon G. Restoration of cytokine imbalance by immunotherapy. Clin Exp Allergy 1998; 28:917–20.

[34] Hamid QA, Schotman E, Jacobson MR, et al. Increases in IL-12 messenger RNA + cells accompany inhibition of allergen-induced late skin responses after successful grass pollen immunotherapy. J Allergy Clin Immunol 1997;99:254–60.

[35] Benjaponpitak S, Oro A, Maguire P, et al. The kinetics of change in cytokine production by CD4 T cells during conventional allergen immunotherapy. J Allergy Clin Immunol 1999;103: 468–75.

[36] Ebner C, Siemann U, Bohle B, et al. Immunological changes during specific immunotherapy of grass pollen allergy: reduced lymphoproliferative responses to allergen and shift from TH2 to TH1 in T-cell clones specific for Phl p 1, a major grass pollen allergen. Clin Exp Allergy 1997;27:1007–15.

[37] Secrist H, Chelen CJ, Wen Y, et al. Allergen immunotherapy decreases interleukin 4 production in CD4 + T cells from allergic individuals. J Exp Med 1993;178:2123–30.

[38] Medicines CoSo. Desensitising vaccines: an allergist's view. BMJ 1986;293:1169–70.

[39] Canonica GW, Passalacqua G. Noninjection routes for immunotherapy. J Allergy Clin Immunol 2003;111:437–48 [quiz 49].

[40] Deuschl H, Johansson GO. Hyposensitization of patients with allergic rhinitis by intranasal administration of chemically modified grass pollen allergen. A pilot study. Acta Allergol 1977; 32:248–62.

[41] Nickelsen JA, Goldstein S, Mueller U, et al. Local intranasal immunotherapy for ragweed allergic rhinitis. I. Clinical response. J Allergy Clin Immunol 1981;68:33–40.

[42] Georgitis JW, Reisman RE, Clayton WF, et al. Local intranasal immunotherapy for grass-allergic rhinitis. J Allergy Clin Immunol 1983;71:71–6.

[43] Andri L, Senna GE, Betteli C, et al. Local nasal immunotherapy in allergic rhinitis to Parietaria. A double-blind controlled study. Allergy 1992;47:318–23.

[44] Andri L, Senna G, Betteli C, et al. Local nasal immunotherapy for Dermatophagoides-induced rhinitis: efficacy of a powder extract. J Allergy Clin Immunol 1993;91:987–96.

[45] D'Amato G, Lobefalo G, Liccardi G, et al. A double-blind, placebo-controlled trial of local nasal immunotherapy in allergic rhinitis to Parietaria pollen. Clin Exp Allergy 1995;25: 141–8.

[46] Andri L, Senna G. Local nasal immunotherapy. Allergy 1995;50:190.

[47] Andri L, Senna G, Betteli C, et al. Local nasal immunotherapy with extract in powder form is effective and safe in grass pollen rhinitis: a double-blind study. J Allergy Clin Immunol 1996;97:34–41.

[48] Passalacqua G, Albano M, Riccio AM, et al. Local nasal immunotherapy: experimental evidences and general considerations. Allergy 1997;52:10–6.

[49] Nickelsen JA, Georgitis JW, Mueller UR, et al. Local nasal immunotherapy for ragweed-allergic rhinitis. III. A second year of treatment. Clin Allergy 1983;13:509–19.

[50] Nickelsen JA, Goldstein S, Mueller U, et al. Local intranasal immunotherapy for ragweed allergic rhinitis. II. Immunologic response. J Allergy Clin Immunol 1981;68:41–5.

[51] Tsitoura DC, DeKruyff RH, Lamb JR, et al. Intranasal exposure to protein antigen induces immunological tolerance mediated by functionally disabled CD4 + T cells. J Immunol 1999; 163:2592–600.

[52] Winkler B, Bolwig C, Seppala U, et al. Allergen-specific immunosuppression by mucosal treatment with recombinant Ves v 5, a major allergen of Vespula vulgaris venom, in a murine model of wasp venom allergy. Immunology 2003;110:376–85.

[53] Bagnasco M, Mariani G, Passalacqua G, et al. Absorption and distribution kinetics of the

major Parietaria judaica allergen (Par j 1) administered by noninjectable routes in healthy human beings. J Allergy Clin Immunol 1997;100:122–9.

[54] Passalacqua G, Altrinetti V, Mariani G, et al. Pharmacokinetics of radiolabelled Par j 1 administered intranasally to allergic and healthy subjects. Clin Exp Allergy 2005;35:880–3.

[55] Rebien W, Puttonen E, Maasch HJ, et al. Clinical and immunological response to oral and subcutaneous immunotherapy with grass pollen extracts. A prospective study. Eur J Pediatr 1982;138:341–4.

[56] Taudorf E, Weeke B. Orally administered grass pollen. Allergy 1983;38:561–4.

[57] Cooper PJ, Darbyshire J, Nunn AJ, et al. A controlled trial of oral hyposensitization in pollen asthma and rhinitis in children. Clin Allergy 1984;14:541–50.

[58] Mosbech H, Dreborg S, Madsen F, et al. High dose grass pollen tablets used for hyposensitization in hay fever patients. A one-year double blind placebo-controlled study. Allergy 1987;42:451–5.

[59] Urbanek R, Burgelin KH, Kahle S, et al. Oral immunotherapy with grass pollen in entero-soluble capsules. A prospective study of the clinical and immunological response. Eur J Pediatr 1990;149:545–50.

[60] Moller C, Dreborg S, Lanner A, et al. Oral immunotherapy of children with rhinoconjunctivitis due to birch pollen allergy. A double blind study. Allergy 1986;41:271–9.

[61] Taudorf E, Laursen LC, Lanner A, et al. Oral immunotherapy in birch pollen hay fever. J Allergy Clin Immunol 1987;80:153–61.

[62] Taudorf E, Laursen L, Lanner A, et al. Specific IgE, IgG, and IgA antibody response to oral immunotherapy in birch pollinosis. J Allergy Clin Immunol 1989;83:589–94.

[63] Giovane AL, Bardare M, Passalacqua G, et al. A three-year double-blind placebo-controlled study with specific oral immunotherapy to Dermatophagoides: evidence of safety and efficacy in paediatric patients. Clin Exp Allergy 1994;24:53–9.

[64] Leng X, Fu YX, Ye ST, et al. A double-blind trial of oral immunotherapy for Artemisia pollen asthma with evaluation of bronchial response to the pollen allergen and serum-specific IgE antibody. Ann Allergy 1990;64:27–31.

[65] Litwin A, Flanagan M, Entis G, et al. Oral immunotherapy with short ragweed extract in a novel encapsulated preparation: a double-blind study. J Allergy Clin Immunol 1997;100:30–8.

[66] Sollid LM. Coeliac disease: dissecting a complex inflammatory disorder. Nat Rev Immunol 2002;2:647–55.

[67] MacPherson G, Milling S, Yrlid U, et al. Uptake of antigens from the intestine by dendritic cells. Ann N Y Acad Sci 2004;1029:75–82.

[68] Bousquet J, Scheinmann P, Guinnepain MT, et al. Sublingual-swallow immunotherapy (SLIT) in patients with asthma due to house-dust mites: a double-blind, placebo-controlled study. Allergy 1999;54:249–60.

[69] La Rosa M, Ranno C, Andre C, et al. Double-blind placebo-controlled evaluation of sublingual-swallow immunotherapy with standardized Parietaria judaica extract in children with allergic rhinoconjunctivitis. J Allergy Clin Immunol 1999;104:425–32.

[70] Wilson DR, Torres LI, Durham SR. Sublingual immunotherapy for allergic rhinitis. Cochrane Database Syst Rev 2003;2:CD002893.

[71] Clavel R, Bousquet J, Andre C. Clinical efficacy of sublingual-swallow immunotherapy: a double-blind, placebo-controlled trial of a standardized five-grass-pollen extract in rhinitis. Allergy 1998;53:493–8.

[72] Vourdas D, Syrigou E, Potamianou P, et al. Double-blind, placebo-controlled evaluation of sublingual immunotherapy with standardized olive pollen extract in pediatric patients with allergic rhinoconjunctivitis and mild asthma due to olive pollen sensitization. Allergy 1998;53:662–72.

[73] Bousquet J, Van Cauwenberge P, Khaltaev N. Allergic rhinitis and its impact on asthma. J Allergy Clin Immunol 2001;108:S147–334.

[74] Pajno GB, Morabito L, Barberio G, et al. Clinical and immunologic effects of long-term sublingual immunotherapy in asthmatic children sensitized to mites: a double-blind, placebo-controlled study. Allergy 2000;55:842–9.

[75] Marogna M, Spadolini I, Massolo A, et al. Clinical, functional, and immunologic effects of sublingual immunotherapy in birch pollinosis: a 3-year randomized controlled study. J Allergy Clin Immunol 2005;115:1184–8.
[76] Smith H, White P, Annila I, et al. Randomized controlled trial of high-dose sublingual immunotherapy to treat seasonal allergic rhinitis. J Allergy Clin Immunol 2004;114:831–7.
[77] Baena-Cagnani CE, Passalacqua G, Baena-Cagnani RC, et al. Sublingual immunotherapy in pediatric patients: beyond clinical efficacy. Curr Opin Allergy Clin Immunol 2005;5:173–7.
[78] Khinchi MS, Poulsen LK, Carat F, et al. Clinical efficacy of sublingual and subcutaneous birch pollen allergen-specific immunotherapy: a randomized, placebo-controlled, double-blind, double-dummy study. Allergy 2004;59:45–53.
[79] Moingeon P, Batard T, Fadel R, et al. Immune mechanisms of allergen-specific sublingual immunotherapy. Allergy 2006;61:151–65.
[80] Garcia BE, Sanz ML, Gato JJ, et al. IgG4 blocking effect on the release of antigen-specific histamine. J Investig Allergol Clin Immunol 1993;3:26–33.
[81] Mothes N, Heinzkill M, Drachenberg KJ, et al. Allergen-specific immunotherapy with a monophosphoryl lipid A-adjuvanted vaccine: reduced seasonally boosted immunoglobulin E production and inhibition of basophil histamine release by therapy-induced blocking antibodies. Clin Exp Allergy 2003;33:1198–208.
[82] Marcucci F, Sensi L, Frati F, et al. Sublingual tryptase and ECP in children treated with grass pollen sublingual immunotherapy (SLIT): safety and immunologic implications. Allergy 2001;56:1091–5.
[83] Passalacqua G, Albano M, Fregonese L, et al. Randomised controlled trial of local allergoid immunotherapy on allergic inflammation in mite-induced rhinoconjunctivitis. Lancet 1998;351:629–32.
[84] Marcucci F, Sensi L, Frati F, et al. Effects on inflammation parameters of a double-blind, placebo controlled one-year course of SLIT in children monosensitized to mites. Allergy 2003;58:657–62.
[85] Silvestri M, Spallarossa D, Battistini E, et al. Changes in inflammatory and clinical parameters and in bronchial hyperreactivity asthmatic children sensitized to house dust mites following sublingual immunotherapy. J Investig Allergol Clin Immunol 2002;12:52–9.
[86] Passalacqua G, Albano M, Riccio A, et al. Clinical and immunologic effects of a rush sublingual immunotherapy to Parietaria species: A double-blind, placebo-controlled trial. J Allergy Clin Immunol 1999;104:964–8.
[87] Rolinck-Werninghaus C, Kopp M, et al. Lack of detectable alterations in immune responses during sublingual immunotherapy in children with seasonal allergic rhinoconjunctivitis to grass pollen. Int Arch Allergy Immunol 2005;136:134–41.
[88] Lima MT, Wilson D, Pitkin L, et al. Grass pollen sublingual immunotherapy for seasonal rhinoconjunctivitis: a randomized controlled trial. Clin Exp Allergy 2002;32:507–14.
[89] Ippoliti F, De Santis W, Volterrani A, et al. Immunomodulation during sublingual therapy in allergic children. Pediatr Allergy Immunol 2003;14:216–21.
[90] Fenoglio D, Puppo F, Cirillo I, et al. Sublingual specific immunotherapy reduces PBMC proliferations. Allerg Immunol (Paris) 2005;37:147–51.
[91] Ciprandi G, Fenoglio D, Cirillo I, et al. Induction of interleukin 10 by sublingual immunotherapy for house dust mites: a preliminary report. Ann Allergy Asthma Immunol 2005;95:38–44.
[92] Bagnasco M, Passalacqua G, Villa G, et al. Pharmacokinetics of an allergen and a monomeric allergoid for oromucosal immunotherapy in allergic volunteers. Clin Exp Allergy 2001;31:54–60.
[93] Allam JP, Novak N, Fuchs C, et al. Characterization of dendritic cells from human oral mucosa: a new Langerhans' cell type with high constitutive FcepsilonRI expression. J Allergy Clin Immunol 2003;112:141–8.
[94] Novak N, Bieber T, Katoh N. Engagement of Fc epsilon RI on human monocytes induces the production of IL-10 and prevents their differentiation in dendritic cells. J Immunol 2001;167:797–804.

[95] von Bubnoff D, Bezold G, Matz H, et al. Quantification of indoleamine 2,3-dioxygenase gene induction in atopic and non-atopic monocytes after ligation of the high-affinity receptor for IgE, Fc(epsilon)RI and interferon-gamma stimulation. Clin Exp Immunol 2003;132: 247–53.

[96] van Wilsem EJ, Breve J, Savelkoul H, et al. Oral tolerance is determined at the level of draining lymph nodes. Immunobiology 1995;194:403–14.

[97] van Helvoort JM, Samsom JN, Chantry D, et al. Preferential expression of IgG2b in nose draining cervical lymph nodes and its putative role in mucosal tolerance induction. Allergy 2004;59:1211–8.

[98] Drachenberg KJ, Wheeler AW, Stuebner P, et al. A well-tolerated grass pollen-specific allergy vaccine containing a novel adjuvant, monophosphoryl lipid A, reduces allergic symptoms after only four preseasonal injections. Allergy 2001;56:498–505.

[99] Drachenberg KJ, Heinzkill M, Urban E, et al. Efficacy and tolerability of short-term specific immunotherapy with pollen allergoids adjuvanted by monophosphoryl lipid A (MPL) for children and adolescents. Allergol Immunopathol (Madr) 2003;31:270–7.

[100] Repa A, Grangette C, Daniel C, et al. Mucosal co-application of lactic acid bacteria and allergen induces counter-regulatory immune responses in a murine model of birch pollen allergy. Vaccine 2003;22:87–95.

[101] Grangette C, Muller-Alouf H, Goudercourt D, et al. Mucosal immune responses and protection against tetanus toxin after intranasal immunization with recombinant Lactobacillus plantarum. Infect Immun 2001;69:1547–53.

[102] Grangette C, Nutten S, Palumbo E, et al. Enhanced antiinflammatory capacity of a Lactobacillus plantarum mutant synthesizing modified teichoic acids. Proc Natl Acad Sci USA 2005;102:10321–6.

[103] Chapat L, Chemin K, Dubois B, et al. Lactobacillus casei reduces CD8 + T cell-mediated skin inflammation. Eur J Immunol 2004;34:2520–8.

[104] Zuany-Amorim C, Manlius C, Trifilieff A, et al. Long-term protective and antigen-specific effect of heat-killed Mycobacterium vaccae in a murine model of allergic pulmonary inflammation. J Immunol 2002;169:1492–9.

[105] Arkwright PD, David TJ. Effect of Mycobacterium vaccae on atopic dermatitis in children of different ages. Br J Dermatol 2003;149:1029–34.

[106] Pizza M, Giuliani MM, Fontana MR, et al. Mucosal vaccines: non toxic derivatives of LT and CT as mucosal adjuvants. Vaccine 2001;19:2534–41.

[107] Bradney CP, Sempowski GD, Liao HX, et al. Cytokines as adjuvants for the induction of anti-human immunodeficiency virus peptide immunoglobulin G (IgG) and IgA antibodies in serum and mucosal secretions after nasal immunization. J Virol 2002;76:517–24.

[108] Staats HF, Bradney CP, Gwinn WM, et al. Cytokine requirements for induction of systemic and mucosal CTL after nasal immunization. J Immunol 2001;167:5386–94.

[109] Sanders MT, Brown LE, Deliyannis G, et al. ISCOM-based vaccines: the second decade. Immunol Cell Biol 2005;83:119–28.

[110] Hobson P, Barnfield C, Barnes A, et al. Mucosal immunization with DNA vaccines. Methods 2003;31:217–24.

[111] Klavinskis LS, Barnfield C, Gao L, et al. Intranasal immunization with plasmid DNA-lipid complexes elicits mucosal immunity in the female genital and rectal tracts. J Immunol 1999; 162:254–62.

[112] Boisgerault F, Moron G, Leclerc C. Virus-like particles: a new family of delivery systems. Expert Rev Vaccines 2002;1:101–9.

[113] Niikura M, Takamura S, Kim G, et al. Chimeric recombinant hepatitis E virus-like particles as an oral vaccine vehicle presenting foreign epitopes. Virology 2002;293:273–80.

[114] El Azami El Idrissi M, Ladant D, et al. The adenylate cyclase of Bordetella pertussis: a vector to target antigen presenting cells. Toxicon 2002;40:1661–5.

[115] Jeannin P, Renno T, Goetsch L, et al. OmpA targets dendritic cells, induces their maturation and delivers antigen into the MHC class I presentation pathway. Nat Immunol 2000;1:502–9.

[116] Haicheur N, Benchetrit F, Amessou M, et al. The B subunit of Shiga toxin coupled to full-

size antigenic protein elicits humoral and cell-mediated immune responses associated with a Th1-dominant polarization. Int Immunol 2003;15:1161–71.

[117] Goetsch L, Gonzalez A, Plotnicky-Gilquin H, et al. Targeting of nasal mucosa-associated antigen-presenting cells in vivo with an outer membrane protein A derived from Klebsiella pneumoniae. Infect Immun 2001;69:6434–44.

[118] Muller U, Akdis CA, Fricker M, et al. Successful immunotherapy with T-cell epitope peptides of bee venom phospholipase A2 induces specific T-cell anergy in patients allergic to bee venom. J Allergy Clin Immunol 1998;101:747–54.

[119] Verhoef A, Alexander C, Kay AB, et al. T cell epitope immunotherapy induces a CD4 + T cell population with regulatory activity. PLoS Med 2005;2:e78.

[120] Larche M, Wraith DC. Peptide-based therapeutic vaccines for allergic and autoimmune diseases. Nat Med 2005;11:S69–76.

[121] Jakobsen CG, Bodtger U, Poulsen LK, et al. Vaccination for birch pollen allergy: comparison of the affinities of specific immunoglobulins E, G1 and G4 measured by surface plasmon resonance. Clin Exp Allergy 2005;35:193–8.

[122] Jutel M, Jaeger L, Suck R, et al. Allergen-specific immunotherapy with recombinant grass pollen allergens. J Allergy Clin Immunol 2005;116:608–13.

[123] Gafvelin G, Thunberg S, Kronqvist M, et al. Cytokine and antibody responses in birch-pollen-allergic patients treated with genetically modified derivatives of the major birch pollen allergen Bet v 1. Int Arch Allergy Immunol 2005;138:59–66.

[124] Francis JN, Till SJ, Durham SR. Induction of IL-10 + CD4 + CD25 + T cells by grass pollen immunotherapy. J Allergy Clin Immunol 2003;111:1255–61.

[125] Nasser SM, Ying S, Meng Q, et al. Interleukin-10 levels increase in cutaneous biopsies of patients undergoing wasp venom immunotherapy. Eur J Immunol 2001;31:3704–13.

[126] Gardner LM, Thien FC, Douglass JA, et al. Induction of T 'regulatory' cells by standardized house dust mite immunotherapy: an increase in CD4 + CD25 + interleukin-10 + T cells expressing peripheral tissue trafficking markers. Clin Exp Allergy 2004;34:1209–19.

[127] Bjorksten B, Moller C, Broberger U, et al. Clinical and immunological effects of oral immunotherapy with a standardized birch pollen extract. Allergy 1986;41:290–5.

[128] Passalacqua G, Villa G, Altrinetti V, et al. Sublingual swallow or spit? Allergy 2001;56:578.

[129] Bahceciler NN, Arikan C, Taylor A, et al. Impact of sublingual immunotherapy on specific antibody levels in asthmatic children allergic to house dust mites. Int Arch Allergy Immunol 2005;136:287–94.

[130] Haan L, Verweij WR, Holtrop M, et al. Nasal or intramuscular immunization of mice with influenza subunit antigen and the B subunit of Escherichia coli heat-labile toxin induces IgA-or IgG-mediated protective mucosal immunity. Vaccine 2001;19:2898–907.

[131] Hagiwar Y, Tsuji T, Iwasaki T, et al. Effectiveness and safety of mutant Escherichia coli heat-labile enterotoxin (LT H44A) as an adjuvant for nasal influenza vaccine. Vaccine 2001;19:2071–9.

[132] Pajak B, Garze V, Davies G, et al. The adjuvant OM-174 induces both the migration and maturation of murine dendritic cells in vivo. Vaccine 2003;21:836–42.

[133] Baldridge JR, Yorgensen Y, Ward JR, et al. Monophosphoryl lipid A enhances mucosal and systemic immunity to vaccine antigens following intranasal administration. Vaccine 2000;18:2416–25.

[134] Mason KW, Zhu D, Scheuer CA, et al. Reduction of nasal colonization of nontypeable Haemophilus influenzae following intranasal immunization with rLP4/rLP6/UspA2 proteins combined with aqueous formulation of RC529. Vaccine 2004;22:3449–56.

[135] Gallichan WS, Woolstencroft RN, Guarasci T, et al. Intranasal immunization with CpG oligodeoxynucleotides as an adjuvant dramatically increases IgA and protection against herpes simplex virus-2 in the genital tract. J Immunol 2001;166:3451–7.

[136] Santeliz JV, Van Nest G, Traquina P, et al. Amb a 1-linked CpG oligodeoxynucleotides reverse established airway hyperresponsiveness in a murine model of asthma. J Allergy Clin Immunol 2002;109:455–62.

[137] Fukushima A, Yoo YC, Yoshimatsu K, et al. Effect of MDP-Lys(L18) as a mucosal immuno-

adjuvant on protection of mucosal infections by Sendai virus and rotavirus. Vaccine 1996;14: 485–91.

[138] Boussiotis VA, Tsai EY, Yunis EJ, et al. IL-10-producing T cells suppress immune responses in anergic tuberculosis patients. J Clin Invest 2000;105:1317–25.

[139] McGuirk P, McCann C, Mills KH. Pathogen-specific T regulatory 1 cells induced in the respiratory tract by a bacterial molecule that stimulates interleukin 10 production by dendritic cells: a novel strategy for evasion of protective T helper type 1 responses by Bordetella pertussis. J Exp Med 2002;195:221–31.

[140] Bracci L, Canini I, Puzelli S, et al. Type I IFN is a powerful mucosal adjuvant for a selective intranasal vaccination against influenza virus in mice and affects antigen capture at mucosal level. Vaccine 2005;23:2994–3004.

[141] Kutzler MA, Robinson TM, Chattergoon MA, et al. Communization with an optimized IL-15 plasmid results in enhanced function and longevity of CD8 T cells that are partially independent of CD4 T cell help. J Immunol 2005;175:112–23.

[142] van Overvelt L, Moingeon P. T cell adjuvants and novel strategies for their identification. In: Schijns V, O'Hagan D, editors. Immunopotentiators in Modern Vaccines. Surrey (UK): Academic Press; 2005.

[143] Durrer P, Gluck U, Spyr C, et al. Mucosal antibody response induced with a nasal virosome-based influenza vaccine. Vaccine 2003;21:4328–34.

[144] Felnerova D, Viret JF, Gluck R, et al. Liposomes and virosomes as delivery systems for antigens, nucleic acids and drugs. Curr Opin Biotechnol 2004;15:518–29.

[145] de Jonge MI, Hamstra HJ, Jiskoot W, et al. Intranasal immunisation of mice with liposomes containing recombinant meningococcal OpaB and OpaJ proteins. Vaccine 2004;22:4021–8.

[146] Hu KF, Lovgren-Bengtsson K, Morein B. Immunostimulating complexes (ISCOMs) for nasal vaccination. Adv Drug Deliv Rev 2001;51:149–59.

[147] Waeckerle-Men Y, Groettrup M. PLGA microspheres for improved antigen delivery to dendritic cells as cellular vaccines. Adv Drug Deliv Rev 2005;57:475–82.

[148] Ball JM, Hardy ME, Atmar RL, et al. Oral immunization with recombinant Norwalk virus-like particles induces a systemic and mucosal immune response in mice. J Virol 1998;72:1345–53.

[149] Ball JM, Graham DY, Opekun AR, et al. Recombinant Norwalk virus-like particles given orally to volunteers: phase I study. Gastroenterology 1999;117:40–8.

[150] Takamura S, Niikura M, Li TC, et al. DNA vaccine-encapsulated virus-like particles derived from an orally transmissible virus stimulate mucosal and systemic immune responses by oral administration. Gene Ther 2004;11:628–35.

[151] Shi W, Liu J, Huang Y, et al. Papillomavirus pseudovirus: a novel vaccine to induce mucosal and systemic cytotoxic T-lymphocyte responses. J Virol 2001;75:10139–48.

[152] Bonifaz LC, Bonnyay DP, Charalambous A, et al. In vivo targeting of antigens to maturing dendritic cells via the DEC-205 receptor improves T cell vaccination. J Exp Med 2004; 199:815–24.

ELSEVIER
SAUNDERS

Immunol Allergy Clin N Am
26 (2006) 307–319

IMMUNOLOGY
AND ALLERGY
CLINICS
OF NORTH AMERICA

Targeting Dendritic Cells in Allergen Immunotherapy

Natalija Novak, MD

Department of Dermatology, University of Bonn, Sigmund-Freud-Strasse 25, 53105 Bonn, Germany

Dendritic cells (DCs) as gatekeepers of our immune system are located at the border zones of the body's internal environment. DCs play a major role in antigen presentation and T-cell priming and are therefore crucial in determining the nature of emerging immune responses. DCs have a paradigmatic role in the immune system because they are strong inducers of (1) allergic–immunogenic reactions that lead to the development and maintenance of allergic diseases, and (2) anti-allergic, tolerogenic reactions that lead to the rapid dampening or complete inhibition of allergic immune responses [1,2].

An allergic reaction is defined as a hyper-reactivity toward normally non-immunogenic substances. The spectrum of these substances ranges from food allergens such as peanuts, egg, milk, soy, and codfish, to aeroallergens such as birch or grass pollen, house dust mites, and cat dander, to natural rubber latex and hymenoptera venom [3–5]. The most severe variant of allergic reactions is life-threatening anaphylactic shock, which is a sudden and severe allergic reaction that occurs within minutes after allergen exposure, progresses rapidly, and can lead to death within a couple of minutes. In the past decades, allergic/atopic diseases such as allergic rhinitis, allergic asthma, and atopic dermatitis have shown an increased incidence that has led to a decreased quality of life for affected individuals [6,7].

Therefore, several therapeutic strategies have been developed to calm the symptoms of allergic diseases. Because of their bivalent character and ability to take up antigens, DCs represent attractive targets for antiallergic treatment

This work was supported by grants from the Deutsche Forschungsgemeinschaft DFG NO 454/2-3, DFG NO454/1-3 and grants from the University of Bonn, BONFOR. N. Norak is supported by a Heisenberg Fellowship of the DFG.

E-mail address: Natalija.Novak@ukb.uni-bonn.de

doi:10.1016/j.iac.2006.02.010   *immunology.theclinics.com*

regimens [8]. Classical allergen immunotherapy represents one of the most recently established therapeutic strategies [9].

What do we know about the mode of action of allergen immunotherapy?

In general, therapeutic strategies used for treating allergic diseases can be subdivided into two major forms: (1) short-term therapeutic strategies that treat the acute symptoms of allergic diseases, and (2) long-term therapeutic strategies, such as allergen-specific immunotherapy, that have the goal of efficient long-term down-regulation of the reactivity toward specific allergens.

Allergen-specific immunotherapy has been shown to be efficient, especially for individuals who have allergic rhinitis or hymenoptera allergy [4,9]. In this treatment regimen, increasing doses of the allergen are applied subcutaneously or sublingually [10–12]. Within weeks an allergen-specific IgG response develops whereby newly formed allergen–IgG complexes are assumed to inhibit further allergen-mediated effector cell activation through IgE receptor/IgG receptor coactivation [9,13,14].

Nevertheless, little is known about the exact immunologic mechanism leading to the therapeutic response of immunotherapy. Recent data support antigen-

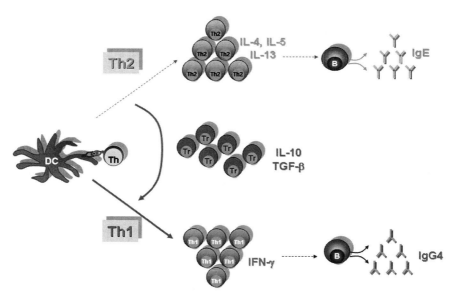

Fig. 1. Mechanisms of action of allergen immunotherapy. Allergen immunotherapy leads to a shift of Th2 immune responses predominated by IL-4–, IL-5–, and IL-13–producing T cells and IgE production by B cells to modified Th2 immune responses and Th1 immune responses in which IFN-γ–producing T cells prevail and B cells start to produce protective IgG4. In parallel, regulatory T cells with high IL-10 and TGF-β–producing properties are induced and might contribute to the mechanisms described.

specific tolerance induction as a leading immunologic mechanism in immunotherapy that inhibits concomitant early and late responses to allergenic substances. Immunotherapy accompanies increased B-cell production of inhibitory IgG subtypes such as IgG_2 and IgG_4, and an increase of allergen-specific IgA [9]. Furthermore, immunotherapy induces a shift from Th2-type immune responses, which predominate in allergic diseases and are characterized by high T-cell production of interleukin (IL)-4, IL-5, and IL-13, to Th1-type immune responses, which are characterized by high T-cell production of interferon (IFN)-γ [15]. In another recently discovered mechanism, immunotherapy induces IL-10 and transforming growth factor (TGF)-β production by T cells and enhances the suppressive activity of regulatory $CD4^+$ $CD25^+$ T-cell subtypes (Fig. 1) [16].

Why are dendritic cells attractive targets for allergen immunotherapy?

DCs are located at the interface of the body and the environment, such as the skin, respiratory tract, and mucosal sites [2]. Therefore, DCs are easily accessible for immunotherapeutic substances applied through subcutaneous injections or administered to mucosal surfaces such as the sublingual or intranasal mucous membranes. Obviously, DCs not only are one of the first cell types to come in contact with naturally occurring allergens in patients who have allergic diseases but also gain early access to allergenic compounds applied for therapeutic purposes through immunotherapy. As another attractive feature, DCs are capable of taking up allergens and presenting these allergens to antigen-specific T cells [17]. Thus, DCs prime T cells into activating proallergic or suppressive, antiallergic T-cell subtypes [18]. Most importantly, DCs in the skin and oral and nasal mucosa of patients who have allergic diseases have been shown to bear the high-affinity IgE receptor (FcϵRI) in high amounts on their cell surface [19–21]. As a characteristic feature of individuals who have allergies, the FcϵRI on DCs is occupied partly by IgE molecules, and the pattern of allergen-specific IgE molecules bound to the cell surface of DCs might comply with the sensitization pattern of these patients [20,22].

DCs are capable of taking up allergens through FcϵRI-bound IgE molecules, internalizing these allergens and presenting the processed allergen peptides to T cells after migrating to the peripheral lymphoid organs [23]. Presumably, allergens applied for the purpose of immunotherapy are also taken up by DCs and presented to T cells. Furthermore, variations in the maturation stage and grade of activation of DCs, the composition of DC subtypes at the different sites of the body, and the dosage of allergens applied, in combination with many other currently unidentified factors, critically modulate the nature of the immune response induced by DCs through immunotherapy [24].

One of the most striking properties of DCs in the context of immunotherapy is their bivalent character: DCs are paradigmatic players in the allergic cascade that on one hand are able to mediate immunogenic reactions leading to allergic inflammation and on the other hand are capable of inducing antiallergic, tolerogenic immune responses [25].

Which tolerogenic properties of dendritic cells might be relevant in allergen immunotherapy?

Different studies provide evidence that DCs are critically involved in the induction of tolerance against allergens, which is a major mode of action of immunotherapy. However, the detailed mechanisms converting DCs into tolerogenic DCs in immunotherapy are far from being known. Although increasing insights into the biology of DCs show that these cells may have a critical involvement in the mechanism contributing to the therapeutic response to immunotherapy, most hypotheses concerning the role of DCs as facilitators of immunotherapy remain speculative. Therefore, experimental data acquired from ex vivo–mechanisms isolated DCs under subcutaneous and sublingual immunotherapy are needed to support these assumptions.

One of the most important mechanisms in this context might be enhanced IL-10 production mirrored by increased local IL-10 levels and IL-10 serum levels of patients undergoing immunotherapy, because IL-10 is known to enforce phenotypic and functional properties of regulatory DCs by creating regulatory DC subtypes [26,27]. IL-10, for instance, reduces the stimulatory capacity of DC toward T cells and modulates the maturation stage of differentiating DCs, keeping them in an immature stage [18,28]. As a secondary phenomenon, IL-10 induces several tolerogenic properties of DCs, such as increased expression of inhibitory FcγRIIB or increased immunoglobulin-like transcript receptors ILT2, ILT3, ILT4, and ILT5 [29], which are known to suppress T-cell responses while downregulating the expression of costimulatory molecules [28].

Looking closer at the immunologic synapse between DCs and T cells, several studies show that the down-regulatory effect of DCs on T cells occurs partially in a cell contact–dependent manner and is mediated by second signals transferred by way of surface molecule interactions between these cells [30].

In this context, in vitro experiments show that the expansion of regulatory T cells is dependent on B7 costimulation and coinhibition by way of DCs [30]. Within the family of B7 costimulatory molecules on DCs, the costimulatory molecules CD80 and CD86 are well characterized and mediate signals through CD28 and CD152/cutaneous-lymphocyte antigen (CTLA)-4 to T cells. As certain types of opponents, the surface molecules B7-H1, B7-H2, B7-H3, B7-H4, and B7-DC belong to the coinhibitory B7 molecule family expressed by DCs [30,31]. One approach cross-linked the coinhibitory molecule B7-DC on DCs, resulting in diminished allergen responsiveness in a mouse model and indicating a critical role of these molecules in allergen-specific tolerance induction [32]. Moreover, another recently described member of the B7 family, the inducible costimulator ligand (B7-H2/ICOS-L), has been shown to be involved in the induction of regulatory T cells [33]. In a mouse model, the interaction of inducible costimulator (ICOS) on T cells and ICOS-L/B7-H2 on pulmonary DCs led to the development of IL-10–producing regulatory T cells that inhibit airway hyper-reactivity, which is a cardinal feature of asthma [34–36]. However, whether B7 molecules expressed by DCs might be relevant for the induction of regulatory T cells in immunotherapy is unclear.

Is the high-affinity receptor for IgE (FcεRI) on dendritic cells a key structure in allergen immunotherapy?

The detection of FcεRI on antigen-presenting DC has brought new insights into the distribution and function of this immunoglobulin receptor. FcεRI has been shown to be expressed in a trimeric form, consisting of the IgE-binding α-chain and the γ-chain dimer responsible for signal transduction, in antigen-presenting cells such as monocytes, Langerhans cells (LCs), and other DC sub-types [19].

The function of FcεRI on DCs is still not elucidated in detail, but FcεRI on DCs is known to play opposing roles. On one hand, FcεRI on DCs such as LCs and inflammatory dendritic epidermal cells (IDECs) in the epidermis of atopic dermatitis is involved in the induction of proinflammatory cytokine production and recruitment of more inflammatory cells to the skin [37]. Thus, FcεRI-bearing DCs in the skin perpetuate the allergic inflammation. In contrast, recent published data suggest that FcεRI is also involved in tolerogenic processes [38]. In this context, on ligation of FcεRI on monocytes and DCs, FcεRI has been shown to trigger production of the anti-inflammatory cytokine IL-10 [39]. Furthermore, this production of IL-10 endogenously induces the generation of DCs with a lower stimulatory capacity toward T cells [39]. Consequently, increased IL-10 production of DCs after FcεRI-mediated allergen challenge under immunother-apy might be another putative mechanism in which DCs might contribute not only to the increased IL-10 levels observable in patients undergoing immuno-therapy but also to the overbalance of tolerogenic immune responses after al-lergen application under immunotherapy. As another tolerogenic mechanism that might be relevant in immunotherapy, FcεRI engagement of monocytes in-duces the overexpression of indoleamine 2,3-dioxygenase (IDO), the immuno-suppressive enzyme involved in the catabolism of the essential amino acid tryptophan to kynurenine and other potentially toxic metabolites [40–43]. In-duction of IDO and prevention of the activation of CD4$^+$ T cells has been shown to be mediated through CTLA-4 activation in in vitro studies [42,43].

Conversely, contact and activation of T cells by way of IDO-expressing DCs increases the CTLA-4 expression and regulatory capacities of T cells [42,43]. Presumably, the tolerogenic properties of FcεRI-bearing DCs might be encour-aged through repeated allergen challenge and FcεRI activation of DCs under immunotherapy, leading to an increase in IDO-expressing tolerogenic DCs, and allergen-specific tolerance perpetuated by regulatory T cells as another putative mechanism of immunotherapy [43,44].

How do the different routes of allergen immunotherapy target dendritic cells?

The classical and most established model for immunotherapy is the subcutaneous immunotherapy for insect sting allergy. In addition, subcutaneous immunotherapy has been used for treating several other allergic sensitizations, such as birch pollen or grass pollen allergy in individuals who have single sensitizations but also allergy to house dust mites and other aeroallergens. Although the mechanisms contributing to the shift from a high reactivity toward allergens to a state of unresponsiveness and tolerance are not completely elucidated, an immune response shift from Th2 to Th1 and a predominant IL-10 production by regulatory T cells of the Tr1 type and T-cell anergy combined with lower allergen-specific IgE and increase of allergen-specific IgG have been shown to be crucial for the process of tolerance induction underlying the therapeutic effect of subcutaneous immunotherapy [9,45–49]. Little information about changes at the local sites of subcutaneous allergen application [50,51] or the DC phenotype and function under immunotherapy exists to confirm that DCs have a key role as natural silencers in subcutaneous immunotherapy.

Apparently the route through which an allergen enters the body affects the nature of the resulting immune responses. One reason is the unique composition of the micromilieu at different sites of the body. In comparison to the classical routes of allergen application in immunotherapy, through compartments such as the skin, the mucosal sites such as the oral mucosa have been shown to represent immunoprivileged compartments that are somewhat capable of maintaining a state of immunologic unresponsiveness to subsequent allergen challenge under physiologic conditions [52]. This effect might be achieved through induction of regulatory T cells with suppressive properties, anergy, or deletion of immunoresponsive cells [52]. Therefore, immunotherapeutic strategies that use alternative routes of application, through immunoprivileged organs such as the oral mucosa, have recently gained increasing interest and hold promise as alternative modes of immunotherapy that may help increase safety by decreasing the risk for anaphylactic side reactions. The key cells perpetuating the state of tolerance in the oral mucosa are believed to be DCs. Their dampening function on the immune response is achieved partially through their expression of coinhibitory IgG receptors such as FcγRIIB observed in murine models [53]. Signaling through these receptors after coactivation of FcϵRI and FcγRIIB induces intracellular signaling through immunoreceptor tyrosine–based inhibition motifs and inhibits the outcome of an allergic immune response by antagonizing the activation signals mediated through immunoreceptor tyrosine–based activation motifs of FcϵRI [14,54].

In the context of allergen challenge, human oral mucosal LCs (oLCs) have recently been shown to display characteristic features, which differ in individuals who have allergies compared with those who do not [21,55]. In contrast to their counterparts in the skin, oLCs express higher levels of IgE-occupied FcϵRI [21]. Furthermore, oLCs express higher levels of major histocompatibility complex I and II molecules and costimulatory molecules such as CD80, CD86, or CD40 than do skin DCs and are therefore much more potent stimulators of T cells [21]. On the functional level, oLCs produce favorably anti-inflammatory cytokines such as TGF-β or IL-10 after allergen challenge in vitro, indicating their ability to induce tolerogenic mechanisms (Allam and Novak, unpublished data, 2005). These LCs express enhanced amounts of IgG receptors [21] and coinhibitory molecules such as B7-H1 and B7-H2 on their cell surface (Allam and Novak, unpublished data, 2005), which are responsible for the DC–T-cell contact–dependent induction of inhibitory regulatory T cells and the maintenance of peripheral tolerance toward allergens (Fig. 2). As another important feature that classifies them as tolerogenic DCs, oLCs induce high amounts of IL-10– and TGF-β–producing T cells after allergen challenge and secrete chemokines capable of recruiting regulatory T cells in vitro (see Fig. 2). Although oLCs express C-type lectins such as CD205, CD206, and CD209 in lower quantities on their cell surface than do LCs in the nasal mucosa [55], oLCs bear higher amounts of the lipopolysaccharide receptor CD14 on their cell surface compared with nasal

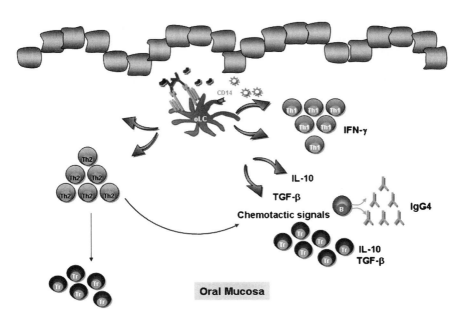

Fig. 2. Summary of the tolerogenic properties of oLCs as putative target cells of sublingual allergen immunotherapy. oLCs express high levels of FcεRI and the lipopolysaccharide receptor CD14 on their cell surface. Costimulation of FcεRI and CD14 might favor the priming of IFN-γ–producing T cells of the Th1 type. FcεRI allergen challenge induces IL-10 and TGF-β production by oLCs combined with the activation of IL-10 and TGF-β–producing regulatory T cells (Tr). Secondary signals mediated through inhibitory B7 molecules such as B7-H2 expressed in high amounts on oLCs might induce allergen-specific tolerance through regulatory T cells.

mucosal LCs or skin LCs (see Fig. 2) [55]. Because bacterial products are often used as adjuvants to boost immune responses of the Th1 type, the expression of CD14 on oLCs makes them attractive targets for adjuvants added to allergen preparations to increase therapeutic effects in immunotherapy.

Are dendritic cells attractive targets for adjuvants of allergen immunotherapy?

Since several studies proved that the therapeutic effect of immunotherapy accompanies a shift of Th2 toward modified Th2 or Th1 responses, immuno-therapy strategies have been developed to coadminister adjuvants with a high capacity to trigger Th1 immune responses and transfer the immune response from innate to adaptive immunity. Most of these adjuvants are bacterial products, such as monophosphoryl lipid A (MPL) or synthetic oligonucleotides containing unmethylated CpG dinucleotides [56,57]. Structures belonging to innate immu-nity, such as the pattern recognition receptors expressed by DCs, play a key role as target structures for these strategies. Some of these adjuvants have been shown to modulate the maturation stage, phenotype, and stimulatory capacity of targeted DCs toward T cells in vitro [58–60]. Under immunotherapy, these adjuvants might bind to phylogenically conserved transmembrane proteins expressed by DCs, such as Toll-like receptor 9 binding to the adjuvant CpG or the lipopoly-saccharide receptor CD14 binding to the adjuvant MPL [59,61–65], and force a rapid shift of Th2 to Th1 immune responses to increase the therapeutic benefit of immunotherapy.

How does anti-IgE treatment target dendritic cells?

An alternative approach to allergen immunotherapy is to reduce the amount of IgE molecules in the sera of the patients, using anti-IgE antibodies to reduce the number of allergen-specific IgE molecules bound to FcεRI on DCs. These strategies have the goal of preventing the earliest steps of allergic reactions by reducing the frequency of IgE–FcεRI receptor interaction. In summary, treatment with anti-IgE antibodies results in a significant reduction of free IgE molecules in the sera of individuals who have allergies [66]. Because the amount of IgE receptors expressed on the cell surface of DCs correlates with the IgE serum levels, the therapeutic reduction of IgE in the sera of the patients accompanies a decrease of the amount of FcεRI expressed on DCs [66]. This down-regulation of FcεRI expressed on DCs reduces the probability of IgE–FcεRI-binding to effector cells of allergic diseases. Anti-IgE treatment has been shown to reduce the total number of myeloid CD11c$^+$ DCs in the peripheral blood of patients treated during the grass pollen season [67]. The advantage of this strategy is that any type of IgE molecule can be targeted. The disadvantage is that although the efficacy of anti-

IgE antibodies has been proven in different clinical studies [66,68], the application of this treatment regimen is limited to a concomitant long-term therapy and can not be used for the treatment of acute allergic reactions.

Summary

What are the future perspectives for dendritic cells as targets for antiallergic treatment strategies?

In summary, DCs play a paradigmatic role in our immune system and are therefore attractive targets of allergy immunotherapeutic strategies, which take advantage of the capability of DCs to act as natural silencers of allergic diseases [24,69,70]. The outstanding features qualifying DCs as target cells for allergen immunotherapy include their accessibility for immunotherapy preparations because of their localization at the border zones of the immune system, their capability to selectively take up allergens by way of IgE receptors on their cell surface, and the expression of a broad spectrum of inhibitory receptors on their cell surface, in combination with a high number of expressed surface structures appropriate for adjuvants of allergen immunotherapy. Furthermore, their capacity to induce exclusively allergic immune responses of the late type after FcεRI-receptor allergen challenge favors DCs as safe targets for allergen immunotherapy. Therefore, using DCs as a route for allergen immunotherapy represents a clever way to use physiologic methods of allergen challenge without increased risk for unwanted anaphylactic side effects.

Future approaches will be aimed at optimizing the routes of allergen immunotherapy, specifically focusing on DC subtypes with a high tolerogenic potential, such as DCs located in the oral mucosa; adjustment of the optimal allergen dosage and frequency of application in combination with the optimal choice of adjuvants; and use of allergen–adjuvant combinations [71].

Approaches that target DCs directly will be further established, such as the administration of B7-DC cross-linking antibodies, which have been used successfully in treating allergic hyper-responsiveness in animal models [32], or the use of chimeric fusion proteins [72] to concomitantly challenge activating FcεRI and inhibitory FcγRIIB receptors, which have already been shown to display inhibitory effects on human DCs [73] in vitro. Other approaches targeting DCs will include different vaccination strategies that use genetically modified allergen derivates or allergen hybrid molecules [74–76] to lower the risk for anaphylactic side reactions while increasing the efficacy of these treatment strategies. However, future studies will have to focus on the phenotypic and functional changes of DCs under immunotherapy to close the gap of knowledge about the exact role of DCs in immunotherapy. These studies might help to finally prove the hypothesis of DCs as efficient silencers and promising candidate cells for immunotherapy.

References

[1] Novak N, Allam JP, Betten H, et al. The role of antigen presenting cells at distinct anatomic sites: they accelerate and they slow down allergies. Allergy 2004;59:5–14.

[2] Rossi M, Young JW. Human dendritic cells: potent antigen-presenting cells at the crossroads of innate and adaptive immunity. J Immunol 2005;175:1373–81.

[3] Holt PG, Thomas WR. Sensitization to airborne environmental allergens: unresolved issues. Nat Immunol 2005;6:957–60.

[4] Golden DB. Insect sting allergy and venom immunotherapy: a model and a mystery. J Allergy Clin Immunol 2005;115:439–47.

[5] Sicherer SH, Leung DY. Advances in allergic skin disease, anaphylaxis, and hypersensitivity reactions to foods, drugs, and insects. J Allergy Clin Immunol 2005;116:153–63.

[6] Kay AB. Allergy and allergic diseases. First of two parts. N Engl J Med 2001;344:30–7.

[7] Kay AB. Allergy and allergic diseases. Second of two parts. N Engl J Med 2001;344:109–13.

[8] Wallet MA, Sen P, Tisch R. Immunoregulation of dendritic cells. Clin Med Res 2005;3:166–75.

[9] Till SJ, Francis JN, Nouri-Aria K, et al. Mechanisms of immunotherapy. J Allergy Clin Immunol 2004;113:1025–34.

[10] Bousquet J, Lockey R, Malling HJ. Allergen immunotherapy: therapeutic vaccines for allergic diseases. A WHO position paper. J Allergy Clin Immunol 1998;102:558–62.

[11] Lockey RF. "ARIA": global guidelines and new forms of allergen immunotherapy. J Allergy Clin Immunol 2001;108:497–9.

[12] Marogna M, Spadolini I, Massolo A, et al. Clinical, functional, and immunologic effects of sublingual immunotherapy in birch pollinosis: a 3-year randomized controlled study. J Allergy Clin Immunol 2005;115:1184–8.

[13] Gehlhar K, Schlaak M, Becker W, et al. Monitoring allergen immunotherapy of pollen-allergic patients: the ratio of allergen-specific IgG4 to IgG1 correlates with clinical outcome. Clin Exp Allergy 1999;29:497–506.

[14] Daeron M, Latour S, Malbec O, et al. The same tyrosine-based inhibition motif, in the intra-cytoplasmic domain of Fc gamma RIIB, regulates negatively BCR-, TCR-, and FcR-dependent cell activation. Immunity 1995;3:635–46.

[15] Jutel M, Pichler WJ, Skrbic D, et al. Bee venom immunotherapy results in decrease of IL-4 and IL-5 and increase of IFN-gamma secretion in specific allergen-stimulated T cell cultures. J Immunol 1995;154:4187–94.

[16] Jutel M, Akdis M, Budak F, et al. IL-10 and TGF-beta cooperate in the regulatory T cell response to mucosal allergens in normal immunity and specific immunotherapy. Eur J Immunol 2003;33:1205–14.

[17] Villadangos JA, Schnorrer P, Wilson NS. Control of MHC class II antigen presentation in dendritic cells: a balance between creative and destructive forces. Immunol Rev 2005;207:191–205.

[18] Lutz MB, Schuler G. Immature, semi-mature and fully mature dendritic cells: which signals induce tolerance or immunity? Trends Immunol 2002;23:445–9.

[19] Novak N, Tepel C, Koch S, et al. Evidence for a differential expression of the Fcepsilon-RIgamma chain in dendritic cells of atopic and nonatopic donors. J Clin Invest 2003;111:1047–56.

[20] Novak N, Allam JP, Hagemann T, et al. Characterization of FcepsilonRI-bearing CD123 blood dendritic cell antigen-2 plasmacytoid dendritic cells in atopic dermatitis. J Allergy Clin Immunol 2004;114:364–70.

[21] Allam JP, Novak N, Fuchs C, et al. Characterization of dendritic cells from human oral mucosa: a new Langerhans' cell type with high constitutive FcepsilonRI expression. J Allergy Clin Immunol 2003;112:141–8.

[22] Bieber T, de la Salle H, Wollenberg A, et al. Human epidermal Langerhans cells express the high affinity receptor for immunoglobulin e (fc epsilon ri). J Exp Med 1992;175:1285–90.

[23] Novak N, Kraft S, Bieber T. Unraveling the mission of FcepsilonRI on antigen-presenting cells. J Allergy Clin Immunol 2003;111:38–44.

[24] Rutella S, Lemoli RM. Regulatory T cells and tolerogenic dendritic cells: from basic biology to clinical applications. Immunol Lett 2004;94:11–26.

[25] Steinman RM. The control of immunity and tolerance by dendritic cell. Pathol Biol (Paris) 2003;51:59–60.

[26] Jonuleit H, Schmitt E. The regulatory T cell family: distinct subsets and their interrelations. J Immunol 2003;171:6323–7.

[27] Roncarolo MG, Levings MK, Traversari C. Differentiation of T regulatory cells by immature dendritic cells. J Exp Med 2001;193:F5–9.

[28] Mosmann TR. Regulation of immune responses by t cells with different cytokine secretion phenotypes: role of a new cytokine, cytokine synthesis inhibitory factor (il10). Int Arch Allergy Appl Immunol 1991;94:110–5.

[29] Velten FW, Duperrier K, Bohlender J, et al. A gene signature of inhibitory MHC receptors identifies a BDCA3(+) subset of IL-10-induced dendritic cells with reduced allostimulatory capacity in vitro. Eur J Immunol 2004;34:2800–11.

[30] Greenwald RJ, Freeman GJ, Sharpe AH. The B7 family revisited. Annu Rev Immunol 2005;23: 515–48.

[31] Yamazaki S, Iyoda T, Tarbell K, et al. Direct expansion of functional CD25+ CD4+ regulatory T cells by antigen-processing dendritic cells. J Exp Med 2003;198:235–47.

[32] Radhakrishnan S, Iijima K, Kobayashi T, et al. Blockade of allergic airway inflammation following systemic treatment with a B7-dendritic cell (PD-L2) cross-linking human antibody. J Immunol 2004;173:1360–5.

[33] Bellinghausen I, Klostermann B, Bottcher I, et al. Importance of the inducible costimulator molecule for the induction of allergic immune responses and its decreased expression on T helper cells after venom immunotherapy. Immunology 2004;112:80–6.

[34] Akbari O, Freeman GJ, Meyer EH, et al. Antigen-specific regulatory T cells develop via the ICOS-ICOS-ligand pathway and inhibit allergen-induced airway hyperreactivity. Nat Med 2002;8:1024–32.

[35] Stock P, Akbari O, Berry G, et al. Induction of T helper type 1-like regulatory cells that express Foxp3 and protect against airway hyper-reactivity. Nat Immunol 2004;5:1149–56.

[36] Witsch EJ, Peiser M, Hutloff A, et al. ICOS and CD28 reversely regulate IL-10 on re-activation of human effector T cells with mature dendritic cells. Eur J Immunol 2002;32:2680–6.

[37] Novak N, Valenta R, Bohle B, et al. FcepsilonRI engagement of Langerhans cell-like dendritic cells and inflammatory dendritic epidermal cell-like dendritic cells induces chemotactic signals and different T-cell phenotypes in vitro. J Allergy Clin Immunol 2004;113:949–57.

[38] Novak N, Kraft S, Bieber T. IgE receptors. Curr Opin Immunol 2001;13:721–6.

[39] Novak N, Bieber T, Katoh N. Engagement of fcepsilonri on human monocytes induces the production of il-10 and prevents their differentiation in dendritic cells. J Immunol 2001;67: 797–804.

[40] Von Bubnoff D, Matz H, Frahnert C, et al. Fc epsilon RI induces the tryptophan degradation pathway involved in regulating T cell responses. J Immunol 2002;169:1810–6.

[41] Mellor A. Indoleamine 2,3 dioxygenase and regulation of T cell immunity. Biochem Biophys Res Commun 2005;338(1):20–4.

[42] Boasso A, Herbeuval JP, Hardy AW, et al. Regulation of indoleamine 2,3-dioxygenase and tryptophanyl-tRNA-synthetase by CTLA-4-Fc in human CD4+ T cells. Blood 2005;105: 1574–81.

[43] Munn DH, Sharma MD, Lee JR, et al. Potential regulatory function of human dendritic cells expressing indoleamine 2,3-dioxygenase. Science 2002;297:1867–70.

[44] Boasso A, Herbeuval JP, Hardy AW, et al. Regulation of indoleamine 2,3-dioxygenase and tryptophanyl-tRNA-synthetase by CTLA-4-Fc in human CD4+ T cells. Blood 2005;105: 1574–81.

[45] Akdis CA, Blaser K. IL-10-induced anergy in peripheral T cell and reactivation by micro-environmental cytokines: two key steps in specific immunotherapy. FASEB J 1999;13:603–9.

[46] Akdis CA, Blesken T, Akdis M, et al. Role of interleukin 10 in specific immunotherapy. J Clin Invest 1998;102:98–106.

[47] Bellinghausen I, Metz G, Enk AH, et al. Insect venom immunotherapy induces interleukin-10 production and a th2-to-th1 shift, and changes surface marker expression in venom-allergic subjects. Eur J Immunol 1997;27:1131–9.

[48] Nasser SM, Ying S, Meng Q, et al. Interleukin-10 levels increase in cutaneous biopsies of patients undergoing wasp venom immunotherapy. Eur J Immunol 2001;31:3704–13.

[49] Nouri-Aria KT, Wachholz PA, Francis JN, et al. Grass pollen immunotherapy induces mucosal and peripheral IL-10 responses and blocking IgG activity. J Immunol 2004;172:3252–9.

[50] Eberlein-Konig B, Jung C, Rakoski J, et al. Immunohistochemical investigation of the cellular infiltrates at the sites of allergoid-induced late-phase cutaneous reactions associated with pollen allergen-specific immunotherapy. Clin Exp Allergy 1999;29:1641–7.

[51] Jung CM, Funk A, Rakoski J, et al. Immunohistochemical analysis of late local skin reactions during rush venom immunotherapy. Allergy 1997;52:717–26.

[52] Kelsall BL, Leon F. Involvement of intestinal dendritic cells in oral tolerance, immunity to pathogens, and inflammatory bowel disease. Immunol Rev 2005;206:132–48.

[53] Samsom JN, van Berkel LA, van Helvoort JM, et al. Fc gamma RIIB regulates nasal and oral tolerance: a role for dendritic cells. J Immunol 2005;174:5279–87.

[54] Kepley CL, Cambier JC, Morel PA, et al. Negative regulation of FcepsilonRI signaling by FcgammaRII costimulation in human blood basophils. J Allergy Clin Immunol 2000;106: 337–48.

[55] Allam JP, Niederhagen B, Büchler M, et al. Comparative analysis of nasal and oral mucosal myeloid Dendritic Cells. Allergy 2006;61:166–72.

[56] Freytag LC, Clements JD. Mucosal adjuvants. Vaccine 2005;23:1804–13.

[57] Jain S, Yap WT, Irvine DJ. Synthesis of protein-loaded hydrogel particles in an aqueous two-phase system for coincident antigen and CpG oligonucleotide delivery to antigen-presenting cells. Biomacromolecules 2005;6:2590–600.

[58] Kuchtey J, Chefalo PJ, Gray RC, et al. Enhancement of dendritic cell antigen cross-presentation by CpG DNA involves type I IFN and stabilization of class I MHC mRNA. J Immunol 2005; 175:2244–51.

[59] Ismaili J, Rennesson J, Aksoy E, et al. Monophosphoryl lipid A activates both human dendritic cells and T cells. J Immunol 2002;168:926–32.

[60] De BG, Moulin V, Pajak B, et al. The adjuvant monophosphoryl lipid A increases the function of antigen-presenting cells. Int Immunol 2000;12:807–15.

[61] Mothes N, Heinzkill M, Drachenberg KJ, et al. Allergen-specific immunotherapy with a monophosphoryl lipid A-adjuvanted vaccine: reduced seasonally boosted immunoglobulin E production and inhibition of basophil histamine release by therapy-induced blocking antibodies. Clin Exp Allergy 2003;33:1198–208.

[62] Bohle B, Jahn-Schmid B, Maurer D, et al. Oligodeoxynucleotides containing CpG motifs induce IL-12, IL-18 and IFN-gamma production in cells from allergic individuals and inhibit IgE synthesis in vitro. Eur J Immunol 1999;29:2344–53.

[63] Tighe H, Takabayashi K, Schwartz D, et al. Conjugation of immunostimulatory DNA to the short ragweed allergen amb a 1 enhances its immunogenicity and reduces its allergenicity. J Allergy Clin Immunol 2000;106:124–34.

[64] Marshall JD, Abtahi S, Eiden JJ, et al. Immunostimulatory sequence DNA linked to the Amb a 1 allergen promotes T(H)1 cytokine expression while downregulating T(H)2 cytokine expression in PBMCs from human patients with ragweed allergy. J Allergy Clin Immunol 2001;108:191–7.

[65] Tulic MK, Fiset PO, Christodoulopoulos P, et al. Amb a 1-immunostimulatory oligodeoxynucleotide conjugate immunotherapy decreases the nasal inflammatory response. J Allergy Clin Immunol 2004;113:235–41.

[66] Milgrom H, Fick Jr RB, Su JQ, et al. Treatment of allergic asthma with monoclonal anti-IgE antibody. rhuMAb-E25 Study Group. N Engl J Med 1999;341:1966–73.

[67] Feuchtinger T, Bartz H, von BA, et al. Treatment with omalizumab normalizes the number of myeloid dendritic cells during the grass pollen season. J Allergy Clin Immunol 2003;111:428–30.

[68] Leung DY, Sampson HA, Yunginger JW, et al. Effect of anti-IgE therapy in patients with peanut allergy. N Engl J Med 2003;348:986–93.

[69] Hackstein H, Thomson AW. Dendritic cells: emerging pharmacological targets of immunosuppressive drugs. Nat Rev Immunol 2004;4:24–34.

[70] O'Neill DW, Adams S, Bhardwaj N. Manipulating dendritic cell biology for the active immunotherapy of cancer. Blood 2004;104:2235–46.

[71] Marcucci F, Sensi L, Di CG, et al. Dose dependence of immunological response to sublingual immunotherapy. Allergy 2005;60:952–6.

[72] Zhu D, Kepley CL, Zhang K, et al. A chimeric human-cat fusion protein blocks cat-induced allergy. Nat Med 2005;11:446–9.

[73] Kepley CL, Zhang K, Zhu D, et al. FcepsilonRI-FcgammaRII coaggregation inhibits IL-16 production from human Langerhans-like dendritic cells. Clin Immunol 2003;108:89–94.

[74] Linhart B, Hartl A, Jahn-Schmid B, et al. A hybrid molecule resembling the epitope spectrum of grass pollen for allergy vaccination. J Allergy Clin Immunol 2005;115:1010–6.

[75] Hufnagl K, Winkler B, Focke M, et al. Intranasal tolerance induction with polypeptides derived from 3 noncross-reactive major aeroallergens prevents allergic polysensitization in mice. J Allergy Clin Immunol 2005;116:370–6.

[76] Reisinger J, Horak F, Pauli G, et al. Allergen-specific nasal IgG antibodies induced by vaccination with genetically modified allergens are associated with reduced nasal allergen sensitivity. J Allergy Clin Immunol 2005;116:347–54.

ELSEVIER
SAUNDERS

Immunol Allergy Clin N Am
26 (2006) 321–332

IMMUNOLOGY
AND ALLERGY
CLINICS
OF NORTH AMERICA

Peptide Immunotherapy

Mark Larché, PhD

Department of Allergy and Clinical Immunology, Faculty of Medicine, Imperial College,
Sir Alexander Fleming Building, Room 360, South Kensington, London SW7 2AZ, UK

Specific allergen immunotherapy is clinically effective and has an extended duration of action following cessation of treatment [1]; however, the therapeutic use of proteins to which the patient is sensitized results in frequent allergic adverse events, most commonly related to cross-linking of allergen-specific IgE on mast cells and basophils. Several strategies aimed at reducing the allergenicity of the treatment preparation while maintaining immunogenicity have been described. Many are discussed elsewhere in this issue. The use of short soluble synthetic peptides for the treatment of allergic disease offers the potential to avoid IgE-mediated allergic reactions while targeting T-cell epitopes and inducing modulation of allergen-specific responses. Synthetic peptides have been evaluated in several experimental animal models and more recently in human studies. Peptides are inexpensive to produce and easy to purify, standardize, and store. Short peptides lack the tertiary structure of the native protein but retain the ability to stimulate T cells.

In vitro and in vivo experimental models

The concept of therapeutic, antigen-specific targeting of T cells for the prevention and treatment of immunologic diseases developed from in vitro studies documenting the effects of high-dose peptide presentation between T cells. CD4+ helper T-cell clones were rendered refractory to antigen stimulation following pretreatment with supraoptimal concentrations of specific peptide [2]. Because antigen-presenting cells were absent, presentation of peptide to T-cell receptors

---

The author is an Asthma UK Senior Research Fellow.
E-mail address: m.larche@imperial.ac.uk

most likely occurred through binding to major histocompatibility complex (MHC) class II molecules on T cells and recognition of antigen in a "nonprofessional" context. Subsequent studies have confirmed the ability of nonprofessional antigen-presenting cells to induce T-cell tolerance [3].

Peptide-induced, antigen-specific nonresponsiveness, also known as tolerance, has been demonstrated in numerous murine models of autoimmunity and allergy. Initial experiments demonstrated that it was possible to induce systemic tolerance to peptides administered in incomplete Freund's adjuvant during the neonatal period [4,5]. Several studies have focused on the prevention and treatment of experimental autoimmune encephalomyelitis (EAE), a model of multiple sclerosis. High-dose intravenous peptide therapy resulted in T-cell clonal deletion and protection against disease [6]. EAE was also prevented by intraperitoneal administration of peptides from myelin basic protein (MBP). Peptide therapy blocked the progression of disease and decreased severity [7]. Intranasal, but not oral, administration of an MBP peptide led to protection from EAE [8]. More recently in a T-cell receptor transgenic model of EAE, MBP peptides were administered intranasally, leading to protection from disease that was dependent on deletion of effector T cells and the presence of interleukin-10 (IL-10) [9,10].

Peptide treatment has also been evaluated in murine models of experimental arthritis. Neonatal and adult rats were protected from collagen-induced arthritis by administration of peptides from type II collagen [11]. In a separate study, 50 μg of an immunodominant T-cell epitope of type II collagen was given intranasally for 4 days before induction of collagen-induced arthritis. Peptide treatment delayed the onset of disease and reduced severity. The treatment effect was associated with induction of IgG1 antibodies rather than IgG2b [12]. Prakken and colleagues [13] administered a peptide from heat shock protein (hsp60) to rats either intranasally (3×100 μg) or subcutaneously (2×300 μg). Both treatments protected the animals from the development of adjuvant arthritis induced by heat-killed mycobacterium tuberculosis.

Nonobese diabetic (NOD) mice were protected from diabetes by subcutaneous administration of 100 μg of a peptide of the insulin B chain in adjuvant or intranasal peptide (240 μg total peptide dose) [14]. Bockova and colleagues [15] used two hsp60 peptides to prevent the development of diabetes in NOD mice following subcutaneous administration in adjuvant. Glutamate decarboxylase (GAD65) peptides given intranasally reduced GAD-specific interferon-γ (IFN-γ) responses, increased IL-5 responses, and protected mice from disease. CD4+ cells from treated mice blocked adoptive transfer of disease to NOD *scid/scid* mice [16].

Fewer in vivo studies of peptide therapy have been performed in allergen sensitization models. Briner and colleagues [17] sensitized mice intraperitoneally with the major cat allergen Fel d 1. Treatment of mice with two allergen-derived polypeptides resulted in decreased production of IL-2 and allergen-specific IgG. Hoyne and colleagues [18] primed mice intraperitoneally with the major house dust mite allergen Der p 2 and then administered Der p 2 peptides intranasally. Peptide therapy downregulated T-cell and antibody responses to the native protein. In a model of tree pollen allergy, the dominant T-cell epitope of the major birch pollen allergen Bet v 1 was administered to CBA/J mice prophylactically and therapeutically. T-cell proliferative responses were inhibited by both treatments, but no change in antibody production or isotype was observed [19]. In a murine model of insect venom sensitivity, prophylactic administration of peptides from the bee venom allergen Api m 4 or the hornet venom allergen Dol m 5 resulted in a partial reduction of T-cell proliferation and B-cell antibody responses to subsequent allergen sensitization [20]. In separate studies of insect venom allergy, mice were sensitized with 100 ng of the major bee venom allergen Api m 1 (phospholipase A_2 [PLA_2]) in alum and treated by administration of 600 μg of a mixture of three polypeptides spanning the entire molecule. Mice were protected from anaphylaxis. A significant reduction in specific IgE was observed together with an increase in allergen-specific IgG2a and a reduced Th2:Th1 ratio [21].

Clinical studies

Autoimmunity

Peptide immunotherapy has been evaluated in small clinical studies with varying degrees of success. Most studies have focused on individuals with allergic disease, but some have also been performed in autoimmune disease including type I diabetes, rheumatoid arthritis, and multiple sclerosis. In many autoimmune diseases, it remains unclear which antigens should be selected as targets for intervention. Multiple sclerosis studies have focused on peptides from MBP, whereas two recent studies have evaluated peptides derived from heat shock proteins for the treatment of diabetes and rheumatoid arthritis. Patients with newly diagnosed type I diabetes were treated with 1 mg of peptide by subcutaneous injection at three time points (at study entry, 1 month, and 6 months). The treatment peptide (p277) was derived (and slightly modified) from the heat shock protein hsp60 and was selected on the basis of data obtained in experimental animals. Ten months after treatment, islet cell function had declined in the placebo-treated control group but had been maintained in the peptide-treated group. Peptide treatment was associated with modulation of peripheral blood responses to antigen. T cells produced more IL-13 and IL-10 following culture with antigen, indicating modulation toward a Th2/regulatory phenotype [22].

In patients with rheumatoid arthritis, another peptide (dnaJP1) derived from a heat shock protein of bacteria (dnaJ) was administered orally. Patients received 0.25, 2.5, or 25 mg of peptide daily for 6 months. The numbers of antigen-specific cells did not change following peptide treatment, but there were significant increases in the percentage of T cells producing IL-4 and IL-10 and concomitant reductions in T-cell proliferation, IL-2, IFN-γ, and tumor necrosis factor-α (TNF-α) production [23]. Furthermore, expression of *foxp3* was increased in CD4+ CD25^{bright} T cells. These findings suggest that a regulatory

T-cell response may have been induced by peptide therapy. Clinical data were not reported in this open study.

Patients with multiple sclerosis were treated with a single modified peptide (altered peptide ligand) from MBP in two related studies [24,25]. Patients were treated with up to 50 mg of peptide weekly by subcutaneous injection. The clinical response to peptide treatment was variable, and no definitive improvement in clinical outcomes was observed. Both studies were suspended as a result of treatment-related adverse events. In one study, adverse events were associated with the development of Th2 cells during treatment. Similar reactions in the other study were associated with expansion of peptide-specific Th1 cells displaying increased avidity for peptide-MHC complexes. Clinical deterioration correlated with expansion of antigen-specific Th1 cells during treatment. Subjects treated with lower doses of peptide (5 mg) weekly showed a trend for a reduction compared with baseline in the number and volume of contrast-enhancing lesions following 4 months of treatment.

Cat allergy

The majority of peptide immunotherapy studies in subjects with allergic disease have been performed with peptides from the major allergen of cat dander Fel d 1. Although cat allergy is not as prevalent as house dust mite or grass pollen allergy, the relative simplicity of Fel d 1 and the fact that 95% of cat-allergic subjects make IgE to this molecule have resulted in the selection of cat allergy as a model for the development and evaluation of this form of therapy. Four published studies evaluated the safety and efficacy of peptide immunotherapy for cat allergy using two polypeptides from Fel d 1. An equimolar mixture of the peptides (27 amino acids each in length) or placebo was administered in four subcutaneous injections (over a 2-week period) to 95 cat-sensitive patients in three dose groups (7.5, 75, and 750 μg per injection) [26]. Statistically significant improvements in lung and nasal symptom scores were observed but only in the high-dose group. A prominent placebo effect was observed. Treatment was associated with a significant incidence of adverse events, which occurred a few minutes to several hours after peptide injection. Related in vitro studies demonstrated reduced IL-4 production in peptide-specific T-cell lines following therapy [27].

A reduction in IL-4 production was also reported by Pene and colleagues [28]. Peripheral blood mononuclear cells (PBMCs) were stimulated with cat dander extract in vitro, before and after treatment with the peptide mixture. A significant reduction in IL-4 production was observed in the high-dose group (subjects received individual doses of 750 μg up to a total dose between 1500 and 4500 μg) but not in lower-dose groups. A reduction in allergen PD_{20} (provocative dose of inhaled allergen resulting in a 20% reduction in forced expiratory volume in 1 second [FEV_1]) was also observed in response to high and medium (individual doses of 75 μg up to a total dose between 150 and 450 μg) dose regimens when compared with baseline but not when compared with placebo.

In a double-blind, parallel group study using the same two peptides, Simons and colleagues [29] administered four weekly subcutaneous injections of 250 μg of the peptide mixture or placebo to 42 subjects with cat-allergic rhinitis or asthma. Treatment was associated with late onset symptoms of rhinitis, asthma, and pruritus. In contrast to other studies with the same peptide preparations, PBMC cytokine secretion profiles were no different in peptide-treated and placebo-treated subjects. No changes in early and late phase skin responses to whole allergen challenge were recorded.

In a multicenter study, 133 cat-allergic individuals received eight subcutaneous injections of 750 μg of the same mixture of two Fel d 1 peptides. A significant improvement in pulmonary function was observed but only in individuals with reduced baseline FEV_1 [30]. Improvements in lung function were evident at a single time point (3 weeks) after therapy, and no other significant treatment responses were observed. Several allergic reactions were reported during treatment, including some requiring epinephrine. In common with other studies using these peptides, late onset adverse reactions diminished with successive doses of peptide, indicating that a degree of tolerance had been induced.

More recently, a series of clinical studies have been performed using mixtures of shorter peptides from Fel d 1 [31–36]. Cat-allergic asthmatic volunteers were challenged intradermally with whole cat dander allergen extract before and after a single injection of 5 μg of each of 12 peptides in saline. The peptides spanned approximately 80% of the Fel d 1 molecule and encompassed most of the major T-cell epitopes. Peptide administration significantly reduced the magnitude of the cutaneous late phase reaction to intradermal allergen challenge. Evaluation of PBMC responses to allergen in vitro revealed a reduction in allergen-specific proliferation and a reduction in Th2 cytokines and IFN-γ [31].

Fel d 1 peptide immunotherapy was subsequently evaluated in a small double-blind, placebo-controlled clinical trial [32]. Twenty-four cat-allergic asthmatic subjects with moderate-to-severe asthma were subjected to cutaneous allergen challenge, inhaled methacholine PC_{20}, and inhaled allergen PD_{20}. Quality of life was evaluated by questionnaire (global evaluation to cat exposure). The primary outcome measure of the study was the magnitude of the late phase cutaneous reaction to intradermal challenge with allergen extract. Secondary outcome measures included the early phase cutaneous reaction to allergen challenge, the allergen PD_{20}, and the histamine PC_{20}. Baseline measurements were compared with two posttreatment follow-up evaluations. The first of these was performed 4 to 8 weeks after therapy and the second 3 to 9 months after peptide therapy. Subjects received a total of 90 μg of each of 12 peptides in divided incremental doses starting at 5 μg and administered at 3- to 4-day intervals. Peptide treatment resulted in a statistically significant reduction in the magnitude of early (second follow-up only) and late phase cutaneous reactions (both follow-up assessments) to intradermal challenge with allergen when compared with placebo. Investigation of peripheral blood responses to allergen before and after therapy demonstrated reduced proliferative responses and reduced Th1 and Th2 cytokine production. The reductions in proinflammatory cytokines were associated with an increase in production of IL-10. Subjects treated with peptides felt significantly better able to tolerate exposure to cats after therapy, although this improvement was not statistically significant when compared with responses from the placebo group. In this study of a small number of individuals, no significant improvements were observed in PD_{20} or PC_{20}.

In a small open-label study using a similar peptide preparation delivered at 2-week intervals rather than 3- to 4-day intervals, a significant reduction in airway hyperreactivity (measured by PC_{20}) was observed [33]. Peptides were administered by intradermal injection as in previous studies; however, a lower dosing regimen was applied (0.1, 1.0, 5, 10, and 25 µg). In addition to an improvement in nonspecific airway hyperreactivity, a significant reduction in the magnitude of the cutaneous late phase reaction was observed following allergen challenge in the skin, in keeping with earlier studies. Immunohistochemistry of skin tissue biopsy obtained after allergen challenge revealed a significant increase in the number of CD25+ cells when compared with the number after placebo challenge after peptide immunotherapy. The number of CD4+/IFN-γ+ cells increased significantly after peptide treatment, suggesting that recruitment of Th1 cells to the skin may be an important mechanism. No increases in IL-10+ cells were observed in the skin, but expression of transforming growth factor-β (TGF-β) mRNA appeared to be elevated. For technical reasons, the identity of the cells producing TGF-β could not be determined.

A related study was performed to investigate the effect of peptide immunotherapy on peripheral blood CD4+ responses and CD4+ CD25+ suppression of allergen-stimulated cultures in a double-blind, placebo-controlled trial [35]. Proliferative responses and IL-13 production from PBMCs cultured with allergen in vitro were significantly reduced following peptide therapy as in previous studies. The functional regulatory activity of CD4+ CD25+ cells was assessed by mixing with autologous CD4+ CD25− cells. Peptide immunotherapy did not alter the suppressive activity of CD4+ CD25+ cells in this study, suggesting that naturally occurring regulatory T cells may not have a significant role in the immunologic changes associated with peptide immunotherapy.

The role of antigen-specific inducible regulatory T cells (rather than naturally occurring CD4+ CD25+ cells) was addressed in a subsequent study by mixing CD4+ T cells (the population of cells containing the putative regulatory cells) with CD4− cells [36]. Each population was labeled with a different color fluorescent dye. CD4+ cells were labeled red, whereas CD4− cells were labeled green with cell cycle tracking dye. In an autologous culture system, CD4+ cells from before and after peptide therapy were mixed with CD4− cells from before and after therapy, in all possible combinations. The results demonstrated that antigen-specific proliferative responses of memory T cells were reduced following peptide immunotherapy when compared with baseline samples, and that CD4+ cells isolated after treatment could suppress the proliferative response of baseline CD4− cells. These data suggest that peptide immunotherapy can induce a population of CD4+ T cells with suppressive-regulatory activity.

Insect venom allergy

Phospholipase A_2 (Api m 1) peptides were evaluated in a small open study in which five bee venom–allergic subjects received divided incremental doses of an equimolar mixture of three immunodominant peptides at weekly intervals [37]. Ten subjects treated with conventional bee venom immunotherapy served as a control group. The cumulative peptide dose was 397.1 μg. One week after the last peptide injection, subjects were challenged subcutaneously with 10 μg of whole Api m 1. All five subjects tolerated the challenge without systemic allergic symptoms. One week later, a wild bee sting challenge was performed. Three of five subjects tolerated this challenge without reaction, whereas the remaining two subjects sustained mild systemic allergic reactions. No change was observed in levels of allergen-specific serum IgE or IgG4 during the course of peptide therapy; however, following subcutaneous challenge with the whole allergen 1 week after the last peptide injection, concentrations of both isotypes increased sharply, particularly IgG4. Three to 4 weeks later, serum levels of specific IgG4 were higher than IgE.

Texier and colleagues [38] defined potentially immunodominant T-cell epitopes in Api m 1 by direct binding of peptides to purified MHC class II molecules. Four peptides were identified, three of which were similar to those used previously for therapy by Müller and colleagues. Following a similar clinical protocol, Tarzi and colleagues [39] performed a controlled, open-label, single-blind study of peptide therapy in subjects with mild bee venom allergy. Peptide therapy was well tolerated, and no allergic reactions were observed during treatment. Peripheral blood responses to allergen in vitro showed reduced proliferation of T cells to purified allergen and whole bee venom. Proliferative responses to treatment peptides were also reduced. Th2 cytokine production following culture with allergen was reduced but associated with a concomitant increase in IL-10. Late phase cutaneous reactions to whole bee venom and Api m 1 were significantly reduced following allergen challenge. Serum samples were collected before, during, and after peptide therapy. Allergen-specific IgG, IgG4, and IgE levels were measured at the conclusion of the study. The results revealed a significant but transient increase in allergen-specific IgG and IgG4 following peptide immunotherapy. The functional activity of such an increase remains to be determined.

Using a rush desensitization protocol, Fellrath and colleagues [40] treated bee venom–allergic subjects using three synthetic polypeptides (long synthetic peptides) covering the whole Api m 1 molecule. Patients received approximately 250 μg in incremental divided doses at 30-minute intervals starting with 0.1 μg. Maintenance injections of 100 μg, or in some cases 300 μg, were given on days 4, 7, 14, 42, and 70. A transient increase in T-cell proliferation to the peptides was observed during therapy in the active treatment group. IFN-γ and IL-10 levels but not Th2 cytokines increased. Allergen-specific IgG4 but not IgE levels increased throughout the study period. Peptide-specific IgE was induced in some patients during the study. No significant change in skin sensitivity to intradermal allergen challenge was observed. Peptide therapy was generally well tolerated; however, local and disseminated erythema with occasional hand palm pruritus was observed in two subjects.

Mechanisms of peptide-induced tolerance

Immunologic tolerance in the T-cell compartment is likely to arise through systemic presentation of peptides (which are delivered to the immune system in saline without adjuvant and at very low doses) to naïve T cells by nonprofessional antigen-presenting cells and steady state (quiescent) dendritic cells, both of which are known to induce tolerogenic T-cell responses [41]. Because the peptides are encountered in a noninflammatory environment, the T-cell response will be one of tolerance through expansion of existing allergen-specific regulatory T cells and de novo generation of such cells from the naïve T-cell pool. When peptides are administered by intradermal injection, a significant amount of the injected dose is likely to pass rapidly into the systemic circulation through the capillary bed. Once in the circulation, peptides rapidly reach all tissues and bind to MHC class II molecules of the appropriate specificity. A relatively low plasma dose and high solubility may render peptides "tolerogenic." Recent studies in allergic disease have suggested that cross-linking of IgE on the surface of antigen-presenting cells (eg, by allergen) results in the activation of these cells and the release of cytokines [42]. Peptides may bind to MHC class II molecules on the cell surface without activating the cell. Previous studies have demonstrated the presence of a significant percentage of MHC class II molecules without bound peptides on the surface of immature and steady state dendritic cells [43]. Furthermore, this observation is associated with active HLA-DM, a chaperone and peptide-editing protein capable of loading exogenous peptides into empty MHC class II binding grooves [44]. As a result, when peptide-loaded dendritic cells recycle through lymphoid tissue, they present peptides to T cells while in a quiescent state, resulting in a tolerogenic encounter.

The role of peptide dose in therapy

Little is known about the most effective dose for induction of tolerance through peptide therapy. In mice, tolerogenic peptide doses range from a few micrograms [45] to milligrams [46]. By delivering T-cell epitopes directly to dendritic cells in vivo, it has recently been shown that doses as small as 500 pg can induce tolerance in a murine model [47]. Fundamental differences may exist in the mechanisms of low- and high-dose tolerance. High-dose protocols have been associated with clonal deletion and, to a lesser extent, anergy of antigen-specific cells [6,46,48]. Fewer studies of low-dose tolerance have been performed, but both high- and low-dose models appear to be characterized by the induction of T cells with regulatory activity [49–51].

The route of administration, physical properties, and solubility of the peptide are likely to influence whether tolerance or T-cell activation occurs. Microgram doses of allergen peptides administered intradermally resulted in systemic manifestations of tolerance such as reduced skin reactivity to allergen [31,32]. The same preparation delivered by inhalation (nebulized in saline and inhaled orally) did not induce tolerance [52]. This observation suggests that the route of administration can determine tolerogenicity. A threshold plasma dose of peptide may be required to establish systemic tolerance. Oral or inhaled delivery of peptide may require higher doses than the intradermal or intravenous routes to achieve efficacy. Indeed, a recent study in which tolerance was achieved through oral peptide administration supports this conclusion [23].

Summary

Synthetic peptides representing T-cell epitopes of allergens and autoantigens have been employed to induce antigen-specific tolerance in vivo in experimental models and the clinical setting. Delivery of peptides orally or by injection leads to reduced reactivity to antigen accompanied by the induction of T cells with a regulatory phenotype. In most models, production of IL-10 (and occasionally TGF-β) has been increased, whereas PBMC secretion of Th1 and Th2 cytokines is reduced. Peptide therapy may provide a safe, effective, and economically viable approach for disease-modifying therapy in autoimmune and allergic diseases.

References

[1] Durham SR, Walker SM, Varga EM, et al. Long-term clinical efficacy of grass-pollen immunotherapy. N Engl J Med 1999;341(7):468–75.

[2] Lamb JR, Skidmore BJ, Green N, et al. Induction of tolerance in influenza virus-immune T lymphocyte clones with synthetic peptides of influenza hemagglutinin. J Exp Med 1983; 157(5):1434–47.

[3] Bal V, McIndoe A, Denton G, et al. Antigen presentation by keratinocytes induces tolerance in human T cells. Eur J Immunol 1990;20(9):1893–7.

[4] Gammon G, Dunn K, Shastri N, et al. Neonatal T-cell tolerance to minimal immunogenic peptides is caused by clonal inactivation. Nature 1986;319(6052):413–5.

[5] Clayton JP, Gammon GM, Ando DG, et al. Peptide-specific prevention of experimental allergic encephalomyelitis: neonatal tolerance induced to the dominant T cell determinant of myelin basic protein. J Exp Med 1989;169(5):1681–91.

[6] Critchfield JM, Racke MK, Zuniga-Pflucker JC, et al. T cell deletion in high antigen dose therapy of autoimmune encephalomyelitis. Science 1994;263(5150):1139–43.

[7] Gaur A, Wiers B, Liu A, et al. Amelioration of autoimmune encephalomyelitis by myelin basic protein synthetic peptide-induced anergy. Science 1992;258(5087):1491–4.

[8] Metzler B, Wraith DC. Inhibition of experimental autoimmune encephalomyelitis by inhalation but not oral administration of the encephalitogenic peptide: influence of MHC binding affinity. Int Immunol 1993;5(9):1159–65.

[9] Burkhart C, Liu GY, Anderton SM, et al. Peptide-induced T cell regulation of experimental autoimmune encephalomyelitis: a role for IL-10. Int Immunol 1999;11(10):1625–34.

[10] Anderton SM, Burkhart C, Liu GY, et al. Antigen-specific tolerance induction and the immunotherapy of experimental autoimmune disease. Novartis Found Symp 1998;215:120–31.

[11] Ku G, Kronenberg M, Peacock DJ, et al. Prevention of experimental autoimmune arthritis with a peptide fragment of type II collagen. Eur J Immunol 1993;23(3):591–9.

[12] Staines NA, Harper N, Ward FJ, et al. Mucosal tolerance and suppression of collagen-induced arthritis (CIA) induced by nasal inhalation of synthetic peptide 184-198 of bovine type II collagen (CII) expressing a dominant T cell epitope. Clin Exp Immunol 1996;103(3):368–75.

[13] Prakken BJ, van Der ZR, Anderton SM, et al. Peptide-induced nasal tolerance for a mycobacterial heat shock protein 60 T cell epitope in rats suppresses both adjuvant arthritis and nonmicrobially induced experimental arthritis. Proc Natl Acad Sci USA 1997;94(7):3284–9.

[14] Daniel D, Wegmann DR. Protection of nonobese diabetic mice from diabetes by intranasal or subcutaneous administration of insulin peptide B-(9-23). Proc Natl Acad Sci USA 1996;93(2):956–60.

[15] Bockova J, Elias D, Cohen IR. Treatment of NOD diabetes with a novel peptide of the hsp60 molecule induces Th2-type antibodies. J Autoimmun 1997;10(4):323–9.

[16] Tian J, Atkinson MA, Clare-Salzler M, et al. Nasal administration of glutamate decarboxylase (GAD65) peptides induces Th2 responses and prevents murine insulin-dependent diabetes. J Exp Med 1996;183(4):1561–7.

[17] Briner TJ, Kuo MC, Keating KM, et al. Peripheral T-cell tolerance induced in naive and primed mice by subcutaneous injection of peptides from the major cat allergen Fel d I. Proc Natl Acad Sci USA 1993;90(16):7608–12.

[18] Hoyne GF, O'Hehir RE, Wraith DC, et al. Inhibition of T cell and antibody responses to house dust mite allergen by inhalation of the dominant T cell epitope in naive and sensitized mice. J Exp Med 1993;178(5):1783–8.

[19] Bauer L, Bohle B, Jahn-Schmid B, et al. Modulation of the allergic immune response in BALB/c mice by subcutaneous injection of high doses of the dominant T cell epitope from the major birch pollen allergen Bet v 1. Clin Exp Immunol 1997;107(3):536–41.

[20] King TP, Lu G, Agosto H. Antibody responses to bee melittin (Api m 4) and hornet antigen 5 (Dol m 5) in mice treated with the dominant T-cell epitope peptides. J Allergy Clin Immunol 1998;101(3):397–403.

[21] von Garnier C, Astori M, Kettner A, et al. Allergen-derived long peptide immunotherapy down-regulates specific IgE response and protects from anaphylaxis. Eur J Immunol 2000;30(6):1638–45.

[22] Raz I, Elias D, Avron A, et al. Beta-cell function in new-onset type 1 diabetes and immuno-modulation with a heat-shock protein peptide (DiaPep277): a randomised, double-blind, phase II trial. Lancet 2001;358(9295):1749–53.

[23] Prakken BJ, Samodal R, Le TD, et al. Epitope-specific immunotherapy induces immune deviation of proinflammatory T cells in rheumatoid arthritis. Proc Natl Acad Sci USA 2004;101(12):4228–33.

[24] Kappos L, Comi G, Panitch H, et al. Induction of a non-encephalitogenic type 2 T helper-cell autoimmune response in multiple sclerosis after administration of an altered peptide ligand in a placebo-controlled, randomized phase II trial: the Altered Peptide Ligand in relapsing MS Study Group. Nat Med 2000;6(10):1176–82.

[25] Bielekova B, Goodwin B, Richert N, et al. Encephalitogenic potential of the myelin basic protein peptide (amino acids 83–99) in multiple sclerosis: results of a phase II clinical trial with an altered peptide ligand. Nat Med 2000;6(10):1167–75.

[26] Norman PS, Ohman JL, Long AA, et al. Treatment of cat allergy with T-cell reactive peptides. Am J Respir Crit Care Med 1996;154(6 Pt 1):1623–8.

[27] Marcotte GV, Braun CM, Norman PS, et al. Effects of peptide therapy on ex vivo T-cell responses. J Allergy Clin Immunol 1998;101(4 Pt 1):506–13.

[28] Pene J, Desroches A, Paradis L, et al. Immunotherapy with Fel d 1 peptides decreases IL-4

release by peripheral blood T cells of patients allergic to cats. J Allergy Clin Immunol 1998; 102(4 Pt 1):571–8.

[29] Simons FE, Imada M, Li Y, et al. Fel d 1 peptides: effect on skin tests and cytokine synthesis in cat-allergic human subjects. Int Immunol 1996;8(12):1937–45.

[30] Maguire P, Nicodemus C, Robinson D, et al. The safety and efficacy of ALLERVAX CAT in cat allergic patients. Clin Immunol 1999;93(3):222–31.

[31] Oldfield WL, Kay AB, Larche M. Allergen-derived T cell peptide-induced late asthmatic reactions precede the induction of antigen-specific hyporesponsiveness in atopic allergic asthmatic subjects. J Immunol 2001;167(3):1734–9.

[32] Oldfield WL, Larche M, Kay AB. Effect of T-cell peptides derived from Fel d 1 on allergic reactions and cytokine production in patients sensitive to cats: a randomised controlled trial. Lancet 2002;360(9326):47–53.

[33] Alexander C, Ying S, Kay B, et al. Fel d 1–derived T cell peptide therapy induces recruitment of CD4CD25; CD4 interferon-gamma T helper type 1 cells to sites of allergen-induced late-phase skin reactions in cat-allergic subjects. Clin Exp Allergy 2005;35(1):52–8.

[34] Alexander C, Tarzi M, Larche M, et al. The effect of Fel d 1–derived T-cell peptides on upper and lower airway outcome measurements in cat-allergic subjects. Allergy 2005;60(10):1269–74.

[35] Smith TR, Alexander C, Kay AB, et al. Cat allergen peptide immunotherapy reduces CD4 T cell responses to cat allergen but does not alter suppression by CD4 CD25 T cells: a double-blind placebo-controlled study. Allergy 2004;59(10):1097–101.

[36] Verhoef A, Alexander C, Kay AB, et al. T cell epitope immunotherapy induces a CD4(+) T cell population with regulatory activity. PLoS Med 2005;2(3):e78.

[37] Muller U, Akdis CA, Fricker M, et al. Successful immunotherapy with T-cell epitope peptides of bee venom phospholipase A2 induces specific T-cell anergy in patients allergic to bee venom. J Allergy Clin Immunol 1998;101(6 Pt 1):747–54.

[38] Texier C, Pouvelle S, Busson M, et al. HLA-DR restricted peptide candidates for bee venom immunotherapy. J Immunol 2000;164(6):3177–84.

[39] Tarzi M, Klunker S, Texier C, et al. Induction of interleukin-10 and suppressor of cytokine signaling-3 gene expression following peptide immunotherapy. Clin Exp Allergy 2006;36: 465–74.

[40] Fellrath JM, Kettner A, Dufour N, et al. Allergen-specific T-cell tolerance induction with allergen-derived long synthetic peptides: results of a phase I trial. J Allergy Clin Immunol 2003; 111(4):854–61.

[41] Steinman RM, Hawiger D, Nussenzweig MC. Tolerogenic dendritic cells. Annu Rev Immunol 2003;21:685–711.

[42] Novak N, Bieber T, Katoh N. Engagement of Fc epsilon RI on human monocytes induces the production of IL-10 and prevents their differentiation in dendritic cells. J Immunol 2001; 167(2):797–804.

[43] Santambrogio L, Sato AK, Fischer FR, et al. Abundant empty class II MHC molecules on the surface of immature dendritic cells. Proc Natl Acad Sci USA 1999;96(26):15050–5.

[44] Santambrogio L, Sato AK, Carven GJ, et al. Extracellular antigen processing and presentation by immature dendritic cells. Proc Natl Acad Sci USA 1999;96(26):15056–61.

[45] Chai JG, James E, Dewchand H, et al. Transplantation tolerance induced by intranasal administration of HY peptides. Blood 2004;103(10):3951–9.

[46] Karin N, Mitchell DJ, Brocke S, et al. Reversal of experimental autoimmune encephalomyelitis by a soluble peptide variant of a myelin basic protein epitope: T cell receptor antagonism and reduction of interferon gamma and tumor necrosis factor alpha production. J Exp Med 1994; 180(6):2227–37.

[47] Kretschmer K, Apostolou I, Hawiger D, et al. Inducing and expanding regulatory T cell populations by foreign antigen. Nat Immunol 2005;6:1219–27.

[48] Kearney ER, Pape KA, Loh DY, et al. Visualization of peptide-specific T cell immunity and peripheral tolerance induction in vivo. Immunity 1994;1(4):327–39.

[49] Wraith DC, Nicolson KS, Whitley NT. Regulatory CD4(+) T cells and the control of autoimmune disease. Curr Opin Immunol 2004;16(6):695–701.

[50] Wraith DC, Goldman M, Lambert PH. Vaccination and autoimmune disease: what is the evidence? Lancet 2003;362(9396):1659–66.

[51] Apostolou I, Von Boehmer H. In vivo instruction of suppressor commitment in naive T cells. J Exp Med 2004;199(10):1401–8.

[52] Ali FR, Oldfield WL, Higashi N, et al. Late asthmatic reactions induced by inhalation of allergen-derived T cell peptides. Am J Respir Crit Care Med 2004;169(1):20–6.

ELSEVIER
SAUNDERS

Immunol Allergy Clin N Am
26 (2006) 333–347

IMMUNOLOGY
AND ALLERGY
CLINICS
OF NORTH AMERICA

IgE-Facilitated Antigen Presentation: Role in Allergy and the Influence of Allergen Immunotherapy

Louisa K. Wilcock, BSc, James N. Francis, PhD,
Stephen R. Durham, MD*

Upper Respiratory Medicine, Imperial College, National Heart and Lung Institute, Dovehouse Street, London, SW3 6LY, UK

One mechanism by which antigen-presenting cells (APCs) sample antigens from the local microenvironment is a crude process involving direct phagocytosis or pinocytosis and is independent of surface receptors. This "scavenging" is inefficient and triggers T-cell activation only in the presence of high antigen concentrations [1]. In addition, B cells are able to focus very low concentrations of antigen via specific membrane immunoglobulin into endosomal compartments, a process that results in greatly enhanced cell activation. This receptor-mediated "antigen focusing" may occur at antigen concentrations 10^3 to 10^4 fold lower than by nonspecific uptake [2]. Antigen focusing by B cells amplifies capture of antigen without the requirement for receptor cross-linking. Capture, per se, may not result in activation of the B cell, which also requires subsequent T-cell recognition. After internalization by either mechanism, antigen is degraded into antigenic peptides within endosomal compartments. Peptides subsequently bind to major histocompatibility complex (MHC) class II molecules, and the complexes are loaded onto the cell surface before presentation to antigen-specific T cells [1]. Activation of immune responses in healthy individuals depends on very high antigen concentrations or the presence of B cells with antigen-specific membrane immunoglobulin.

* Corresponding author.
E-mail address: s.durham@imperial.ac.uk (S.R. Durham).

0889-8561/06/$ – see front matter © 2006 Elsevier Inc. All rights reserved.
doi:10.1016/j.iac.2006.02.004   *immunology.theclinics.com*

In allergic individuals, exposure to common inhalant allergens involves minute allergen concentrations at respiratory mucosal surfaces. In patients who have seasonal pollinosis, the quantity of allergen that reaches the nasal mucosa, even at the peak of the pollen season, is estimated to be a few micrograms per year [3]. In normal nonatopic individuals, such small quantities of allergen fail to activate an immune response. In atopic individuals, allergen-specific IgE produced at least in part by plasma cells activated locally within mucosal tissue [4–6] binds to allergen at the mucosal surface in a process referred to as IgE-facilitated allergen presentation (FAP). This process is fundamentally different from antigen focusing mediated by antigen-specific B cells in normal subjects. In contrast to the lack of effect in normal nonatopic subjects, the additional presence of high local IgE allows APCs that express IgE receptors to process extremely low concentrations of antigen. FAP is dependent on the combined presence of allergen, elevated IgE, and the expression of IgE receptors on the surface of APCs.

IgE is a characteristic marker of atopy

IgE is central to allergic inflammation [7]. The abundance of IgE in the target organs of allergy sufferers emphasizes the importance of this immunoglobulin in promoting allergic inflammation [5,8]. IgE has the ability to bind with extremely high affinity to IgE receptors on the surface of mast cells and basophils [7]. The proximity of IgE-producing cells to tissue mast cells enables a continuous supply of antibody for cell surface receptors. Subsequent allergen exposure triggers an immediate local response. IgE promotes IgE receptor expression on effector cells, supports the survival of mast cells in mucosal tissue, and induces positive signals for IgE synthesis [9].

Overproduction of allergen-specific IgE in atopic individuals is a consequence of differential cytokine production. B cells recruited to sites of allergic inflammation encounter inflammatory mediators and Th2 cytokines, in particular, interleukin-4 (IL-4) and IL-13. These cytokines are produced locally by Th2 lymphocytes but also in high concentrations by activated mast cells and basophils [10]. Local IL-4 and IL-13 promote B cells to switch preferentially to IgE synthesis [11]. Circulating immature B cells that encounter antigen in the periphery will present processed epitopes to specific T cells (cognate recognition). Subsequent CD40/CD40L ligation at the T-cell surface results in further IL-4 production by activated Th2 T cells and initiation of heavy-chain constant region gene recombination in favor of IgG4 or IgE antibodies (isotype switching). This process has been shown to occur locally, in nasal [12,13] tissue and in bronchial tissue [14,15], enabling localization of the allergic response to a particular region with associated clinical manifestations. Following isotype switching, B cells differentiate into plasma cells and secrete antigen-specific IgE into the local environment [16]. IgE-mediated responses are inevitably dependent on IgE receptors, which exist in morphologically distinct and independent high- (FcεR1) and low-affinity (FcεRII, CD23) species.

High-affinity IgE receptor mediates immediate hypersensitivity

FcƐRI is expressed widely on the surface of mast cells and basophils and has also been identified on monocytes and dendritic cells [17]. FcƐRI is expressed in trimeric form (FcƐRIαγ_2) on APCs and is upregulated in allergic subjects, whereas it is low or absent in normal individuals [18]. A member of the immunoglobulin super family of proteins, tetrameric (FcƐRI αβγ2) is expressed on mast cells and basophils (Fig. 1) and mediates immediate hypersensitivity reactions [19]. Cross-linking of FcƐRI-bound IgE by allergen induces a cascade of complex signaling events [20] that ultimately results in the release of preformed inflammatory mediators that include histamine, tryptase, and IL-4. The parallel upregulation of CD40 ligand provides a switch factor for B cells and promotes prolonged B-cell survival. IL-4 and IgE upregulate FcƐRI expression, which enables a positive feedback loop for FcƐRI-associated signaling. In contrast, trimeric FcƐRI on APCs is primarily involved in IgE-facilitated antigen presentation [11].

Low-affinity IgE receptor, CD23, has multiple functions

The low-affinity receptor for IgE (FcƐRII/CD23) is a type II integral membrane protein. The active receptor is a trimer that comprises C-type lectin-binding

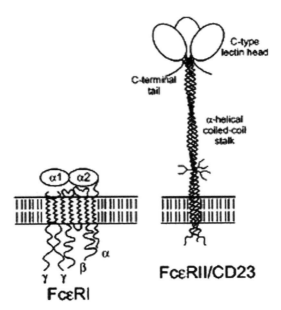

Fig. 1. Schematic representations of the IgE receptors FcƐRI and FcƐRII/CD23. (*Adapted from* Gould HJ, Sutton BJ, Beavil AJ, et al. The biology of IgE and the basis of allergic disease. Annu Rev Immunol 2003;21:582; with permission.)

regions that are attached to the cell membrane surface via α-helical stalks (Fig. 1). The receptor has two isoforms that differ in six of seven amino acids in the intracellular region, resulting in their differential expression and distinct functions. CD23a is expressed exclusively on the B cell surface following activation. CD23b expression is IL-4 inducible and is present on a variety of cells, including B cells, macrophages, monocytes, follicular dendritic cells, and eosinophils [7]. CD23 has a variety of functions. Its ligands include IgE, complement receptors CR1, CR2, and CR4, and vitronectin [7]. In mice, CD23 is involved in negative regulation of IgE synthesis [21]. Membrane CD23 is cleaved by proteases to form soluble CD23 (sCD23), which functions to promote B-cell differentiation in germinal centers via interactions with CD21 on the B-cell surface [7]. CD23 expression is upregulated by IL-13 and IL-4; therefore, it has increased expression among atopic individuals when compared with healthy individuals [22]. An important function of CD23 is its role in IgE-dependent facilitated antigen presentation.

Allergen-IgE complexes are internalized on IgE receptors

IgE-allergen complexes are captured and immobilized on the APC surface by binding to IgE receptors. Fig. 2 illustrates CD23-dependent IgE-FAP as mediated by B cells. The IgE-allergen complexes are internalized to endosomal compartments where the allergen is processed and presented to T cells on MHC class II molecules [23]. There is growing evidence for a role of IgE-FAP in activating allergen-specific T cells in vivo. Expression of the low-affinity receptor CD23 is higher in atopic individuals when compared with nonatopic individuals [22], and CD23, CD40, and HLA are all upregulated on B cells during the pollen season [24]. Interestingly, studies of B-cell lines have shown that CD23 is co-expressed in association with MHC molecules at the surface membrane of B cells [25]. Karagiannis and colleagues [26] described endocytosis of the entire CD23/IgE/allergen complex along with the associated MHC class II molecule. The association of CD23 with MHC molecules is thought to enable more efficient loading of peptide onto MHC in endosomal compartments. In the same study, CD23 was shown to be recycled to the cell surface with the peptide loaded MHC. As well as CD23-mediated IgE-FAP, Maurer and colleagues [27] isolated blood dendritic cells that expressed trimeric FcεRI (FcεRIα$γ_2$). Despite extremely low numbers, these cells were able to efficiently stimulate IgE-dependent T-cell responses. Because FAP is known to occur via CD23 and FcεRI, any cell type expressing these receptors is able to focus allergen for more effective processing, presentation, and activation of T cells in an IgE-dependent fashion [28].

Furthermore, because FcεRI and CD23 are expressed on professional APCs, priming of naïve T cells can occur in addition to the activation of secondary responses. The potential consequences of IgE-FAP are substantial. When occurring between B cells and T cells, activation of the T cell will induce Th2 cytokine expression that further promotes IgE production by B cells. This expression, in turn, would lead to an abundance of IgE in the mucosal tissue, further

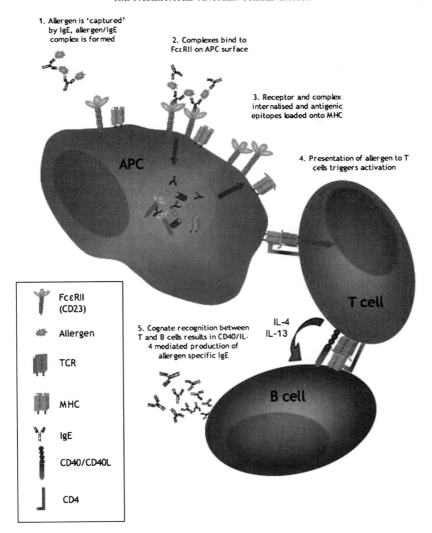

1. Allergen is 'captured' by IgE, allergen/IgE complex is formed

2. Complexes bind to FcεRII on APC surface

3. Receptor and complex internalised and antigenic epitopes loaded onto MHC

4. Presentation of allergen to T cells triggers activation

APC

T cell

5. Cognate recognition between T and B cells results in CD40/IL-4 mediated production of allergen specific IgE

IL-4
IL-13

B cell

FcεRII (CD23)

Allergen

TCR

MHC

IgE

CD40/CD40L

CD4

Fig. 2. CD23-mediated IgE-facilitated allergen presentation. Cartoon depicts IgE-FAP using CD23 on the surface of a B cell and resulting in cognate recognition by allergen-specific T cell. The interaction results in further production of allergen-specific IgE.

perpetuating the cycle of T-cell activation and intensifying the inflammatory response (Fig. 2).

Experimental assessment of IgE-facilitated allergen presentation

The role of IgE and IgE-CD23 interaction in antigen presentation was originally demonstrated in a murine model [29]. Trinitrophenyl (TNP)-specific IgE facilitated the presentation of TNP by mouse B cells at 100-fold less concentrations of TNP than in the presence of TNP alone. These experiments were subsequently confirmed in humans [23].

The addition of antigen-specific IgE was shown to enhance significantly the ability of Epstein-Barr virus (EBV)–transformed B cells to present antigen to T cells with subsequent enhanced T-cell activation and proliferation. CD23-dependent FAP has since been confirmed using monomeric IgE [30] and atopic serum containing polymeric IgE when complexed with allergen [31]. In vitro experiments of IgE-FAP have used EBV-transformed human B-cell lines that express high levels of CD23 and are efficient in processing and presenting antigens to specific T cells, with resulting activation and proliferation [23]. Indicator serum from an atopic individual with high allergen-specific IgE levels is mixed

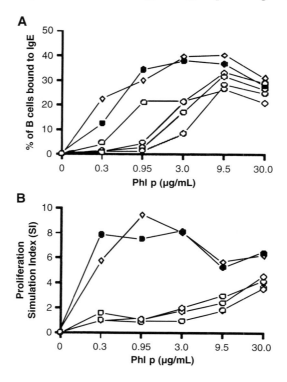

Fig. 3. Allergen-IgE binding to B cells is associated with enhanced antigen presentation to allergen-specific T cells, which is inhibited by sera from immunotherapy patients. Graph shows allergen-dependent binding of IgE in the absence (*filled circles*) or presence (*open circles*) of sera from four grass and one birch (*open diamonds*) immunotherapy patients. IgE-allergen complexes bound to B cells were detected with fluorescently labeled anti-IgE antibody by flow cytometry (*A*), or EBV-transformed B cells were irradiated and used as APCs for an autologous grass pollen–specific T-cell clone, and proliferation was measured after 24 hours by 3[H]-thymidine incorporation (*B*). Data shown are representative of three separate experiments. (*Adapted from* Wachholz PA, Soni NK, Till SJ, et al. Inhibition of allergen-IgE binding to B cells by IgG antibodies after grass pollen immunotherapy. J Allergy Clin Immunol 2003;112:920; with permission.)

with allergen. Subsequent incubation of the allergen-IgE complexes with EBV-transformed B cells results in higher binding of IgE with CD23 [32], with internalization and processing of allergen to generate small peptide epitopes that are expressed at the cell surface in the context of MHC class II. In standardized proliferation assays, the B cells are used to present the allergen peptides to T-cell clones. Elevated T-cell activation is measured as proliferation of clones [31]. Van der Heijden and colleagues [33] showed that Der-p 2 (house dust mite major allergen)–specific T-cell clones proliferated at 100- to 1000-fold lower concentrations of Der-p 2 when the allergen was complexed to high IgE-containing serum compared with uncomplexed allergen. The investigators were able to demonstrate a direct correlation between FAP-mediated T-cell proliferation and the subject's serum IgE levels.

The use of T-cell assays as a readout of efficient IgE-FAP is complex and time-consuming and requires the generation and maintenance of long-term allergen-specific T-cell clones. The assay can be greatly simplified by measuring only the IgE-dependent binding of allergen to CD23 on the surface of B cells, which has been shown to correlate closely with subsequent T-cell activation and proliferation (Fig. 3). In this modified assay, surface binding of the allergen-IgE complexes is performed at low temperatures to prevent internalization of the complex [3], thereby allowing detection by flow cytometry of the allergen-IgE complexes to the B-cell surface. Detection of the allergen-IgE complexes is most easily measured by use of anti-IgE antibodies, although allergen binding may also be confirmed by use of biotinylated allergen [34]. Using sera from subjects with grass pollen allergy, the authors have confirmed that specific IgE levels correlate with the efficiency of allergen-IgE complex binding ($r = 0.79$, $P < .0001$). This association strongly supports a role for IgE-FAP in the pathogenesis of allergic disease in vivo.

Immunotherapy induces changes in humoral responses to allergen

The clinical benefits of specific allergen immunotherapy are well documented [35]. The mechanisms of successful treatment are not fully understood, although immune deviation or the induction of T regulatory cells is likely to be central to disease remission. Chronic antigen exposure results in high-titered IgG4 responses [36], and because immunotherapy involves the long-term administration of high-dose allergen, it is not surprising that levels of IgG4 increase dramatically following treatment [34,37,38]. Far from being a simple bystander effect, IgG4 antibodies induced by immunotherapy have been shown to have functionally relevant "blocking" activity.

The concept of blocking antibodies, whereby competition with IgE for binding to allergen prevents IgE-mediated responses, has existed since Cooke and co-workers [39] demonstrated in 1935 that postimmunotherapy serum prevented inflammation that had been induced by preimmunotherapy serum. In 1968, this inhibitory activity was shown to be elicited by IgG "blocking" antibodies [40], suggesting that these IgG antibodies could inhibit histamine release from sensitized basophils induced by atopic serum. More recently, IgG4 has been shown to be the prominent antibody isotype that is induced by immunotherapy.

In a study of chronic parasitic filarial infection, a significant correlation was demonstrated between high IgG4 titers and patients who were asymptomatic despite chronic infection. IgG1 and not IgG4 levels were associated with allergic responses to the parasite, and depletion of IgG4 from the serum removed blocking activity as defined by basophil histamine release [41]. Serum from post allergen-immunotherapy patients has been shown to inhibit basophil histamine release, a marker of FcεRI-mediated immediate hypersensitivity reactions [42,43]. In a study of modified birch pollen immunotherapy, serum from immunotherapy-treated but not placebo-treated patients could inhibit Bet v 1 (birch pollen major allergen)–mediated basophil histamine release but not grass pollen–mediated release, demonstrating the allergen-specific nature of immunotherapy [43].

IgE-facilitated allergen presentation is inhibited by postimmunotherapy serum

In 1999 van Neerven and colleagues demonstrated the induction of blocking antibodies during immunotherapy that were capable of inhibiting IgE-FAP–mediated T-cell activation [3]. Serum from a patient treated with long-term birch pollen immunotherapy was incubated with birch pollen allergen and serum containing high levels of birch-specific IgE. The inhibition was shown to be allergen-specific, because serum from grass-treated immunotherapy patients was unable to inhibit IgE-facilitated presentation of birch pollen. The researchers showed that this inhibitory activity was present 3 to 6 months after starting treatment. The induction of inhibitory activity following immunotherapy has since been confirmed in other trials [3,34]. van Neerven further demonstrated that blocking IgG antibodies induced by birch immunotherapy and isolated by fractionation could inhibit IgE-FAP–mediated activation of CD4+ T cells [3]. Wachholz and co-workers confirmed these findings using IgG-fractionated sera from grass pollen–immunotherapy patients [34]. Nouri-Aria and colleagues [44] confirmed that immunotherapy induced increases in serum inhibitory activity for allergen-IgE complex binding (Fig. 4) and increases in allergen-specific IgG4 antibody levels. These observations occurred in parallel with increases in IL-10 production. Furthermore, blocking activity for IgE-FAP demonstrated in postimmunotherapy serum co-purified with IgG4-containing fractions [44].

Lack of correlation between IgG4 and clinical improvement

The main argument against a functional role for IgG4 is that the serum levels of the antibody do not correlate well with clinical efficacy. For example, in a trial

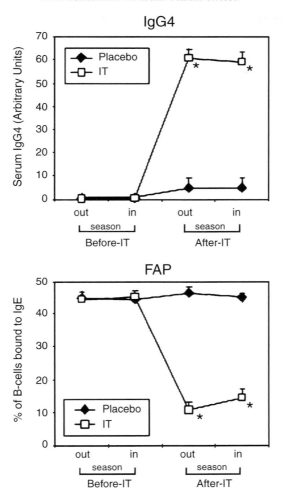

Fig. 4. Increased serum allergen-specific IgG4 concentrations and inhibition of allergen-IgE binding to B cells by sera from immunotherapy-treated but not placebo-treated patients before (*Before IT*) and after 2 years of treatment (*After IT*) before (*out*) and during (*in*) the pollen season. Results are expressed as mean + SE. *$P < .05$ as determined by Wilcoxon matched pairs test. (*Adapted from* Wilcock LK, Wachholz PA, Hae-Won D, et al. Inhibition of IgE-facilitated allergen presentation: a longitudinal study of grass pollen immunotherapy. ACI International 2006, Supplement 2, 244–7, with permission. © 2006 Hogrefe & Huber)

of venom immunotherapy, IgG4 levels were markedly elevated in patients who responded to treatment but also in those who did not [45]. This lack of correlation has been confirmed in trials of immunotherapy with venom [46] and inhalant allergens [47]. More recently, the role of IgG4 as a blocking antibody induced by immunotherapy has been reviewed. The findings suggest that impure or irregular allergen extracts used for determining IgG titers fail to distinguish true blocking antibodies and may be responsible for the reported lack of positive correlations [48].

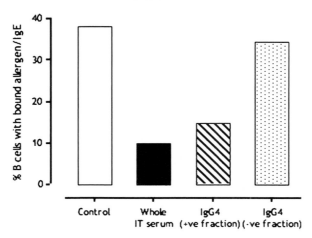

Fig. 5. Serum obtained following grass pollen immunotherapy was separated by affinity chromatography. The IgG4 fraction, the eluted fraction from which IgG4 had been removed, and the whole serum were compared for their ability to inhibit the binding of allergen-IgE complexes to B cells, as detected by flow cytometry (*Adapted from* Nouri-Aria KT, Wachholz PA, Francis JN, et al. Grass pollen immunotherapy induces mucosal and peripheral IL-10 responses and blocking IgG activity. J Immunol 2004;172:3257.)

The authors recently demonstrated that IgG4 contributes most of the inhibitory activity contained within postimmunotherapy sera [44]. Serum from one patient who had received 2 years of grass pollen immunotherapy was fractionated to separate IgG4. The IgG4 fraction was able to inhibit the binding of allergen and IgE with a similar capacity as whole serum (Fig. 5). In contrast, the fraction in which IgG4 had been removed displayed dramatically reduced inhibitory activity. Further studies involving larger numbers of patients are required to confirm these findings. Nonetheless, these data support a role for IgG4 as the principal inhibitory activity in postimmunotherapy serum.

IgA as a blocking antibody

IgA is also increased in response to allergen immunotherapy [38]. IgA is the predominant antibody isotype at mucosal surfaces; the active antibody is polymeric and is associated with a secretory component. IgA functions as a sequestering agent by binding to antigens and preventing their passage into the tissue where activation of immune responses may occur. IgA from nasal secretions of immunotherapy patients has been shown along with IgG to block IgE-mediated basophil histamine release [49]. To investigate the potential role of IgA in blocking facilitated antigen presentation, the authors fractionated the serum from three immunotherapy patients for IgA and IgG. The fraction containing IgG was able to inhibit binding of allergen-IgE complexes to EBV-transformed B cells. In contrast, IgA displayed no inhibitory activity in its polymeric or secretory form (C. Pilette, unpublished observations, 2005).

IL-10 induces isotype switching to IgG4

The induction of T regulatory cells is a recognized feature of allergen immunotherapy, along with the associated production of the regulatory cytokine IL-10. IL-10 induces anergy by blocking co-stimulation; however, a secondary function that has more relevance to IgE-FAP is its ability to induce isotype switching to IgG4 antibodies [50]. The authors recently showed that grass pollen immunotherapy induced local increases in IL-10–positive cells in the nasal mucosa. This induction was associated with increases in IgG4 and blocking activity for IgE-FAP [44]. Further evidence comes from Satoguina and colleagues [51] who demonstrated that when T regulatory-1 (Tr-1) cells producing IL-10 were added to B-cell cultures, they induced preferential production of IgG4. Increased production of IL-10 seems to be a consistent feature of allergen immunotherapy [38], and it can be concluded that increases in IgG4 may be at least partially explained by the associated increases in IL-10. Time course studies before and after immunotherapy may further test the possible causal association between these events.

IgG4-blocking activity may result from direct competition with IgE

The mechanism by which IgG4 blocks IgE-facilitated antigen presentation is not completely understood. The lack of correlation between IgG4 levels and clinical correlates of successful treatment may indicate that a distinct subpopulation of IgG4 antibodies is important. Chronic antigen stimulation induces high titered IgG4 responses that may not have a fundamental role in inhibiting IgE-mediated responses. In contrast, a component of T regulatory/IL-10 induced "high-affinity" IgG4 may comprise the major inhibitory component. This effect is supported by data showing an increase in the binding capacity of IgG4 and a concurrent decrease in the binding capacity of IgE following ragweed immunotherapy [52]. In contrast, a separate study by Jakobsen and coworkers [53] reported that immunotherapy with birch pollen had no effects on the affinities of IgG4, IgE, or IgG1 as measured by surface plasmon resonance. Blocking IgG4 antibodies may compete directly with IgE for epitopes. IgG4 is functionally monovalent; therefore, it does not have the capacity to cross-link antigen [36]. IgG4 is also noninflammatory in that it is unable to activate complement or bind with high affinity to Fcγ receptors. It is therefore likely that IgG4 is only able to compete with IgE for binding of allergen and is unlikely to have other inflammatory and potentially deleterious effects other than inhibition of IgE-mediated allergic responses and possibly helminthic infections.

In addition to the concept of IgG4 as a scavenging receptor competing with IgE for allergen binding, inhibitory activity may result from the binding and co-aggregation of FcεRI with adjacent FcγRIIb on the surface of effector cells. FcγRII receptor signaling via the inhibitory cytoplasmic domain has been shown to block IgE-mediated degranulation of human basophils [54] and mast cells [55]. It is suggested that IgE bound to its receptor may bind allergen complexed to (immunotherapy-induced) allergen-specific IgG, and that this results in the co-aggregation of IgG receptors, with subsequent postreceptor inhibitory signaling events downregulating IgE-mediated responses [56].

Clinical relevance of IgE-facilitated allergen presentation inhibition

The presence of IgE bound to the high-affinity receptor on the Langerhans cells of patients with atopic dermatitis [57], the high expression of the low-affinity receptor among atopic individuals [58], and its differential expression during the pollen season [24] all point toward a role for IgE-FAP in local Th2 cell activation and associated allergic responses.

The potential role of IgG4-blocking antibodies in preventing IgE-mediated pathology is apparent. IgG4 antibodies are known to block FcεRI-mediated immediate hypersensitivity reactions and may be important in preventing the early phase responses of allergic disease. The role of IgG4-blocking antibodies in inhibiting IgE-FAP also proposes a role in the inhibition of late phase allergic responses as mediated by T cells. Inhibition of this pathway could also prevent the overproduction of IgE antibodies. Paradoxically, IgE initially increases after immunotherapy with subsequent blunting of seasonal increases, followed by a gradual and prolonged fall in IgE after 3 to 5 years to below baseline IgE levels. Long-lived IgE-producing plasma cells may be responsible for the persistence of IgE in the serum despite long-term immunotherapy. Nevertheless, the effects of IgE could be minimized by parallel elevations in "functional" high-affinity IgG4 antibodies that block IgE-mediated responses and prevent the induction of new IgE-producing cells.

Current data concerning the contribution that IgE-FAP has in allergic disease suggest that this is an important process that contributes to activation and exacerbation of inflammatory pathways. The role of blocking antibodies in inhibiting this process in vivo is now emerging.

References

[1] Trombetta ES, Mellman I. Cell biology of antigen processing in vitro and in vivo. Annu Rev Immunol 2005;23:975–1028.

[2] Lanzavecchia A. Receptor-mediated antigen uptake and its effect on antigen presentation to class II-restricted T lymphocytes. Annu Rev Immunol 1990;8:773–93.

[3] Van Neerven RJ, Wikborg T, Lund G, et al. Blocking antibodies induced by specific allergy

vaccination prevent the activation of CD4+ T cells by inhibiting serum IgE-facilitated allergen presentation. J Immunol 1999;163:2944–52.

[4] Takhar P, Smurthwaite L, Coker HA, et al. Allergen drives class switching to IgE in the nasal mucosa in allergic rhinitis. J Immunol 2005;174:5024–32.

[5] Coker HA, Durham SR, Gould HJ. Local somatic hypermutation and class switch recombination in the nasal mucosa of allergic rhinitis patients. J Immunol 2003;171:5602–10.

[6] Smurthwaite L, Walker SN, Wilson DR, et al. Persistent IgE synthesis in the nasal mucosa of hay fever patients. Eur J Immunol 2001;31:3422–31.

[7] Gould HJ, Sutton BJ, Beavil AJ, et al. The biology of IgE and the basis of allergic disease. Annu Rev Immunol 2003;21:579–628.

[8] Durham SR, Gould HJ, Hamid QA. Local IgE production in nasal allergy. Int Arch Allergy Immunol 1997;113:128–30.

[9] Prussin C, Metcalfe DD. IgE, mast cells, basophils, and eosinophils. J Allergy Clin Immunol 2003;111:S486–94.

[10] Banchereau J, Blanchard D, Briere F, et al. Role of cytokines in human B lymphocyte growth and differentiation. Nouv Rev Fr Hematol 1993;35:61–6.

[11] Corry DB, Kheradmand F. Induction and regulation of the IgE response. Nature 1999;402: B18–23.

[12] Durham SR, Gould HJ, Thienes CP, et al. Expression of epsilon germ-line gene transcripts and mRNA for the epsilon heavy chain of IgE in nasal B cells and the effects of topical corticosteroid. Eur J Immunol 1997;27:2899–906.

[13] Cameron L, Gounni AS, Frenkiel S, et al. S epsilon S mu and S epsilon S gamma switch circles in human nasal mucosa following ex vivo allergen challenge: evidence for direct as well as sequential class switch recombination. J Immunol 2003;171:3816–22.

[14] Wilson DR, Merrett TG, Varga EM, et al. Increases in allergen-specific IgE in BAL after segmental allergen challenge in atopic asthmatics. Am J Respir Crit Care Med 2002;165: 22–6.

[15] Ying S, Humbert M, Meng Q, et al. Local expression of epsilon germline gene transcripts and RNA for the epsilon heavy chain of IgE in the bronchial mucosa in atopic and nonatopic asthma. J Allergy Clin Immunol 2001;107:686–92.

[16] KleinJan A, Vinke JG, Severijnen LW, et al. Local production and detection of (specific) IgE in nasal B-cells and plasma cells of allergic rhinitis patients. Eur Respir J 2000;15:491–7.

[17] Bieber T. Fc epsilon RI on antigen-presenting cells. Curr Opin Immunol 1996;8:773–7.

[18] Novak N, Kraft S, Bieber T. Unraveling the mission of Fc epsilon RI on antigen-presenting cells. J Allergy Clin Immunol 2003;111:38–44.

[19] Kinet JP. The high-affinity IgE receptor (Fc epsilon RI): from physiology to pathology. Annu Rev Immunol 1999;17:931–72.

[20] Turner H, Kinet JP. Signalling through the high-affinity IgE receptor Fc[epsi]RI. Nature 1999; 402:24–30.

[21] Getahun A, Hjelm F, Heyman B. IgE enhances antibody and T cell responses in vivo via CD23+ B cells. J Immunol 2005;175:1473–82.

[22] Corominas M, Mestre M, Bas J, et al. CD23 expression on B-lymphocytes and its modulation by cytokines in allergic patients. Clin Exp Allergy 1993;23:612–7.

[23] Pirron U, Schlunck T, Prinz J, et al. IgE-dependent antigen focusing by human B lymphocytes is mediated by the low-affinity receptor for IgE. Eur J Immunol 1990;20:1547–51.

[24] Hakansson L, Heinrich C, Rak S, et al. Activation of B-lymphocytes during pollen season: effect of immunotherapy. Clin Exp Allergy 1998;28:791–8.

[25] Bonnefoy JY, Guillot O, Spits H, et al. The low-affinity receptor for IgE (CD23) on B lymphocytes is spatially associated with HLA-DR antigens. J Exp Med 1988;167:57–72.

[26] Karagiannis SN, Warrack JK, Jennings KH, et al. Endocytosis and recycling of the complex between CD23 and HLA-DR in human B cells. Immunology 2001;103:319–31.

[27] Maurer D, Fiebiger S, Ebner C, et al. Peripheral blood dendritic cells express Fc epsilon RI as a complex composed of Fc epsilon RI alpha- and Fc epsilon RI gamma-chains and can use this receptor for IgE-mediated allergen presentation. J Immunol 1996;157:607–16.

[28] Mudde GC, Bheeka R, Bruijnzeel-Koomen CA. Consequences of IgE/CD23-mediated antigen presentation in allergy. Immunol Today 1995;16:380–3.

[29] Kehry M, Yamashita L. Low-affinity IgE receptor (CD23) function on mouse B cells: role in IgE-dependent antigen focusing. Proc Natl Acad Sci USA 1989;86:7556–60.

[30] Santamaria LF, Bheekha R, van Reijsen FC, et al. Antigen focusing by specific monomeric immunoglobulin E bound to CD23 on Epstein-Barr virus-transformed B cells. Hum Immunol 1993;37:23–30.

[31] van der Heijden FL, van Neerven RJ, van Katwijk M, et al. Serum-IgE-facilitated allergen presentation in atopic disease. J Immunol 1993;150:3643–50.

[32] Richards ML, Marcelletti JF, Katz DH. IgE-antigen complexes enhance Fc epsilon R and Ia expression by murine B lymphocytes. J Exp Med 1988;168:571–87.

[33] van der Heijden FL, Van Neerven RJ, Kapsenberg ML. Relationship between facilitated allergen presentation and the presence of allergen-specific IgE in serum of atopic patients. Clin Exp Immunol 1995;99:289–93.

[34] Wachholz PA, Soni NK, Till SJ, et al. Inhibition of allergen-IgE binding to B cells by IgG antibodies after grass pollen immunotherapy. J Allergy Clin Immunol 2003;112:915–22.

[35] Bousquet J, Lockey R, Malling HJ, et al. Allergen immunotherapy: therapeutic vaccines for allergic diseases. World Health Organization. American Academy of Allergy, Asthma and Immunology. Ann Allergy Asthma Immunol 1998;81:401–5.

[36] Van der Zee JS, van SP, Aalberse RC. Serologic aspects of IgG4 antibodies. II. IgG4 antibodies form small, nonprecipitating immune complexes due to functional monovalency. J Immunol 1986; 137:3566–71.

[37] Muller U, Akdis CA, Fricker M, et al. Successful immunotherapy with T-cell epitope peptides of bee venom phospholipase A2 induces specific T-cell anergy in patients allergic to bee venom. J Allergy Clin Immunol 1998;101:747–54.

[38] Jutel M, Akdis M, Budak F, et al. IL-10 and TGF-beta cooperate in the regulatory T cell response to mucosal allergens in normal immunity and specific immunotherapy. Eur J Immunol 2003; 33:1205–14.

[39] Cooke RA, Barnard JH, Hebald S, et al. Serological evidence of immunity with coexisting sensitization in a type of human allergy (hay fever). J Exp Med 1935;62:733–50.

[40] Lichtenstein LM, Holtzman NA, Burnett LS. A quantitative in vitro study of the chromatographic distribution and immunoglobulin characteristics of human blocking antibody. J Immunol 1968;101:317–24.

[41] Hussain R, Poindexter RW, Ottesen EA. Control of allergic reactivity in human filariasis: predominant localization of blocking antibody to the IgG4 subclass. J Immunol 1992;148:2731–7.

[42] Mothes N, Heinzkill M, Drachenberg KJ, et al. Allergen-specific immunotherapy with a monophosphoryl lipid A-adjuvanted vaccine: reduced seasonally boosted immunoglobulin E production and inhibition of basophil histamine release by therapy-induced blocking antibodies. Clin Exp Allergy 2003;33:1198–208.

[43] Niederberger V, Horak F, Vrtala S, et al. Vaccination with genetically engineered allergens prevents progression of allergic disease. Proc Natl Acad Sci USA 2004;101:14677–82.

[44] Nouri-Aria KT, Wachholz PA, Francis JN, et al. Grass pollen immunotherapy induces mucosal and peripheral IL-10 responses and blocking IgG activity. J Immunol 2004;172:3252–9.

[45] Muller U, Helbling A, Bischof M. Predictive value of venom-specific IgE, IgG and IgG subclass antibodies in patients on immunotherapy with honey bee venom. Allergy 1989;44:412–8.

[46] Ewan PW, Deighton J, Wilson AB, et al. Venom-specific IgG antibodies in bee and wasp allergy: lack of correlation with protection from stings. Clin Exp Allergy 1993;23:647–60.

[47] Djurup R, Malling HJ. High IgG4 antibody level is associated with failure of immunotherapy with inhalant allergens. Clin Allergy 1987;17:459–68.

[48] Flicker S, Valenta R. Renaissance of the blocking antibody concept in type I allergy. Int Arch Allergy Immunol 2003;132:13–24.

[49] Platts-Mills TA, von Maur RK, Ishizaka K, et al. IgA and IgG anti-ragweed antibodies in nasal secretions: quantitative measurements of antibodies and correlation with inhibition of histamine release. J Clin Invest 1976;57:1041–50.

[50] Jeannin P, Lecoanet S, Delneste Y, et al. IgE versus IgG4 production can be differentially regulated by IL-10. J Immunol 1998;160:3555–61.

[51] Satoguina JS, Weyand E, Larbi J, et al. T regulatory-1 cells induce IgG4 production by B cells: role of IL-10. J Immunol 2005;174:4718–26.

[52] Pierson-Mullany LK, Jackola D, Blumenthal M, et al. Altered allergen binding capacities of Amb a 1-specific IgE and IgG4 from ragweed-sensitive patients receiving immunotherapy. Ann Allergy Asthma Immunol 2000;84:241–3.

[53] Jakobsen CG, Bodtger U, Poulsen LK, et al. Vaccination for birch pollen allergy: comparison of the affinities of specific immunoglobulins E, G1 and G4 measured by surface plasmon resonance. Clin Exp Allergy 2005;35:193–8.

[54] Kepley CL, Cambier JC, Morel PA, et al. Negative regulation of Fc epsilon RI signaling by Fc gamma RII costimulation in human blood basophils. J Allergy Clin Immunol 2000;106:337–48.

[55] Kepley CL, Taghavi S, Mackay G, et al. Co-aggregation of Fc gamma RII with Fc epsilon RI on human mast cells inhibits antigen-induced secretion and involves SHIP-Grb2-Dok complexes. J Biol Chem 2004;279:35139–49.

[56] Saxon A, Zhu D, Zhang K, et al. Genetically engineered negative signaling molecules in the immunomodulation of allergic diseases. Curr Opin Allergy Clin Immunol 2004;4:563–8.

[57] Mudde GC, van Reijsen FC, Bruijnzeel-Koomen CA. IgE-positive Langerhans cells and Th2 allergen-specific T cells in atopic dermatitis. J Invest Dermatol 1992;99:103S.

[58] Bujanowski-Weber J, Brings B, Knoller I, et al. Expression of low-affinity receptor for IgE (Fc epsilon RII, CD23) and IgE-BF (soluble CD23) release by lymphoblastoid B-cell line RPMI-8866 and human peripheral lymphocytes of normal and atopic donors. Immunology 1989;66:505–11.

ELSEVIER
SAUNDERS

Immunol Allergy Clin N Am
26 (2006) 349–364

IMMUNOLOGY
AND ALLERGY
CLINICS
OF NORTH AMERICA

Biodegradable PLGA Particles for Improved Systemic and Mucosal Treatment of Type I Allergy

Isabella Schöll, PhD, Tamara Kopp, MD, Barbara Bohle, PhD, Erika Jensen-Jarolim, MD*

Medical University of Vienna, Währinger Gürtel 18-20, 1090 Vienna, Austria

The goal of treatment for numerous diseases is the induction of an appropriate, or the modification of an ongoing, immune response. Therapy for type I allergy also has this goal, whereby the application of specific immunotherapy (SIT) (desensitization or hyposensitization therapy) has remained nearly unchanged since Noon [1] invented the procedure in 1911. In SIT, allergens are applied subcutaneously in increasing doses aiming to counterbalance the Th2-dominated response with IgE-mediated effects. The Th2-promoting adjuvant aluminium hydroxide (alum) is often used for allergen formulation, which may cause several well-known side effects during the treatment, such as the initial boost of IgE [2], sensitization against new allergens [3], and reactions at the injection site [4].

Immunotherapies in general have improved over the past decades, often focusing on producing active substances with a lower risk for side effects. However, some active substances per se are unable to evoke efficient immune responses because of their small molecular size [5,6]. In the allergy field, various techniques have been used to develop hypoallergens [7–11]. Another major concern is that novel sensitizations might be induced when hypoallergens are applied in the context of Th2-promoting adjuvants. Therefore, improved and optimized adjuvants, immune-stimulating substances or motifs, or delivery vehicles are needed.

This work was supported by the Austrian Science Fund SFB F018 #8, #12 and #7, and a TransKoop grant of the Vienniese Fund for the Promotion of Economy (WWFF).

* Corresponding author.
E-mail address: erika.jensen-jarolim@meduniwien.ac.at (E. Jensen-Jarolim).

doi:10.1016/j.iac.2006.02.007   *immunology.theclinics.com*

For the adjuvant effect, three principal mechanisms occur: (1) the antigen is deposited and delivered; (2) antigens are targeted through vehicle delivery systems to cells specialized for antigen uptake and presentation, including macrophages and dendritic cells; and (3) the adjuvant acts as an immunostimulant [5].

Many of the vaccine delivery systems have particulate characteristics. Examples include emulsions such as MF59, a squalene microemulsion [12]; microparticles made of different materials [13–16]; immune-stimulating complexes [17]; and liposomes [18]. These particulate features allow an enhanced uptake by antigen-presenting cells (APCs). Moreover, the transport to secondary lymph organs is facilitated and together these events support an immune response to simultaneously applied antigen [19]. In the past decades, an amazingly high number of novel drug and antigen delivery systems in the form of micro- or nanoparticles have been developed, many of them interesting for allergen immunotherapy [20], and various natural and synthetic polymers have been explored for their suitability for particle production. Among these numerous materials, the polymer of lactic acid and the copolymer of lactic and glycolic acid, poly(D,L-lactic-co-glycolic) acid (PLGA), have been studied extensively because of their biocompatibility and biodegradability [21], and the Food and Drug Administration has approved their use in humans.

The features of PLGA particles

Biodegradability

PLGA particles can be prepared using different well-established techniques, such as spray freeze-drying [22], coacervation, (double) emulsion–solvent evaporation technique [23], or salting-out [24]. Jain [25] reviewed various traditional and novel techniques, such as in situ microencapsulation, for preparing different drug-loaded PLGA devices. The advantage of PLGA is that it is completely biodegradable; it can be broken down through nonenzymatic hydrolytic cleavage when the PLGA device comes into contact with artificial or biologic fluids [26]. PLGA degrades in two stages [27]. During the first process the ester bonds are broken randomly through hydrolysis, and oligomers and monomers are generated. This breakdown leads to a polymer molecular weight decrease. Thereafter, during erosion, microspheres lose mass and the polymer breakdown may be increased through autocatalysis by acidic products [28].

Biocompatibility

PLGA is not only biodegradable but also highly biocompatible because the resulting monomeric units, lactic and glycolic acid, are physiologically occurring substances in the human organism and can be easily metabolized through the Krebs cycle into carbon dioxide and water [29]. Therefore, this material has a long history of use in humans as resorbable surgery sutures, bone fixation material, artificial skin, tracheal replacement, vascular grafts, dental materials, and implants [30]. Furthermore, PLGA polymers are commercially available as clinical products for delivering gonadotropin-releasing hormone analog for treating prostate cancer and endometriosis; human growth hormone for treating growth deficiencies; and doxycycline hyclate for treating chronic adult periodontitis [21]. Clinical trials are underway to test their application with paclitaxel in treating solid tumors, with vapreotide in treating esophageal bleeding varices, and with plasmid DNA encoding for human papillomavirus (HPV) epitopes to cure HPV-associated anal dysplasia and cervical intraepithelial neoplasia [31,32]. Thus, PLGA particles have been used as resorbable and inert carriers for small drug molecules of various classes, such as anticancer agents, antihypertensive agents, and immunomodulators [21]; for macromolecules like peptides, proteins, and hormones; and for protein subunits and DNA [33].

Antigen delivery

PLGA polymers are broadly used because, in addition to their biocompatibility and biodegradability, their use as delivery devices has several advantages. First, the bioerosion rates and thereby the release kinetics can be tailored to the needs of the respective application [34]. This material is able to deposit the entrapped antigen and release it in a delayed continuous or pulsatile manner [35], depending on the particle size [5] and several surface characteristics, thereby mimicking booster applications [36,37] and allowing reduction of numerous injections. Second, the adjuvancy of PLGA is of major interest for vaccines in any field of medicine [38] because it allows reduction or even removal of further adjuvants. Third, the ability of PLGA particles to elicit cellular T-cell responses in addition to antibody responses [39–41] makes them an intriguing weapon also against intracellular infections (caused by bacteria, viruses, or parasites) or cancer. Fourth, they are able to protect the entrapped antigen from enzymatic breakdown and can therefore also be used for oral applications [42]. Along this line, studies have shown that PLGA can evoke systemic and mucosal immune responses [43,44]. Fifth, depending on their size, their surface charge, hydrophobicity, and administration routes, different cells of the immune system can be targeted [45]. For instance, after subcutaneous immunization, microspheres with a diameter of 1 to 10 μm are phagocytosed by macrophages that are recruited to the injection site, and thereby intracellular antigen delivery and subsequent enhanced antibody response is guaranteed. In contrast, particles larger than 10 μm remain as deposit on the injection site and release the antigen in a sustained manner. After intravenous application, particles approximately 200 nm in diameter are phagocytosed by Kupffer cells and end up in the lysosomal part of liver tissue [46]. Applied orally, microspheres smaller than 5 μm are effectively taken up by Peyer's patches and are brought to mesenteric lymph nodes and spleen by macrophages, whereas particles from 5 to 10 μm remain in Peyer's patches for up to 35 days, and microparticles larger than 10 μm were not absorbed at any point in the gastrointestinal tract (GIT) [47].

On the cellular level, the particle size, surface properties, antigen type and loading, and release kinetics of PLGA particles may also influence the outcome of parenteral immunizations [48]. For example, particles smaller than 10 μm can be directly taken up by APCs and result in major histocompatibility complex (MHC) II–restricted or cytotoxic T-lymphocyte (CTL) responses [49]. These small PLGA particles deliver the encapsulated antigen to APCs through uptake in either phagolysosomes or cytosol [33,50]. The first mechanism leads to presentation of antigen epitopes on MHC II. The CTL responses mirror the second mechanism, in which antigens can be processed and presented like endogenous antigens on MHC I. This feature is important because alum, for instance, is not capable of eliciting such CD8$^+$ responses. PLGA particles larger than 10 μm may also release the antigen extracellularly, thereby stimulating a secondary immune response through interaction with circulating or B-cell–bound immunoglobulins [48]. Whether B cells can also phagocytose microparticles and process and present the encapsulated antigen is not certain. Apart from the size of the particles, a high antigen load could be responsible for the induction of T helper 2 (Th2) responses with simultaneous poor affinity maturation during the secondary response [51]. Antigen release during an initial burst, and thereafter in pulses, can be advantageous when memory cells display longevity, whereas a continuous release may be necessary to restimulate memory cells [52].

The advantageous features and flexible preparation that allows PLGA particles to be tailored to respective needs led to their application as carriers for several protein antigens [43,53–63] and plasmid DNA [44]. They were capable of stimulating systemic and mucosal immunity [43] on not only the humoral but also the cellular level. They displayed their function through different application routes, such as peroral, intranasal, intramuscular, intratracheal, intradermal, intraduodenal, and intraperitoneal [64–70].

Use of PLGA in the treatment of allergy: first steps

Apart from early published studies on the entrapment of ovalbumin (OVA) or bovine serum albumin as model antigens [37,43,71–78], Sharif and colleagues [79,80] in 1994 were the first to attempt to use PLGA particles as carriers for allergens and in 1995 to encapsulate mite allergen extract. This group prepared the microparticles by double emulsion technique, rendering a mean size of 1 μm, and characterized the effect of the encapsulation process on the integrity and activity of the allergens. When the mite extract was released again, the proteins showed small alterations in the isoelectric focusing pattern. However, these changes only slightly affected the capability to inhibit IgE-binding to the extract or IgG-binding to mite allergen Der p 1. The authors therefore suggested that the encapsulation and release processes do not adversely affect the mite proteins, making them suitable for hyposensitization therapy.

Approximately 6 years later the idea of allergen in PLGA particles resurfaced. The food allergen β-lactoglobulin (BLG) from milk was entrapped in PLGA

[62,81] to induce tolerance in mice through a single feeding of encapsulated antigen. Five days after feedings, mice were immunized intraperitoneally with BLG and OVA adsorbed to alum. Evaluated on day 28, anti-BLG IgE was suppressed in a concentration-dependent manner in serum and intestinal contents of mice pretreated with different amounts of BLG encapsulated in PLGA microspheres (mean diameter of 7.8 μm). These feedings showed that 0.5 μg of entrapped BLG was enough to reach the same suppression as 5 mg of soluble BLG. In these studies, 0.5 μg of PLGA-BLG per gram of mouse reduced IgE in serum and intestinal secretions (2.39 and 1.48 titres, respectively) compared with gavage with unloaded particles or free BLG (approximately 3.6 and 2.2 titres, respectively). This suppression was specific for BLG because no changes were seen regarding OVA-specific IgE. The delayed-type hypersensitivity, evaluated as thickness measurements of the footpad after intradermal administration, was reduced in the BLG-particle group treated with 0.5 μg per gram of mouse and in the group treated with free BLG (5 mg per gram of mouse). This high dose of soluble antigen was required because the dose was shown to be essential for tolerance induction [82]. In these studies, the greatest benefit of PLGA particles was the drastically reduced dose of allergen necessary to induce tolerance.

PLGA for parenteral or oral applications of allergens: immunogenicity

Two working groups independently encapsulated *Olea europaea* pollen extract [83], the major olive pollen allergen Ole e 1 [84], through double-emulsion method. The main focus of these studies was the in vitro characterization of this delivery system with the prospect of using it for either parenteral [83] or oral immunization [84]. In the latter study, the size of the particles ranged from 0.5 to 2 μm, thereby making them suitable for optimal uptake by Peyer's patches. A protein load of 6 to 7 μg/mg polymer was reached. The release pattern of allergen from these particle preparations showed a biphasic shape with an initial burst (around 47% of entrapped allergens were released within the first hour) followed by a continuous slow release (74% of the encapsulated amount were released after 42 days). Entrapment of fluorescence-labeled allergen showed that Ole e 1 was distributed close to the surface of the microparticles, possibly causing the initial burst release. The authors discussed this scheme as optimal for mucosal application because of the limited exposure time of particles to the mucosal surface and the high dose required to prime an immune response. In addition to these in vitro experiments, intraperitoneal immunization was performed [85]. The main antibody type induced by PLGA-allergen was the Th1 isotype IgG2a, whereas the predominant antibodies were IgE and IgG1 in the group immunized with Ole e 1 adsorbed to alum. Accordingly, splenocytes from PLGA-immunized mice stimulated with Ole e 1 mainly produced interferon (INF)-γ, in contrast to mice immunized with allergen plus alum, which synthesized high levels of interleukin (IL)-4.

PLGA for parenteral and oral allergen applications: therapeutic potential

The true therapeutic potential of PLGA particles was shown for the first time in mice with the major birch pollen (BP) allergen Bet v 1 [86,87] and BP extract [88–91]. When Bet v 1 entrapped in PLGA particles (PLGA–Bet v 1) was compared with Bet v 1 adsorbed to alum, similar levels of allergen-specific IgG1 titres were achieved. The most important difference between the two protocols was the different sensitization potential: particle-treated mice did not develop type I skin sensitivity, whereas 100% of animals in the alum-treated group showed a positive result. In allergic mice, an ongoing Th2-dominated response could be redirected to a Th1-biased profile with a single subcutaneous shot of PLGA-Bet v 1. Accordingly, spleen cell cultures of the PLGA-Bet v 1 group produced high levels of IFN-γ and some IL-10 on stimulation with Bet v 1, but only low levels of IL-4. The group treated with alum showed even higher amounts of these cytokines but, unfortunately, also an increase of IL-4.

To evaluate the safety of the PLGA polymer in vivo, we subcutaneously applied 100 μL nanoparticle solution and 100 μL of alum without any additional proteins to naïve mice. As can be seen in Fig. 1, no granuloma formation occurred at the site of the PLGA particle shot but the administration of alum induced a granuloma after 12 to 24 hours, which was clearly visible and could be confirmed in histologic examinations of the immunization sites. These two

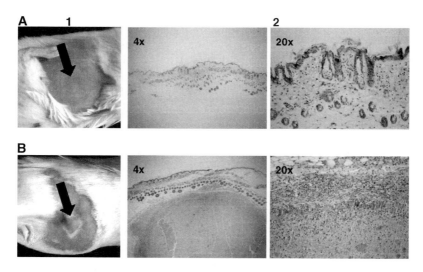

Fig. 1. PLGA nanoparticles are readily degraded in vivo and do not induce inflammation in mice. Empty PLGA particles (*A*, 100 μL) were applied subcutaneously in untreated mice (n=6). At the injection sites (*arrow*) no symptoms of inflammation were induced (*1*) and no granuloma formation or infiltration with inflammatory cells was seen in histology (*2*, magnification 4× and 20×). In contrast, alum (*B*, 100 μL) applied in the same mice induced granuloma formation after 12 to 24 hours, which remained two more months until biopsies were taken (*1*, photograph of shaved mouse skin; *2*, histologic analysis 4× and 20×). Representative tests are shown.

solutions were not only applied in mice but (with informed consent) also in healthy volunteers. PLGA nanoparticles were also clearly readily degradable and did not induce any inflammation, whereas alum led to classical inflammatory symptoms and to granulomas, which were visualized through ultrasonic skin measurement (Fig. 2).

To estimate the putative effects of PLGA in humans, we isolated human peripheral blood mononuclear cells in patients allergic to BP and stimulated them with PLGA nanoparticles with or without entrapped Bet v 1, with Bet v 1 alone or Bet v 1 in alum. The stimulation indices shown in Fig. 3 indicate that empty nanospheres were already able to induce cell proliferation, which was further underlined by the levels of IFN-γ detected in the supernatants of these cultures (Fig. 4). In a prophylactic setting with empty PLGA microspheres, Jilek and colleagues [92] also saw an effect of plain particles. They treated mice with plain microspheres or microspheres filled with plasmid DNA encoding for the whole bee venom phospholipase A2. The particle preparations were able to induce a transient IgG2a-response during a subsequent sensitization and to evoke IL-10 production in stimulated splenocytes. Although in our in vivo mouse model the plain nanospheres had no effect on the allergen-specific immune response (in neither the prophylactic nor the therapeutic protocol) [86], our in

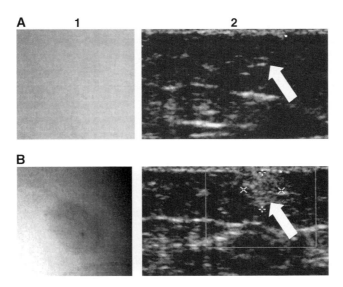

Fig. 2. PLGA nanoparticles are biocompatible after subcutaneous application in humans (n=2). Empty PLGA nanoparticles (A, 100 μL) were injected popliteal subcutaneously. Neither inflammatory symptoms at the skin surface (1) nor subcutaneous granuloma formation, evaluated through ultrasonic measurement (2), could be observed. However, the application of alum (B, 100 μL) induced itching, swelling, redness, and heat at the application site after 12 to 24 hours (1). After 14 days, granulomas were apparent in ultrasonic scans (2) and were still present after several months. Arrows indicate site of injection.

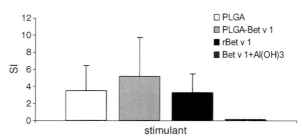

Fig. 3. PLGA nanoparticles induce T-cell proliferation in PBMC of patients allergic to BP (n=3). Peripheral blood mononuclear cells from patients allergic to BP were isolated and 2×10^5 cells per 200 μL were stimulated with either plain PLGA nanoparticles (PLGA, 100 μL), PLGA filled with rBet v 1 (PLGA–Bet v 1, 5.85 μg Bet v 1 per 100 μL suspension), recombinant Bet v 1 (rBet v 1, 5.85 μg/100 μL), or Bet v 1 adsorbed to alum (Bet v 1 + Al(OH)$_3$, 5.85 μg/100 μL suspension). The empty and filled particles induced a proliferation of cells that was at least as high as with the recombinant allergen. In contrast, alum seemed to severely damage the cells because no proliferation could be induced at all. Proliferation was measured as ^{3}H-thymidine incorporation, and mean values + SD of stimulation indices (SI) are given. No statistical analysis was performed because of the small patient number. SI represents counts per minutes with stimulant divided by counts per minutes with medium.

vitro results with splenocytes indicate that they may additionally act through antigen-independent immune modulation.

Because of better patient compliance and convenience, multiple efforts have been made to construct oral vaccines for the treatment of type I allergy. PLGA microparticles are able to protect an encapsulated antigen from acidic and proteolytic degradation in the gut [42,87,91]. Therefore, they could also be used for oral administration of antigens [93]. Orally applied PLGA particles are readily absorbed by Peyer's patches, where they are taken up by so-called "membranous

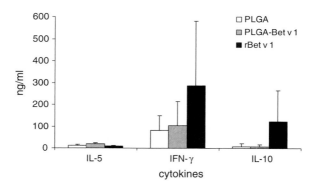

Fig. 4. In patients allergic to BP, the stimulation of peripheral blood mononuclear cells with PLGA particles mainly induces IFN-γ production. The examination of the supernatants of the stimulated cells in enzyme-linked immunosorbent assay showed that PLGA particles, even when plain, were able to induce a Th1-biased cytokine pattern, dominated by high amounts of IFN-γ and very low levels of IL-5 and IL-10 (stimulated as described in legend of Fig. 3). Mean values + SD are given.

cells," transcytosed, and transported to the lymphoid tissue where they encounter APCs and induce antibody responses [94].

To examine whether PLGA particles can also be used for oral application of allergens, we used BP extract for encapsulation in microspheres [88]. These microparticles had a mean diameter of 4.8 μm, allowing uptake by cells of the GIT. An average load of 40 μg BP protein per milligram of microparticles was achieved, with 60% of this protein actually still capable of binding a specific monoclonal antibody after 2 hours of simulated gastric digestion. In this study, we especially aimed at targeting the microparticles to specific sites of the intestine to prolong their persistence and thereby enhance antigen delivery. For targeting the sialylic residues on enterocytes, wheat germ agglutinin (WGA) was coupled to microspheres. Feeding these BP allergen-loaded and WGA-functionalized PLGA to naïve mice induced an antigen-specific IgG response in serum. In a subsequent study, the targeting was directed toward the intestinal immune induction sites, the Peyer's patches covered by membranous cells. These cells express α-L-fucose moieties, which can be targeted by the lectin from *Aleuria aurantia* (AAL), the edible orange peel mushroom [91]. In an immunization protocol, feedings of naïve mice with AAL-coated PLGA induced mainly IgG2a

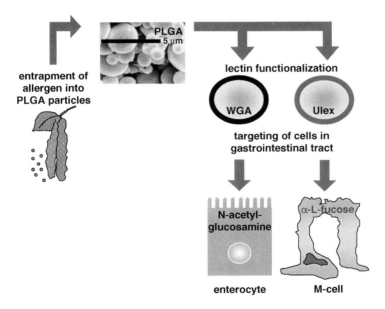

Fig. 5. For the oral application, PLGA particles are targeted through lectins to the sugar coats of the intestinal cells. Allergen can be entrapped in PLGA microparticles through the spray-drying technique [88]. A heterologous size distribution among the particles guarantees a release pattern, which mimics booster applications of the allergen. To target particles to the enterocytes, wheat germ agglutinin (WGA) can be attached through covalent binding. To target membranous cells (M-cells), particles can be directed to α-L-fucose residues on their surface through lectins (eg, *Aleuria aurantia* lectin of the edible mushroom orange cup). The result is a Th1-biased immune response similar to that of bacterial and viral pathogens, which use M-cells for their invasion.

[90]. These preparations, compared with WGA-functionalized microspheres (Fig. 5), were further examined for their therapeutic capacity through oral treatments of BP-sensitized mice [91]. Here, the membranous cell–targeted PLGA induced higher IgG2a titers than WGA or noncoated particles. The efficacy of this targeting approach was also reflected in the higher proliferation capacity of BP-stimulated splenocytes of these mice and by the fact that IFN-γ was only found in splenocyte supernatants from mice treated with AAL-functionalized PLGA targeted to membranous cells. This efficacy indicates that targeting of the intestinal immune induction sites is necessary to (1) avoid immune ignorance and (2) to modulate an ongoing Th2-type response toward Th1.

The differentiation of membranous cells in vitro is possible in a coculture model of CaCo-2 cells with Raji-lymphoma B-cells [95]. When the transport of the PLGA microspheres across this epithelium was studied, an increased cellular uptake and transcytosis was observed even against gravitation with AAL-grafted PLGA [89]. There is structural similarity of AAL to the neuraminidases of several pathogens such as *Salmonella typhimurium* [96], which invade humans through membranous cells.

Ongoing studies and future prospective

Clinical studies with PLGA-entrapped allergens will prove whether these experimental concepts can be translated into practical application. Further approaches are presently designed to target APCs, such as dendritic cells of the immune system, with PLGA and encapsulated peptides [97–104]. Furthermore, several growth factors [57,105,106] and cytokines have been prepared in PLGA and additional hydrogels and scaffolds, such as transforming growth factor β [107], IL-2 [108], granulocyte-monocyte colony-stimulating factor [109], and IFN-α [110]. Although the initial ideas for these approaches were focused on treating other diseases, the preliminary results may also serve as prototypes for incorporation of other cytokines in treating allergic disorders.

Summary

Numerous studies with different antigens and our experiments indicate that PLGA represents a controlled release system for allergens, which allows reduction of necessary booster shots in parenteral immunizations. In the treatment of type I allergy, ongoing Th2 responses can be modified by PLGA-entrapped allergens, at least in the murine model and probably also in humans, as we conclude from our in vitro studies. Furthermore, this material is highly biocompatible and biodegradable because it does not evoke granuloma formation or inflammatory symptoms in mice and humans after subcutaneous application. It protects the entrapped antigen from degradation at the mucosal sites. Therefore, nanospheres at the parenteral route and microspheres targeted to membranous cells in oral applications can be realistic perspectives for counter-balancing an allergic immune response in the near future.

References

[1] Noon L. Prophylactic inoculation against hay fever. Lancet 1911;i:1572–3.

[2] Jarolim E, Poulsen LK, Stadler BM, et al. A long-term follow-up study of hyposensitization with immunoblotting. J Allergy Clin Immunol 1990;85(6):996–1004.

[3] Ball T, Sperr WR, Valent P, et al. Induction of antibody responses to new B cell epitopes indicates vaccination character of allergen immunotherapy. Eur J Immunol 1999;29(6):2026–36.

[4] Gupta RK, Rost BE, Relyveld E, et al. Adjuvant properties of aluminum and calcium compounds. Pharm Biotechnol 1995;6:229–48.

[5] Lima KM, Rodrigues Jr JM. Poly-DL-lactide-co-glycolide microspheres as a controlled release antigen delivery system. Braz J Med Biol Res 1999;32(2):171–80.

[6] Hanly WC, Artwohl JE, Bennett BT. Review of polyclonal antibody production procedures in mammals and poultry. ILAR J 1995;37(3):93–118.

[7] Akdis CA, Blaser K. Regulation of specific immune responses by chemical and structural modifications of allergens. Int Arch Allergy Immunol 2000;121(4):261–9.

[8] Bhalla PL. Genetic engineering of pollen allergens for hayfever immunotherapy. Expert Rev Vaccines 2003;2(1):75–84.

[9] Holm J, Gajhede M, Ferreras M, et al. Allergy vaccine engineering: epitope modulation of recombinant Bet v 1 reduces IgE binding but retains protein folding pattern for induction of protective blocking-antibody responses. J Immunol 2004;173(8):5258–67.

[10] Ferreira F, Wallner M, Breiteneder H, et al. Genetic engineering of allergens: future therapeutic products. Int Arch Allergy Immunol 2002;128(3):171–8.

[11] Swoboda I, De Weerd N, Bhalla PL, et al. Mutants of the major ryegrass pollen allergen, Lol p 5, with reduced IgE-binding capacity: candidates for grass pollen-specific immunotherapy. Eur J Immunol 2002;32(1):270–80.

[12] Singh M, O'Hagan D. Advances in vaccine adjuvants. Nat Biotechnol 1999;17(11):1075–81.

[13] Edman P, Sjoholm I. Acrylic microspheres in vivo V: immunological properties of immobilized asparaginase in microparticles. J Pharm Sci 1982;71(5):576–80.

[14] Krauland AH, Bernkop-Schnurch A. Thiomers: development and in vitro evaluation of a peroral microparticulate peptide delivery system. Eur J Pharm Biopharm 2004;57(2):181–7.

[15] Rydell N, Sjoholm I. Oral vaccination against diphtheria using polyacryl starch microparticles as adjuvant. Vaccine 2004;22(9–10):1265–74.

[16] van der Lubben IM, Verhoef JC, van Aelst AC, et al. Chitosan microparticles for oral vaccination: preparation, characterization and preliminary in vivo uptake studies in murine Peyer's patches. Biomaterials 2001;22(7):687–94.

[17] Cox JC, Sjolander A, Barr IG. ISCOMs and other saponin based adjuvants. Adv Drug Deliv Rev 1998;32(3):247–71.

[18] Kersten GF, Crommelin DJ. Liposomes and ISCOMS as vaccine formulations. Biochim Biophys Acta 1995;1241(2):117–38.

[19] O'Hagan DT, Valiante NM. Recent advances in the discovery and delivery of vaccine adjuvants. Nat Rev Drug Discov 2003;2(9):727–35.

[20] Schöll I, Boltz-Nitulescu G, Jensen-Jarolim E. Review of novel particulate antigen delivery systems with special focus on treatment of type I allergy. J Control Release 2005;104:1–27.

[21] Bala I, Hariharan S, Kumar MN. PLGA nanoparticles in drug delivery: the state of the art. Crit Rev Ther Drug Carrier Syst 2004;21(5):387–422.

[22] Johnson OL, Cleland JL, Lee HJ, et al. A month-long effect from a single injection of microencapsulated human growth hormone. J Pharm Sci 1996;85(12):1346–9.

[23] Cleland JL. Solvent evaporation processes for the production of controlled release

biodegradable microsphere formulations for therapeutics and vaccines. Pharm Res 1998; 15(2):357–61.

[24] Allemann E, Leroux JC, Gurny R, et al. In vitro extended-release properties of drug-loaded poly(DL-lactic acid) nanoparticles produced by a salting-out procedure. Pharm Res 1993; 10(12):1732–7.

[25] Jain RA. The manufacturing techniques of various drug loaded biodegradable poly(lactide-co-glycolide) (PLGA) devices. Biomaterials 2000;21(23):2475–90.

[26] Tamber H, Johansen P, Merkle HP, et al. Formulation aspects of biodegradable polymeric microspheres for antigen delivery. Adv Drug Deliv Rev 2005;57(3):357–76.

[27] Göpferich A. Mechanisms of polymer degradation and erosion. Biomaterials 1996;17(2): 103–14.

[28] Fu K, Pack DW, Klibanov AM, et al. Visual evidence of acidic environment within degrading poly(lactic-co-glycolic acid) (PLGA) microspheres. Pharm Res 2000;17(1):100–6.

[29] Bazile DV, Ropert C, Huve P, et al. Body distribution of fully biodegradable [14C]-poly(lactic acid) nanoparticles coated with albumin after parenteral administration to rats. Biomaterials 1992;13(15):1093–102.

[30] Ueda H, Tabata Y. Polyhydroxyalkanonate derivatives in current clinical applications and trials. Adv Drug Deliv Rev 2003;55(4):501–18.

[31] Klencke B, Matijevic M, Urban RG, et al. Encapsulated plasmid DNA treatment for human papillomavirus 16-associated anal dysplasia: a Phase I study of ZYC101. Clin Cancer Res 2002;8(5):1028–37.

[32] Sheets EE, Urban RG, Crum CP, et al. Immunotherapy of human cervical high-grade cervical intraepithelial neoplasia with microparticle-delivered human papillomavirus 16 E7 plasmid DNA. Am J Obstet Gynecol 2003;188(4):916–26.

[33] Panyam J, Labhasetwar V. Biodegradable nanoparticles for drug and gene delivery to cells and tissue. Adv Drug Deliv Rev 2003;55(3):329–47.

[34] Thomasin C, Corradin G, Men Y, et al. Tetanus toxoid and synthetic malaria antigen containing poly(lactide)/poly(lactide-co-glycolide) microspheres: importance of polymer degradation and antigen release for immune response. J Control Release 1996;41(1–2):131–45.

[35] Sah H, Chien YW. Prolonged immune response evoked by a single subcutaneous injection of microcapsules having a monophasic antigen release. J Physiol Pharmacol 1999;50(3):419–28.

[36] Cleland JL. Single-administration vaccines: controlled-release technology to mimic repeated immunizations. Pharm Res 1999;16(2):232–40.

[37] Igartua M, Hernandez RM, Esquisabel A, et al. Enhanced immune response after subcutaneous and oral immunization with biodegradable PLGA microspheres. J Control Release 1998; 56(1–3):63–73.

[38] Nakaoka R, Tabata Y, Ikada Y. Adjuvant effect of biodegradable poly(DL-lactic acid) granules capable for antigen release following intraperitoneal injection. Vaccine 1996;14(17–18): 1671–6.

[39] Partidos CD, Vohra P, Jones D, et al. CTL responses induced by a single immunization with peptide encapsulated in biodegradable microparticles. J Immunol Methods 1997;206(1–2): 143–51.

[40] Men Y, Tamber H, Audran R, et al. Induction of a cytotoxic T lymphocyte response by immunization with a malaria specific CTL peptide entrapped in biodegradable polymer microspheres. Vaccine 1997;15(12–13):1405–12.

[41] Audran R, Peter K, Dannull J, et al. Encapsulation of peptides in biodegradable microspheres prolongs their MHC class-I presentation by dendritic cells and macrophages in vitro. Vaccine 2003;21(11–12):1250–5.

[42] O'Hagan DT, Palin K, Davis SS, et al. Microparticles as potentially orally active immunological adjuvants. Vaccine 1989;7(5):421–4.

[43] Maloy KJ, Donachie AM, O'Hagan DT, et al. Induction of mucosal and systemic immune responses by immunization with ovalbumin entrapped in poly(lactide-co-glycolide) microparticles. Immunology 1994;81(4):661–7.

[44] Jones DH, Corris S, McDonald S, et al. Poly(DL-lactide-co-glycolide)-encapsulated plasmid

DNA elicits systemic and mucosal antibody responses to encoded protein after oral administration. Vaccine 1997;15(8):814 – 7.

[45] Tabata Y, Ikada Y. Macrophage phagocytosis of biodegradable microspheres composed of L-lactic acid/glycolic acid homo- and copolymers. J Biomed Mater Res 1988;22(10):837 – 58.

[46] Rodrigues Jr JM, Croft SL, Fessi H, et al. The activity and ultrastructural localization of primaquine-loaded poly (d,l-lactide) nanoparticles in Leishmania donovani infected mice. Trop Med Parasitol 1994;45(3):223 – 8.

[47] Eldridge JH, Staas JK, Chen D, et al. New advances in vaccine delivery systems. Semin Hematol 1993;30(4, Suppl 4):16 – 24 [discussion 5].

[48] Johansen P, Men Y, Merkle HP, et al. Revisiting PLA/PLGA microspheres: an analysis of their potential in parenteral vaccination. Eur J Pharm Biopharm 2000;50(1):129 – 46.

[49] Men Y, Audran R, Thomasin C, et al. MHC class I- and class II-restricted processing and presentation of microencapsulated antigens. Vaccine 1999;17(9–10):1047 – 56.

[50] Panyam J, Zhou WZ, Prabha S, et al. Rapid endo-lysosomal escape of poly(DL-lactide-co-glycolide) nanoparticles: implications for drug and gene delivery. FASEB J 2002;16(10): 1217 – 26.

[51] Constant SL, Bottomly K. Induction of Th1 and Th2 CD4 + T cell responses: the alternative approaches. Annu Rev Immunol 1997;15:297 – 322.

[52] Swain SL, Hu H, Huston G. Class II-independent generation of CD4 memory T cells from effectors. Science 1999;286(5443):1381 – 3.

[53] Lima KM, Rodrigues Jr JM. Poly-DL-lactide-co-glycolide microspheres as a controlled release antigen delivery system. Infect Immun 2001;69(9):5305 – 12.

[54] O'Hagan DT, Jeffery H, Roberts MJ, et al. Controlled release microparticles for vaccine development. J Drug Target 1993;1(3):245 – 9.

[55] Hilbert AK, Fritzsche U, Kissel T. Biodegradable microspheres containing influenza A vaccine: immune response in mice. Vaccine 1999;17(9–10):1065 – 73.

[56] Jones DH, McBride BW, Jeffery H, et al. Protection of mice from Bordetella pertussis respiratory infection using microencapsulated pertussis fimbriae. Vaccine 1995;13(18):1741 – 9.

[57] Lam XM, Duenas ET, Cleland JL. Encapsulation and stabilization of nerve growth factor into poly(lactic- co-glycolic) acid microspheres. J Control Release 1999;58(2):223 – 32.

[58] Moore A, McGuirk P, Adams S, et al. Immunization with a soluble recombinant HIV protein entrapped in biodegradable microparticles induces HIV-specific CD8 + cytotoxic T lymphocytes and CD4 + Th1 cells. Vaccine 1996;14(16):1523 – 30.

[59] Rosas JE, Hernandez RM, Gascon AR, et al. Biodegradable PLGA microspheres as a delivery system for malaria synthetic peptide SPf66. Vaccine 2001;19(31):4445 – 51.

[60] Sturesson C, Artursson P, Ghaderi R, et al. Encapsulation of rotavirus into poly(lactide-co-glycolide) microspheres. J Control Release 1999;59(3):377 – 89.

[61] Vordermeier HM, Coombes AG, Jenkins P, et al. Synthetic delivery system for tuberculosis vaccines: immunological evaluation of the M. tuberculosis 38 kDa protein entrapped in biodegradable PLG microparticles. Vaccine 1999;17(15–16):1814 – 9.

[62] Pecquet S, Leo E, Fritsche R, et al. Oral tolerance elicited in mice by beta-lactoglobulin entrapped in biodegradable microspheres. Vaccine 2000;18(13):1196 – 202.

[63] Singh M, Kazzaz J, Chesko J, et al. Anionic microparticles are a potent delivery system for recombinant antigens from Neisseria meningitidis serotype B. J Pharm Sci 2004;93(2): 273 – 82.

[64] Sau K, Reid RH, McQueen C, et al. Intraduodenal immunization with microencapsulated CFA/ II induces a delayed, anti-CFA/II, IgG antibody-secreting spleen cell response. Adv Exp Med Biol 1995;371B:1469 – 74.

[65] Carcaboso AM, Hernandez RM, Igartua M, et al. Enhancing immunogenicity and reducing dose of microparticulated synthetic vaccines: single intradermal administration. Pharm Res 2004;21(1):121 – 6.

[66] Vajdy M, O'Hagan DT. Microparticles for intranasal immunization. Adv Drug Deliv Rev 2001;51(1–3):127 – 41.

[67] Challacombe SJ, Rahman D, O'Hagan DT. Salivary, gut, vaginal and nasal antibody re-

362 SCHÖLL et al

sponses after oral immunization with biodegradable microparticles. Isr J Med Sci 1980;16(12): 849–52.

[68] Conway MA, Madrigal-Estebas L, McClean S, et al. Protection against Bordetella pertussis infection following parenteral or oral immunization with antigens entrapped in biodegradable particles: effect of formulation and route of immunization on induction of Th1 and Th2 cells. Arzneimittelforschung 1986;36(8):1206–9.

[69] Israel ZR, Gettie A, Ishizaka ST, et al. Combined systemic and mucosal immunization with microsphere- encapsulated inactivated simian immunodeficiency virus elicits serum, vaginal, and tracheal antibody responses in female rhesus macaques. AIDS Res Hum Retroviruses 1999;15(12):1121–36.

[70] Spiers ID, Eyles JE, Baillie LW, et al. Biodegradable microparticles with different release profiles: effect on the immune response after a single administration via intranasal and intramuscular routes. J Pharm Pharmacol 2000;52(10):1195–201.

[71] Gutierro I, Hernandez RM, Igartua M, et al. Influence of dose and immunization route on the serum Ig G antibody response to BSA loaded PLGA microspheres. Vaccine 2002;20(17–18): 2181–90.

[72] Gutierro I, Hernandez RM, Igartua M, et al. Size dependent immune response after sub-cutaneous, oral and intranasal administration of BSA loaded nanospheres. Vaccine 2002; 21(1–2):67–77.

[73] O'Hagan DT, Rahman D, McGee JP, et al. Biodegradable microparticles as controlled release antigen delivery systems. Immunology 1991;73(2):239–42.

[74] O'Hagan DT, Jeffery H, Roberts MJ, et al. Controlled release microparticles for vaccine development. Vaccine 1991;9(10):768–71.

[75] Uchida T, Martin S, Foster TP, et al. Dose and load studies for subcutaneous and oral delivery of poly(lactide-co-glycolide) microspheres containing ovalbumin. Biol Pharm Bull 1994;17(9): 1272–6.

[76] Challacombe SJ, Rahman D, Jeffery H, et al. Enhanced secretory IgA and systemic IgG antibody responses after oral immunization with biodegradable microparticles containing antigen. Exp Neurol 1995;134(1):126–34.

[77] Uchida T, Goto S, Foster TP. Particle size studies for subcutaneous delivery of poly(lactide-co-glycolide) microspheres containing ovalbumin as vaccine formulation. Chem Pharm Bull (Tokyo) 1995;43(9):1569–73.

[78] Bennewitz NL, Babensee JE. The effect of the physical form of poly(lactic-co-glycolic acid) carriers on the humoral immune response to co-delivered antigen. Biomaterials 2005;26(16): 2991–9.

[79] Sharif S, Wheeler AW, O'Hagan DT. Investigation of the structural and immunologic integrity of an allergen entrapped in poly (lactide-co-glycolide) microparticles. In: 21st International Symposium on Controlled Release of Bioactive Materials. Nice (France): Controlled Release Society; 1994. p. 292–5.

[80] Sharif S, Wheeler AW, O'Hagan DT. Biodegradable microparticles as a delivery system for the allergens of *Dermatophagoides pteronyssinus* (house dust mite): I: preparation and characterization of microparticles. Int J Pharm 1995;119:239–46.

[81] Fattal E, Pecquet S, Couvreur P, et al. Biodegradable microparticles for the mucosal delivery of antibacterial and dietary antigens. Int J Pharm 2002;242(1–2):15–24.

[82] Friedman A, Weiner HL. Induction of anergy or active suppression following oral tolerance is determined by antigen dosage. Proc Natl Acad Sci USA 1994;91(14):6688–92.

[83] Igartua M, Hernandez RM, Gutierro I, et al. Preliminary assessment of the immune response to Olea europaea pollen extracts encapsulated into PLGA microspheres. Pharm Dev Technol 2001;6(4):621–7.

[84] Batanero E, Barral P, Villalba M, et al. Biodegradable poly (DL-lactide glycolide) micro-particles as a vehicle for allergen-specific vaccines: a study performed with Ole e 1, the main allergen of olive pollen. J Org Chem 2002;67(7):2369–71.

[85] Batanero E, Barral P, Villalba M, et al. Encapsulation of Ole e 1 in biodegradable microparti-

cles induces Th1 response in mice: a potential vaccine for allergy. J Control Release 2003; 92(3):395–8.

[86] Schöll I, Weissenböck A, Förster-Waldl E, et al. Allergen-loaded biodegradable poly(d,l–lactic-co-glycolic) acid nanoparticles down-regulate an ongoing Th2 response in the BALB/c mouse model. Clin Exp Allergy 2004;34(2):315–21.

[87] Schöll I, Gusenbauer C, Gabor F, et al. Biodegradable nanospheres as allergen delivery-system in immunizations of Balb/c mice. In: Bienenstock J, Ring J, Togias AG, editors. Allergy, frontiers and futures (Proceedings of the 24th Symposium of the Collegium Internationale Allergologicum). Göttingen: Hogrefe & Huber; 2004. p. 324–6.

[88] Walter F, Schöll I, Untersmayr E, et al. Functionalisation of allergen-loaded microspheres with wheat germ agglutinin for targeting enterocytes. Biochem Biophys Res Commun 2004;315(2): 281–7.

[89] Roth-Walter F, Bohle B, Schöll I, et al. Targeting antigens to murine and human M-cells with Aleuria aurantia lectin-functionalized microparticles. Immunol Lett 2005;100(2):182–8.

[90] Roth-Walter F, Schöll I, Untersmayr E, et al. Mucosal targeting of allergen-loaded microspheres by Aleuria aurantia lectin. Vaccine 2005;23(21):2703–10.

[91] Roth-Walter F, Schöll I, Untersmayr E, et al. M cell targeting with Aleuria aurantia lectin as a novel approach for oral allergen immunotherapy. J Allergy Clin Immunol 2004;114(6):1362–8.

[92] Jilek S, Walter E, Merkle HP, et al. Modulation of allergic responses in mice by using biodegradable poly(lactide-co-glycolide) microspheres. J Allergy Clin Immunol 2004;114(4): 943–50.

[93] Jung T, Kamm W, Breitenbach A, et al. Biodegradable nanoparticles for oral delivery of peptides: is there a role for polymers to affect mucosal uptake? Eur J Pharm Biopharm 2000; 50(1):147–60.

[94] Shalaby WS. Development of oral vaccines to stimulate mucosal and systemic immunity: barriers and novel strategies. Clin Immunol Immunopathol 1995;74(2):127–34.

[95] Gullberg E, Leonard M, Karlsson J, et al. Expression of specific markers and particle transport in a new human intestinal M-cell model. Biochem Biophys Res Commun 2000;279(3):808–13.

[96] Wimmerova M, Mitchell E, Sanchez JF, et al. Crystal structure of fungal lectin: six-bladed beta-propeller fold and novel fucose recognition mode for Aleuria aurantia lectin. J Biol Chem 2003;278(29):27059–67.

[97] Sun H, Pollock KG, Brewer JM. Analysis of the role of vaccine adjuvants in modulating dendritic cell activation and antigen presentation in vitro. Vaccine 2003;21(9–10):849–55.

[98] Newman KD, Elamanchili P, Kwon GS, et al. Uptake of poly(D,L-lactic-co-glycolic acid) microspheres by antigen-presenting cells in vivo. J Biomed Mater Res 2002;60(3):480–6.

[99] Yoshida M, Babensee JE. Poly(lactic-co-glycolic acid) enhances maturation of human monocyte-derived dendritic cells. J Biomed Mater Res A 2004;71(1):45–54.

[100] Waeckerle-Men Y, Gander B, Groettrup M. Delivery of tumor antigens to dendritic cells using biodegradable microspheres. Methods Mol Med 2005;109:35–46.

[101] Waeckerle-Men Y, Groettrup M. PLGA microspheres for improved antigen delivery to dendritic cells as cellular vaccines. Adv Drug Deliv Rev 2005;57(3):475–82.

[102] Jilek S, Merkle HP, Walter E. DNA-loaded biodegradable microparticles as vaccine delivery systems and their interaction with dendritic cells. Adv Drug Deliv Rev 2005;57(3):377–90.

[103] Ribeiro S, Hussain N, Florence AT. Release of DNA from dendriplexes encapsulated in PLGA nanoparticles. Int J Pharm 2005;298(2):354–60.

[104] Lutsiak ME, Robinson DR, Coester C, et al. Analysis of poly(D,L-lactic-co-glycolic acid) nanosphere uptake by human dendritic cells and macrophages in vitro. Pharm Res 2002; 19(10):1480–7.

[105] Jones AJ, Putney S, Johnson OL, et al. Recombinant human growth hormone poly(lactic-co-glycolic acid) microsphere formulation development. Adv Drug Deliv Rev 1997;28(1): 97–119.

[106] Yang Z, Birkenhauer P, Julmy F, et al. Sustained release of heparin from polymeric particles for inhibition of human vascular smooth muscle cell proliferation. Vaccine 1999;18(3–4): 209–15.

[107] DeFail AJ, Chu CR, Izzo N, et al. Controlled release of bioactive TGF-beta (1) from microspheres embedded within biodegradable hydrogels. Biomaterials 2006;27(8):1579–85.

[108] Thomas TT, Kohane DS, Wang A, et al. Microparticulate formulations for the controlled release of interleukin-2. J Pharm Sci 2004;93(5):1100–9.

[109] Mandal B, Kempf M, Merkle HP, et al. Immobilisation of GM-CSF onto particulate vaccine carrier systems. Int J Pharm 2004;269(1):259–65.

[110] Sanchez A, Tobio M, Gonzalez L, et al. Biodegradable micro- and nanoparticles as long-term delivery vehicles for interferon-alpha. Eur J Pharm Sci 2003;18(3–4):221–9.

ELSEVIER
SAUNDERS

Immunol Allergy Clin N Am
26 (2006) 365–377

IMMUNOLOGY
AND ALLERGY
CLINICS
OF NORTH AMERICA

Bacillus Calmette-Guerin, *Mycobacterium bovis*, as an Immunomodulator in Atopic Diseases

Isil Barlan, MD[a],*, Nerin N. Bahceciler, MD[a],
Mübeccel Akdis, MD[b], Cezmi A. Akdis, MD[b]

[a]*Division of Pediatric Allergy and Immunology, Marmara University Hospital, 81190 Uskudar,
Istanbul, Turkey*
[b]*Swiss Institute of Allergy and Asthma Research, CH-7270 Davos, Switzerland*

The increase in the prevalence of atopic diseases in Western societies over the past few decades [1,2] cannot solely be explained by genetic factors, because substantial shifts in the genome do not occur over a few generations. Changes in diagnostic procedures or exposure to conventional etiologic factors of asthma and atopy are also unable to explain most of this increase. An attractive explanation is offered by the hygiene hypothesis, which states that a relative lack of infections early in life could promote the development of allergic diseases in genetically predisposed individuals [1,2]. In line with this hypothesis, the reduced frequency, less severity, and prevention of infections with certain vaccinations and the frequent use of antibiotics could prevent the development of allergic disease [3].

A breakthrough in understanding the regulation of allergic immune responses came with the discovery of different T-cell effector subsets termed *T helper 1* (Th1) and *T helper 2* (Th2) [4]. Research in the last decade has highlighted the key role played by Th2 cells in orchestrating the chronic inflammation in allergic diseases. Th2 cells preferentially produce interleukin-4 (IL-4), IL-5, IL-9, and IL-13, whereas Th1 cells produce IL-2, interferon-γ (IFN-γ), and tumor necrosis factor (TNF). Because Th1 and Th2 responses are to a certain degree antagonistic, it is possible that certain infections that predominantly evoke Th1 re-

The authors' laboratories are supported by Swiss National Science Foundation grants 32-100266 and 32-105865, the Global Allergy and Asthma European Network (GA²LEN), and Tubitak grant SGAG-1432.

* Corresponding author.
    E-mail address: isilbarlan@marmara.edu.tr (I. Barlan).

doi:10.1016/j.iac.2006.02.002
immunology.theclinics.com

sponses might limit allergic Th2 responses. A further subtype of T cells with immunosuppressive functions and cytokine profiles distinct from Th1 and Th2 cells termed *T regulatory* (T_{Reg}) has been described [5], and evidence for their existence in humans has been demonstrated [6]. Recent studies have shown that, in addition to Th1 cells, T_{Reg} cells are able to inhibit the development of allergic Th2 responses and play a major role in allergen-specific immunotherapy [6–8]. Mycobacteria elicit particularly strong protective Th1 immune responses; however, it remains to be elucidated whether some of the mycobacterial components trigger T_{Reg} cells. Mycobacterial lipoproteins bind to dendritic cell and macrophage bound Toll-like receptors (TLRs), and this interaction leads to prominent synthesis of IL-12 and Th1 switching [9].

Bacillus Calmette-Guerin, *Mycobacterium bovis*, tuberculin reactivity and atopy

In their hallmark study in 1997, Shirakawa and coworkers [10] demonstrated an inverse association among Japanese school children between exposure to mycobacteria and the subsequent development of atopy, which provided epidemiologic evidence in favor of the hygiene hypothesis and mycobacterial exposure. These results have been debated in an attempt to determine to what extent the results are explained by exposure to mycobacteria, bacillus Calmette-Guerin (BCG) vaccination, or unknown host factors [11,12]. Tuberculin reactivity has been found to be unreliable as a marker of exposure to *Mycobacterium tuberculosis*, because considerable genetic variations have been recognized in tuberculin reactivity [13]. The accuracy and sensitivity of skin testing is influenced by several factors. The technique of administering, placement, and interpretation, as well as different characteristics of patients' skin and age, can introduce some degree of variability. In addition, false-positive reactions can occur owing to cross-reactivity occurring as a result of previous infections with a nontuberculosis mycobacteria or prior immunization with BCG.

Analysis of health records of children in Guinea-Bissau, West Africa, has demonstrated that vaccinating African children early in life significantly reduces the prevalence of atopy, as demonstrated by skin prick test positivity to common airborne allergens later in life. Nevertheless, in that study, the BCG response pattern was not assessed [14]. Furthermore, the study demonstrated that the greatest reduction in atopy was achieved in children who were vaccinated during the first week of life. In addition, a protective effect of early BCG vaccination was demonstrated for wheezing, atopic sensitization, and symptoms of allergic rhinitis up to the first 24 months of life, but the effect was not sustained thereafter [15].

A prospective international study evaluated the effect of BCG vaccination at birth on the development of atopy, asthma, and allergic diseases at the age of 2 and 5 years by administering an International Study of Asthma and Allergies in Childhood (ISAAC) questionnaire and skin prick testing. That study showed a protective effect of the BCG vaccine in young children against the development of allergic symptoms but not IgE sensitization in Turkey and Thailand where BCG is still in routine use [16].

Recently, additional support for the protective role of *M tuberculosis* infection came from a study carried out cross-sectionally in South Africa. In that study, purified protein derivative (PPD) positivity reduced the prevalence of allergic rhinitis and influenced skin prick test reactivity in children [17]. In contrast, a retrospective study performed on children from Sweden found no reduction in atopic disease associated with BCG among children born in Sweden [18], whereas among immigrant children, many born in Asia and South America, BCG was associated with a lower prevalence of atopic disease, providing evidence that ethnicity might affect the susceptibility to the immunomodulatory effects of vaccination. In this retrospective study by Alm and coworkers, it was not clear whether the controls were recruited from allergic families, and there was no skin testing to rule out the existence of any atopic status. The discrepancy between these studies could partially be due to the difference in the timing of BCG vaccination, natural exposure to mycobacteria in early infancy, and genetic background.

Diseases of *Mycobacterium tuberculosis* and atopy

It is important to distinguish between BCG vaccination and mycobacterial infection. An inverse association between the prevalence of tuberculosis in a given country and the prevalence of atopic disorders has been reported repeatedly [19,20]. The relationship between tuberculosis notification rates and the prevalence of symptoms of asthma, allergic rhinoconjuctivitis, and atopic eczema was investigated in 85 centers from 23 countries in which standardized data were available [19]. These centers were located in Europe, as well as the United States, Canada, Australia, and New Zealand. Tuberculosis notification rates were significantly inversely associated with the lifetime prevalence of wheezing and asthma. An increase in the tuberculosis rates of 25 cases per 100,000 persons was associated with an absolute decrease of 4.7% in the prevalence of wheeze. Symptoms of allergic rhinoconjunctivitis in the previous 12 months were also inversely associated with tuberculosis notification rates. Another retrospective study evaluated the occurrence of allergic disease among Finnish adults who had tuberculosis in the first two decades of life. Tuberculosis was inversely associated with allergies and asthma in women, but the opposite trend was observed in men [21]. Because the incidence of tuberculosis is approximately 10 times greater in Japan when compared with Scandinavian countries, exposure of children to environmental mycobacteria was not similar.

Species of atypical mycobacteria and atopy

Environmental saprophytic mycobacteria that have been present throughout evolutionary history may be involved in shaping of the immune response to avirulent microorganisms. The level of exposure to environmental atypical mycobacteria would vary to a great extent between countries in different regions. Through its powerful immunoregulatory effects, exposure to those mycobacteria may exert a protective effect on the development of childhood allergic disease. On the other hand, in a recent study in which the relationship between childhood atopy or allergic disease and previous infection with four species of atypical mycobacteria (*Aviumin C, Gordonin, Chelonin, and Ranin I*) was cross-sectionally examined in Crete [22], the findings did not lend support to the suggestion that infection with atypical mycobacteria is protective against childhood allergic disease.

Toll-like receptors and mycobacteria

TLRs are believed to represent key receptors for the recognition of mycobacterial antigens and activation of macrophages and dendritic cells, as well as other cells of innate immunity, thereby modulating the adaptive immune response [23,24]. Mycobacterial products released by the sequestered bacilli, such as phosphatidyl-myoinositol mannosides, lipomannan, lipoarabinomannan, and lipoproteins, and other factors may contribute to continued macrophage and dendritic cell activation through pathogen pattern recognition receptors such as TLRs and others.

Several investigations have been performed on the interaction between mycobacteria and the innate immune system. It is known that mycobacterial lipoproteins bind particularly to TLR2, which leads to prominent synthesis of IL-12 and associated Th1 switching and secretion of IFN-γ and TNF-α [9], the cytokines shown to downregulate Th2 immune mechanisms in vivo and in vitro [25–29]. In this context, a mycobacterial muramyl-tripeptide analogue, which triggers TLR2, has been shown to suppress Th2 cytokines, IgE, and lung eosinophilia while enhancing IFN-γ, IL-12, and IL-10 [30].

In addition to TLR2, TLR4 and, more recently, TLR1/ TLR6 that heterodimerase with TLR2 have been implicated in the recognition of mycobacterial antigens [31,32]. A soluble heat-stable mycobacterial fraction distinct from the mycobacterial cell wall lipoarabinomannan signals through TLR2, whereas heat-labile cell-associated ones signal through TLR4 (Fig. 1) [33].

Use of bacillus Calmette-Guerin, *Mycobacterium bovis*, in experimental models of atopy

Underlying mechanisms of the impact of mycobacterial antigens on IgE sensitization and asthma have been investigated in several models. In one study, high IgE responder Balb/c mice were infected with BCG 14 days before the start of sensitization with ovalbumin (OVA). BCG immunization markedly hindered the development of IgE/IgG1 antibody responses, IL-4 and IL-10 secretion in

mycobacterial lipoproteins   **lung eosinophilia**

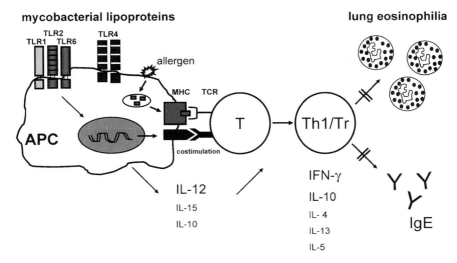

Fig. 1. Interaction of mycobacterial products and the innate immune system. Mycobacterial components are recognized by TLR2 in association with TLR1/TLR6, or by TLR4, which affects the differentiation of naive T cells (T) mainly to Th1-like cells (Th1/Tr) with the help of IL-12, TNF-γ, IL-15, as well as IL-10 release from antigen-presenting cells (APC). The generated T-cell response is dominated by high quantities of IFN-γ and IL-10 production and relatively low quantities of IL-4, IL-5, and IL-13 production, which leads to suppressed lung eosinophilia and IgE production from B cells.

splenocytes, airway hyperresponsiveness, eosinophilic influx into the airway, and IL-4 and IL-5 levels in bronchoalveolar lavage fluid. In parallel, a marked rise in anti-OVA–specific IgG2a antibody and Con A–induced IFN-γ production from splenocytes was detected [34].

In a murine model of allergen-induced airway eosinophilia, intranasal BCG infection 4 weeks before allergen airway challenge resulted in a 90% to 95% reduction in eosinophilia within the lungs in a comparison with uninfected controls. This effect was associated with reduced IL-5 production by T cells from the draining lymph nodes. Furthermore, BCG-induced inhibition of airway eosinophilia was strongly reduced in IFN-γ receptor–deleted mice and could be partially reversed by intranasal IL-5 application. The suppressive effect of BCG infection on the allergen-specific Th2 response was localized to the lung and did not influence blood eosinophil or allergen-specific IgG1 and IgE serum levels [35]. The exact mechanism by which IFN-γ mediates this effect has not been established.

Additional experimental data on the inverse link between mycobacteria and atopy came from studies in which exposure to mycobacteria had prominent Th2-limiting effects [34–38]. In one of these experiments, intranasal BCG inhibited pulmonary eosinophilia and synthesis of IL-5 by splenocytes in an IFN-γ–dependent mechanism [35]. Intravenous BCG promoted IFN-γ synthesis and inhibited secretion of IL-4, IL-5, IgE, and IgG1 and airway eosinophilia [34]. Similarly, subcutaneous injection of heat-killed BCG suppressed serum total IgE [37] and chronic changes of allergic airway inflammation [38].

Bacillus Calmette-Guerin as a therapeutic agent in allergic disease

BCG administration to asthmatic children allergic to house dust mites revealed a decline in serum IgE levels but no effect on IL-2, IL-4, IL-5, and IFN-γ production from peripheral blood mononuclear cells (PBMCs) [39]. Another randomized controlled trial of BCG vaccination in human asthma demonstrated a significant improvement in pulmonary function and the need for asthma medication [40] with no apparent suppressive effect on the Th2 immune response. BCG revaccination further improved lung function and resulted in an apparent increase in the IFN-γ/IL-4 ratio in a subsequent study by the same group [41].

Intradermal BCG vaccination in atopic children induced IFN-γ mRNA expression in PBMCs, although there was no expression before. Additionally, all subjects were found to develop an appropriate tuberculin skin test response 8 weeks after the vaccination, which contradicts the suggestion that atopic children have a decreased ability to mount a delayed-type hypersensitivity response [42]. Based on these initial findings, a trial with repeated intradermal injections of heat-killed BCG in adult asthma was initiated; however, it was prematurely halted owing to the occurrence of severe local reactions [43].

Bacillus Calmette-Guerin/recombinant bacillus Calmette-Guerin as adjuvants in specific immunotherapy

Bacillus Calmette-Guerin

Besides causing disease, mycobacteria have long been recognized for having powerful immunologic adjuvant activity, augmenting cell-mediated and humoral immune responses. The experimental research on improving immunotherapy involves a combination of standardized or purified/cloned allergens with an appropriate adjuvant, which may consist of live or killed microorganisms as a vaccine vector, molecular immunostimulants such as those carrying CpG sequences, or plasmids encoding protective cytokines. BCG has been selected as a vaccine vector because it offers the following unique advantages [44–47]:

- It lends itself to the development of a multi-allergen vaccine, as would be required for downregulation of specific allergies.
- Live attenuated BCG has been used for immunization worldwide since 1948, with a low incidence of serious complications.
- BCG has been shown to be a potent adjuvant in experimental animals and humans, particularly in relation to induction of Th1 cells.

- BCG is heat stable and inexpensive.
- It can be administered by the oral route.
- It can be given at or any time after birth and is unaffected by maternal antibodies.
- Sensitization to tuberculoproteins lasts for 5 to 50 years.
- Various in vitro studies of human and murine systems show that BCG-reactive CD4+ T cells are potent inducers of IFN-γ [48].

Recently, the authors investigated whether the administration of BCG as an adjuvant to allergen-specific sublingual immunotherapy (SLIT) had any additive effect on clinical, laboratory, and immunologic parameters in children with asthma sensitized to house dust mites. The results demonstrated a higher in vitro production of IFN-γ from the PBMCs of SLIT and SLIT + BCG groups when compared with controls who never received immunotherapy. This increase was well correlated with the improvement in bronchial hyperreactivity, clinical parameters, and decrease in eosinophil counts in both groups. Meanwhile, in vitro production of IL-12 was found to be higher in the BCG-receiving group, not resulting in any further improvement in the clinical outcome measures [49]. Similarly, immunotherapy with *Dermatophagoides pteronyssinus* in conjunction with BCG did not alter lung functions, nonspecific hyperreactivity, and allergen-specific IgE in asthmatic patients sensitized to house dust mites [50].

Recombinant bacillus Calmette-Guerin

Vaccination of mice with a single dose of recombinant BCG (rBCG) resulted in higher amounts of IFN-γ and IL-2 and lower amounts of IL-5 from splenocytes, as well as less serum IgE levels, in a comparison with controls [51]. In a recent study, the anti-Th2 effect of the IL-18–producing BCG strain (rBCG) was compared with that of nonrecombinant BCG when administered concomitantly with the antigen OVA in a murine model of pulmonary allergic inflammation. Lymph nodes from the rBCG-treated mice produced less OVA-induced IL-5 and more IFN-γ than those of mice immunized with nonrecombinant BCG. In addition, there was a strong reduction in bronchoalveolar lavage fluid eosinophilia in the rBCG-injected group [52]. These advances suggest the potential of live BCG or other mycobacteria administered by themselves or in the form of recombinant organisms for expressing desirable allergens as an adjuvant in the management of allergic diseases.

Perspectives

Based on the evidence obtained from humans and animal models, there seems to be a discrepancy regarding the preventive and therapeutic effects of BCG on atopic diseases. Several factors may cause this conflict.

Timing of vaccination

Pregnancy is known to be characterized by intrauterine Th2 predominance, which clearly is essential for prevention of fetal allograft rejection [53]. Although the development of atopy in the newborn is determined by a variety of factors, an intense Th1 stimulus such as BCG vaccination right after birth could contribute to switching away from the Th2 environment of the placental unit. One may speculate that any mycobacterial inhibition of atopy in humans should have its maximum impact early in life before the establishment of a predominant Th2 response. The study by Aaby and coworkers provided further evidence for less atopy in infants receiving BCG in Guinea-Bissau, particularly in the first week of life [14]. The results of another international prospective study further support the role of early BCG vaccination in preventing allergy by history [16]. Omenaas and coworkers [54] report that PPD reactivity in young adults receiving BCG as late as 14 years of age is not associated with atopy.

The route of delivery

Following inhalation, mycobacteria are phagocytosed primarily by alveolar macrophages. Although evidence suggests that systemic delivery is efficient in suppressing allergic responses [33,37], alternative noninvasive routes such as intranasal administration have given promising results. In support of this possibility, intranasal infection with BCG suppressed the accumulation of eosinophils into the airways, proving to be superior to intraperitoneal or subcutaneous routes [35]. Similarly, intranasal BCG treatment was superior to the intraperitoneal route in reversing antigen-induced asthma symptoms, bronchoalveolar lavage and peribronchial eosinophilia, as well as bronchoalveolar lavage fluid levels of IL-5 [55].

Genetic contribution and ethnicity

Results from immigrant and African children raise the possibility that BCG vaccination prevents atopy only in certain ethnic groups [14]. In humans, the association or linkage of *NRAMP1* with susceptibility to infectious diseases as well as atopy and autoimmune disease has been demonstrated [56,57]. The immune response to mycobacteria is known to be under control of *NRAMP1*, and polymorphisms in the genomic region of *NRAMP1* have been suggested to be associated with the risk of atopy in BCG-vaccinated children [56]. In addition, *NRAMP1* affects the efficiency of *Mycobacterium vaccae* in diminishing the allergic response in a mouse model, providing a link between genes, environment, and allergic asthma [58,59].

In an asthma family–based cohort from northeastern Quebec, five genetic variations of *NRAMP1* were tested for the candidacy of asthma susceptibility. No significant association was observed between *NRAMP1* variants (5′Can, 274C > T, 469 + 14G > C, D543N, and 1729 + del4) and asthma, atopy, or serum

IgE levels. These results demonstrate that despite direct involvement of Nramp1 in a murine asthma model, in human populations, *NRAMP1* is not likely to be a major contributor to the genetic etiology of asthma and asthma-related phenotypes [60].

Exposure to environmental mycobacteria

Previous observations have shown that prior exposure to live environmental mycobacteria primes the host immune system against mycobacterial antigens shared with BCG, modulating immune responses generated by the vaccine [61]. BCG is highly efficient at preventing tuberculosis in neonates vaccinated before exposure to environmental mycobacteria occurs [62]. In contrast, BCG has been demonstrated to be particularly ineffective and fails to protect against pulmonary tuberculosis in adults in southern India, where various environmental mycobacteria are ubiquitously found [63]. Several studies have suggested that immunization with a fast-growing saprophytic mycobacteria, *M vaccae*, prevents or treats allergic and asthmatic manifestations more efficiently than BCG in murine models [2,37,38,64].

Most of the evidence available to date suggests a need for an improved mycobacterial vaccine administered early in life. Because switching away from the Th2 immune response by inducing Th1 is unable to explain the underlying mechanisms of action of mycobacterial antigens, it may be worthwhile to investigate whether T_{Reg} cells are induced in response to different mycobacterial strains including BCG. Although there is some evidence that exposure to environmental mycobacteria might have a role in the prevention of allergic diseases, further studies are required to identify the dose, time, and strain differences. In addition, studies should also focus on the purification and characterization of certain mycobacterial components in the development of Th1- or T_{Reg}-type immune response.

Supporting this concept, it has been demonstrated that *M vaccae* can induce CD4+ CD45RB^{low} T_{reg} cells that secrete IL-10 and transforming growth factor-β (TGF-β) [64–66] and upon transfer can protect recipient allergic mice from airway inflammation. Recently, *M vaccae*-induced CD11c+ cells have been shown to have a potential regulatory role at the site of inflammation through secretion of immunomodulatory cytokines such as IL-10, TGF-β, and TNF-α [67].

Summary

Data obtained from human and animal models indicate a discrepancy regarding the preventive and therapeutic effect of BCG in atopic diseases. Among the issues that require clarification are whether the distinction in Th1/Th2 cells described in mice can be fully extrapolated to humans. Other factors involved could be due to genetic variation, the optimal timing, dose, and route of delivery, as well as environmental factors, which affect the degree of natural exposure to pathogenic or saprophytic mycobacteria. Because switching away from the Th2 immune response by inducing Th1 is unable to explain the underlying mechanisms of action of mycobacterial antigens, it may be worthwhile to investigate whether T_{reg} cells are induced in response to different mycobacterial adjuvants.

References

[1] Strachan DP. Hay fever, hygiene, and household size. BMJ 1989;299:1259–60.
[2] Rook GA, Hernandez-Pando R. Immunological and endocrinological characteristics of tuberculosis that provide opportunities for immunotherapeutic intervention. Novartis Found Symp 1998;217:73–87 [discussion: 87–98].
[3] Shaheen SO, Aaby P, Hall AJ, et al. Measles and atopy in Guinea-Bissau. Lancet 1996;347: 1792–6.
[4] Mosmann TR, Sad S. The expanding universe of T-cell subsets: Th1, Th2 and more. Immunol Today 1996;17:138–46.
[5] Taylor A, Verhagen J, Akdis CA, et al. T regulatory cells in allergy and health: a question of allergen specificity and balance. Int Arch Allergy Immunol 2004;135:73–82.
[6] Akdis CA, Blesken T, Akdis M, et al. Role of IL-10 in specific immunotherapy. J Clin Invest 1998;102:98–106.
[7] Akdis M, Verhagen J, Taylor A, et al. Immune responses in healthy and allergic individuals are characterized by a fine balance between allergen-specific T regulatory 1 and T helper 2 cells. J Exp Med 2004;199:1567–75.
[8] Jutel M, Akdis M, Budak F, et al. IL-10 and TGF-β cooperate in regulatory T cell response to mucosal allergens in normal immunity and specific immunotherapy. Eur J Immunol 2003;33: 1205–14.
[9] Brightbill HD, Libraty DH, Krutzik SR, et al. Host defense mechanisms triggered by microbial lipoproteins through toll-like receptors. Science 1999;285:732–6.
[10] Shirakawa T, Enomoto T, Shimazu S, et al. The inverse association between tuberculin responses and atopic disorder. Science 1997;275:77–9.
[11] Gruber C, Paul KP. Tuberculin reactivity and allergy. Allergy 2002;57:277–80.
[12] Martinati LC, Boner AL. The inverse relationship between tuberculin responses and atopic disorder. Allergy 1997;52:1036–7.
[13] Sepulveda RL, Heiba IM, King A, et al. Evaluation of tuberculin reactivity in BCG-immunized siblings. Am J Respir Crit Care Med 1994;149:620–4.
[14] Aaby P, Shaheen SO, Heyes CB, et al. Early BCG vaccination and reduction in atopy in Guinea-Bissau. Clin Exp Allergy 2000;30:644–50.
[15] Gruber C, Kulig M, Bergmann R, et al. Delayed hypersensitivity to tuberculin, total immunoglobulin E, specific sensitization, and atopic manifestation in longitudinally followed early bacille Calmette-Guerin-vaccinated and nonvaccinated children. Pediatrics 2001;107:E36.
[16] Townley RG, Barlan IB, Patino C, et al. The effect of BCG vaccine at birth on the development of atopy or allergic disease in young children. Ann Allergy Asthma Immunol 2004;92: 350–5.
[17] Obihara CC, Beyers N, Gie RP, et al. Inverse association between *Mycobacterium tuberculosis* infection and atopic rhinitis in children. Allergy 2005;60(9):1121–5.
[18] Alm JS, Lilja G, Pershagen G, et al. BCG vaccination does not seem to prevent atopy in children with atopic heredity. Allergy 1998;53:537.
[19] von Mutius E, Pearce N, Beasley R, et al. International patterns of tuberculosis and the prevalence of symptoms of asthma, rhinitis, and eczema. Thorax 2000;55:449–53.
[20] Shirtcliffe P, Weatherall M, Beasley R. An inverse correlation between estimated tuberculosis notification rates and asthma symptoms. Respirology 2002;7:153–5.
[21] Von Hertzen L, Klaukka T, Mattila H, et al. *Mycobacterium tuberculosis* infection and the

subsequent development of asthma and allergic conditions. J Allergy Clin Immunol 1999;104: 1211–4.

[22] Bibakis I, Zekveld C, Dimitroulis I, et al. Childhood atopy and allergic disease and skin test responses to environmental mycobacteria in rural Crete: a cross-sectional survey. Clin Exp Allergy 2005;35(5):624–9.

[23] Stenger S, Modlin RL. Control of *Mycobacterium tuberculosis* through mammalian Toll-like receptors. Curr Opin Immunol 2002;14(4):452–7.

[24] Heldwein KA, Fenton MJ. The role of Toll-like receptors in immunity against mycobacterial infection. Microbes Infect 2002;4(9):937–44.

[25] Ria F, Penna G, Adorini L. Th1 cells induce and Th2 inhibit antigen-dependent IL-12 secretion by dendritic cells. Eur J Immunol 1998;28:2003–16.

[26] Parronchi P, De Carli M, Manetti R, et al. IL-4 and IFN (alpha and gamma) exert opposite regulatory effects on the development of cytolytic potential by Th1 or Th2 human T cell clones. J Immunol 1992;149:2977–83.

[27] Randolph DA, Carruthers CJ, Szabo SJ, et al. Modulation of airway inflammation by passive transfer of allergen-specific Th1 and Th2 cells in a mouse model of asthma. J Immunol 1999; 162:2375–83.

[28] Li XM, Chopra RK, Chou TY, et al. Mucosal IFN-gamma gene transfer inhibits pulmonary allergic responses in mice. J Immunol 1996;157:3216–9.

[29] Gavett SH, O'Hearn DJ, Li X, et al. Interleukin 12 inhibits antigen-induced airway hyper-responsiveness, inflammation, and Th2 cytokine expression in mice. J Exp Med 1995;182: 1527–36.

[30] Akdis CA, Kussebi F, Pulendran B, et al. Inhibition of T helper 2-type responses, IgE production and eosinophilia by synthetic lipopeptides. Eur J Immunol 2003;33:2717–26.

[31] Bulut Y, Faure E, Thomas L, et al. Cooperation of Toll-like receptor 2 and 6 for cellular activation by soluble tuberculosis factor and *Borrelia burgdorferi* outer surface protein A lipoprotein: role of Toll-interacting protein and IL-1 receptor signaling molecules in Toll-like receptor 2 signaling. J Immunol 2001;167(2):987–94.

[32] Hajjar AM, O'Mahony DS, Ozinsky A, et al. Cutting edge: functional interactions between toll-like receptor (TLR) 2 and TLR1 or TLR6 in response to phenol-soluble modulin. J Immunol 2001;166(1):15–9.

[33] Means TK, Wang S, Lien E, et al. Human toll-like receptors mediate cellular activation by *Mycobacterium tuberculosis*. J Immunol 1999;163(7):3920–7.

[34] Herz U, Gerhold K, Gruber C, et al. BCG infection suppresses allergic sensitization and development of increased airway reactivity in an animal model. J Allergy Clin Immunol 1998;102: 867–74.

[35] Erb KJ, Holloway JW, Sobeck A, et al. Infection of mice with *Mycobacterium bovis*-bacillus Calmette-Guerin (BCG) suppresses allergen-induced airway eosinophilia. J Exp Med 1998;187: 561–9.

[36] Wang CC, Rook GA. Inhibition of an established allergic response to ovalbumin in BALB/c mice by killed *Mycobacterium vaccae*. Immunology 1998;93:307–13.

[37] Tukenmez F, Bahceciler NN, Barlan IB, et al. Effect of pre-immunization by killed *Mycobacterium bovis* and *vaccae* on immunoglobulin E response in ovalbumin-sensitized newborn mice. Pediatr Allergy Immunol 1999;10:107–11.

[38] Ozdemir C, Akkoc T, Bahceciler NN, et al. Impact of *Mycobacterium vaccae* immunization on lung histopathology in a murine model of chronic asthma. Clin Exp Allergy 2003;33:266–70.

[39] Barlan IB, Tukenmez F, Bahceciler NN, et al. The impact of in vivo Calmette-Guerin bacillus administration on in vitro IgE secretion in atopic children. J Asthma 2002;39:239–46.

[40] Choi IS, Koh YI. Therapeutic effects of BCG vaccination in adult asthmatic patients: a randomized, controlled trial. Ann Allergy Asthma Immunol 2002;88:584–91.

[41] Choi IS, Koh YI. Effects of BCG revaccination on asthma. Allergy 2003;58:1114–6.

[42] Ozer A, Tukenmez F, Biricik A, et al. Effect of BCG vaccination on cytokine mRNA expression in atopic children with asthma. Immunol Lett 2003;86:29–35.

[43] Shirtcliffe PM, Easthope SE, Weatherall M, et al. Effect of repeated intradermal injections

of heat-inactivated *Mycobacterium bovis* bacillus Calmette-Guerin in adult asthma. Clin Exp Allergy 2004;34:207–12.

[44] Husson RN, James BE, Young RA. Gene replacement and expression of foreign DNA in mycobacteria. J Bacteriol 1990;172(2):519–24.

[45] Aldovini A, Young RA. Development of a BCG recombinant vehicle for candidate AIDS vaccines. Int Rev Immunol 1990;7(1):79–83.

[46] Stover CK, de la Cruz VF, Fuerst TR, et al. New use of BCG for recombinant vaccines. Nature 1991;351(6326):456–60.

[47] Aldovini A, Young RA. Humoral and cell-mediated immune responses to live recombinant BCG-HIV vaccines. Nature 1991;351(6326):479–82.

[48] Wang CC, Rook GA. Inhibition of an established allergic response to ovalbumin in BALB/c mice by killed *Mycobacterium vaccae*. Immunology 1998;93(3):307–13.

[49] Arikan C, Bahceciler NN, Deniz G, et al. Bacillus Calmette-Guerin-induced interleukin-12 did not additionally improve clinical and immunologic parameters in asthmatic children treated with sublingual immunotherapy. Clin Exp Allergy 2004;34:398–405.

[50] Tsai JJ, Peng HJ, Shen HD. Therapeutic effect of bacillus Calmette-Guerin with allergen on human allergic asthmatic patients. J Microbiol Immunol Infect 2002;35:99–102.

[51] Kumar M, Behera AK, Matsuse H, et al. A recombinant BCG vaccine generates a Th1-like response and inhibits IgE synthesis in BALB/c mice. Immunology 1999;97(3):515–21.

[52] Biet F, Duez C, Kremer L, et al. Recombinant *Mycobacterium bovis* BCG producing IL-18 reduces IL-5 production and bronchoalveolar eosinophilia induced by an allergic reaction. Allergy 2005;60(8):1065–72.

[53] Wilczynski JR. Th1/Th2 cytokines balance: yin and yang of reproductive immunology. Eur J Obstet Gynecol Reprod Biol 2005;122(2):136–43.

[54] Omenaas E, Jentoft HF, Vollmer WM, et al. Absence of relationship between tuberculin reactivity and atopy in BCG vaccinated young adults. Thorax 2000;55:454–8.

[55] Hopfenspirger MT, Agrawal DK. Airway hyperresponsiveness, late allergic response, and eosinophilia are reversed with mycobacterial antigens in ovalbumin-presensitized mice. J Immunol 2002;168:2516–22.

[56] Alm JS, Sanjeevi CB, Miller EN, et al. Atopy in children in relation to BCG vaccination and genetic polymorphisms at SLC11A1 (formerly NRAMP1) and D2S1471. Genes Immun 2002; 3:71–7.

[57] Karupiah G, Hunt NH, King NJ, et al. NADPH oxidase, Nramp1 and nitric oxide synthase 2 in the host antimicrobial response. Rev Immunogenet 2000;2:387–415.

[58] Smit JJ, Van Loveren H, Hoekstra MO, et al. The Slc11a1 (Nramp1) gene controls efficacy of mycobacterial treatment of allergic asthma. J Immunol 2003;171:754–60.

[59] Smit JJ, Folkerts G, Nijkamp FP. Mycobacteria, genes and the 'hygiene hypothesis'. Curr Opin Allergy Clin Immunol 2004;4:57–62.

[60] Poon AH, Laprise C, Lemire M, et al. NRAMP1 is not associated with asthma, atopy, and serum immunoglobulin E levels in the French Canadian population. Genes Immun 2005;6(6): 519–27.

[61] Brandt L, Feino Cunha J, Weinreich Olsen A, et al. Failure of the *Mycobacterium bovis* BCG vaccine: some species of environmental mycobacteria block multiplication of BCG and induction of protective immunity to tuberculosis. Infect Immun 2002;70:672–8.

[62] Colditz GA, Brewer TF, Berkey CS, et al. Efficacy of BCG vaccine in the prevention of tuberculosis: meta-analysis of the published literature. JAMA 1994;271:698–702.

[63] Demangel C, Garnier T, Rosenkrands I, et al. Differential effects of prior exposure to environmental mycobacteria on vaccination with *Mycobacterium bovis* BCG or a recombinant BCG strain expressing RD1 antigens. Infect Immun 2005;73:2190–6.

[64] Zuany-Amorim C, Sawicka E, Manlius C, et al. Suppression of airway eosinophilia by killed *Mycobacterium vaccae*-induced allergen-specific regulatory T-cells. Nat Med 2002;8:625–9.

[65] Zuany-Amorim C, Manlius C, Trifilieff A, et al. Long-term protective and antigen-specific effect of heat-killed *Mycobacterium vaccae* in a murine model of allergic pulmonary inflammation. J Immunol 2002;169:1492–9.

[66] Walker C, Sawicka E, Rook GA. Immunotherapy with mycobacteria. Curr Opin Allergy Clin Immunol 2003;3:481–6.
[67] Adams VC, Hunt JR, Martinelli R, et al. *Mycobacterium vaccae* induces a population of pulmonary CD11c+ cells with regulatory potential in allergic mice. Eur J Immunol 2004;34: 631–8.

ELSEVIER
SAUNDERS

Immunol Allergy Clin N Am
26 (2006) 379–385

IMMUNOLOGY
AND ALLERGY
CLINICS
OF NORTH AMERICA

Index

Note: Page numbers of article titles are in **boldface** type.

Changing Your Address?

Make sure your subscription changes too! When you notify us of your new address, you can help make our job easier by including an exact copy of your Clinics label number with your old address (see illustration below.) This number identifies you to our computer system and will speed the processing of your address change. Please be sure this label number accompanies your old address and your corrected address—you can send an old Clinics label with your number on it or just copy it exactly and send it to the address listed below.

We appreciate your help in our attempt to give you continuous coverage. Thank you.

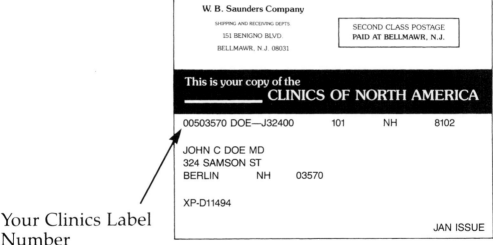

Your Clinics Label Number

Copy it exactly or send your label along with your address to:
W.B. Saunders Company, Customer Service
Orlando, FL 32887-4800
Call Toll Free 1-800-654-2452

Please allow four to six weeks for delivery of new subscriptions and for processing address changes.